Treating Drug Abusers Effectively

Treating Drug Abusers Effectively

Edited by

Joel A. Egertson,

Daniel M. Fox,

and

Alan I. Leshner

A Copublication with the Milbank Memorial Fund

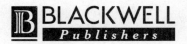

First published 1997
2 4 6 8 10 9 7 5 3 1

Blackwell Publishers Inc.
350 Main Street
Malden, MA 02148
USA

Blackwell Publishers Ltd
108 Cowley Road
Oxford OX4 1JF
UK

Library of Congress Cataloging-in-Publication Data
Treating drug abusers effectively / edited by Joel A. Egertson, Daniel M. Fox, and
  Alan I. Leshner.
      p.   cm.
   Includes bibliographical references and index.
   ISBN 1–57718–041–0.
   1. Drug abuse—Treatment.   I. Egertson, Joel A.   II. Fox, Daniel M.   III.
Leshner, Alan I., 1944–   .
RC566.T72   1996
362.29'18—dc20
                                                                96–27367
                                                                CIP

British Library Cataloguing in Publication Data
A CIP catalogue record for this book is available from the British Library.

Copublished by the Milbank Memorial Fund

Printed in Great Britain by Hartnolls Limited, Bodmin, Cornwall

This book is printed on acid-free paper

Contents

v

Contributors

Barry S. Brown received his Ph.D. in psychology from Western Reserve University. His work in the field of drug abuse has involved both clinical and research activity in correctional and outpatient settings. Most recently he was employed in various research administration positions at the National Institute on Drug Abuse. He is currently a member of the Graduate Faculty of the University of North Carolina at Wilmington and a Collaborating Scientist with the Institute of Behavioral Research at Texas Christian University.

David Cole is professor of law at Georgetown University Law Center, a volunteer staff attorney for the Center for Constitutional Rights, and a consultant for *Legal Times*. He is writing a book on race and the criminal justice system.

Margaret Commons is a research consultant currently working with researchers at Boston University. The focus of her work has been on the financing and delivery of mental health and substance abuse treatment services. She has published articles on the availability of treatment for the homeless mentally ill and on financing mechanisms for publicly-funded services to substance abusers.

Thomas D'Aunno is associate professor in the University of Chicago's School of Social Service Administration. He has published articles in leading management and health care journals. Dr. D'Aunno is on the editorial boards of several journals, including *Administrative Science Quarterly* and *The Journal of Health and Social*

Behavior, and is the current chairman of the Academy of Management Division of Health Care Administration.

Joel A. Egertson is senior advisor to the director of the Medications Development Division, at the National Institute on Drug Abuse (NIDA). He has served in numerous positions in the criminal justice, and alcohol and drug fields. He was a probation officer at Hennepin County Court Services, director of the methadone treatment program at Mount Sinai Hospital in Minneapolis, executive director of the Minnesota State Alcohol and Drug Abuse Authority, manager of field services at the National Center for Alcohol Education (University Research Corporation), a deputy division director at the National Institute on Alcohol Abuse and Alcoholism, and chief of the legislative branch at NIDA before assuming his present position.

Daniel M. Fox is president of the Milbank Memorial Fund. His most recent book is *Power and Illness: The Failure and Future of American Health Policy* (Berkeley: University of California Press, paperback edition, 1995).

Allen C. Goodman is professor and chair of the department of economics at Wayne State University in Detroit. He is currently studying ADM (alcoholism, drug abuse, and mental health) treatment costs, as well as cost and utilization offsets.

Janet R. Hankin is associate professor of sociology and obstetrics at Wayne State University in Detroit. She is currently studying the impacts of alcohol beverage warning labels on antenatal drinking. Other research includes a randomized clinical trial to examine the effectiveness of a cognitive behavioral program designed to prevent antenatal drinking.

Scott W. Henggeler is professor of psychiatry and behavioral sciences and director of the Family Services Research Center at the Medical University of South Carolina. Recent volumes include *Delinquency in Adolescence, Family Therapy and Beyond: A Multisystemic Approach to Treating the Behavior Problems of Children and Adolescents* (with C. M. Borduin), *Pediatric and Adolescent AIDS: Research Findings from the Social Sciences* (with G. B. Melton and J. R. Rodrigue), and *Innovative Services for "Difficult to Treat" Populations* (with A. Santos).

Constance M. Horgan is research professor at the Heller School, Brandeis University, and director of health services research within the Institute for Health Policy at Brandeis University. She is the author of numerous articles on the financing and organization of substance abuse and mental health services.

Alan I. Leshner is director of the National Institute on Drug Abuse, a component of the National Institutes of Health charged with leading the nation's efforts to bring the power of science to bear on drug abuse and addiction. Dr Leshner received his Ph.D. in physiological psychology from Rutgers University, held a variety of senior-level positions at the National Science Foundation, and served as deputy director and acting director of the National Institute of Mental Health. He has been elected a fellow of many professional societies, and has received numerous awards from both professional and lay groups for his national leadership in science, mental illness and mental health, and substance abuse and addiction.

Barry Littman received his bachelor's degree from Harvard University and is a third-year student at Georgetown University Law Center.

Willard G. Manning, Jr. is professor of health services research at the School of Public Health at the University of Minnesota. He is currently involved in an evaluation of the effects of capitation versus traditional fee-for-service Medicaid for mental health services for the Utah Medicaid program, as well as a project looking at the effect of taxes and alcohol control policies on accidents and violence.

Thomas G. McGuire is professor of economics at Boston University, and has been the research director of a training program in economics and mental health at the Heller School at Brandeis University since 1981. He has written or edited three books and more than 100 published articles on health and mental health economics and policy. He has also received an Investigator Award in Health Policy from the Robert Wood Johnson Foundation (joint with Richard Frank) to study reform of the organization and financing of mental health and substance abuse.

A. Thomas McLellan is professor of psychiatry at the Center for Studies on Addiction, University of Pennsylvania School of Medicine.

Eleanor Nishiura is research associate in the Department of Economics at Wayne State University in Detroit. A sociologist with expertise in the analysis of health insurance claims, Ms Nishiura is currently managing studies of ADM (alcoholism, drug abuse, and mental health) treatment costs, as well as cost and utilization offsets.

Richard H. Price is professor of psychology and research scientist in the Survey Research Center, Institute for Social Research, University of Michigan, and director of the Michigan Prevention Research Center, which is concerned with the impact of working life on mental health. Dr. Price is the author or editor of a number of books and articles on mental health and prevention, including *Fourteen Ounces of Prevention, Exploring Choices, Person–Environment Psychology, Psychology and Community Change, Abnormal Psychology in the Human Context, Evaluation and Action in the Social Environment,* and *Prevention in Mental Health.*

D. Dwayne Simpson is director of the Institute of Behavioral Research (IBR) and professor of psychology at Texas Christian University, where he also holds the Saul B. Sells Chair in Psychology. His work includes the first national study of community-based treatment in the United States, widely known as the Drug Abuse Reporting Program (DARP). His publications include over 150 articles and five books in the field of substance abuse. Dr. Simpson's current research focuses on service delivery process and client attributes, and how these factors influence treatment engagement and retention rates, stages of recovery, and long-term outcomes of addicts.

Jody L. Sindelar is associate professor in the School of Epidemiology and Public Health (Economics) and the Institution for Social and Policy Studies at Yale University. She has received a Research Scientist Career Development Award by the National Institute on Alcohol Abuse and Alcoholism, and was also appointed to be a research associate of the National Bureau of Economic Research.

Foreword

The Milbank Memorial Fund is an endowed national foundation that supports nonpartisan analysis, study, and research on significant issues in health policy. The Fund often makes available the results of its work in pamphlets and books, and it publishes as well the *Milbank Quarterly*, a peer-reviewed journal of public health and health-care policy.

This book is the result of collaboration between policymakers in state government and researchers. The collaboration was organized by the Fund and the National Institute of Drug Abuse. The editors describe in their introduction how state officials and academic researchers planned, debated, and reviewed the chapters that comprise the book.

Another result of this project is a report, *Treating Drug Abusers Effectively: Researchers Talk with Policy Makers*, by Harry Nelson, a long-time reporter for the *Los Angeles Times*, who is now a staff journalist for the Fund. Nelson covered the discussions among officials and researchers that led to this book. Participants in these meetings then reviewed the accuracy of the information in Nelson's report. The report is available without charge from the Fund's office in New York City.

The Fund and Blackwell Publishers copublish a series of books that result from projects of the Fund. Each of these books is reviewed for both scientific merit and salience for policy under the direction of the Fund. Then Blackwell conducts an internal review and assumes responsibility for editing, printing, and distributing the book. The Fund and Blackwell also copublish the *Milbank Quarterly*.

Samuel L. Milbank
Chairman

Daniel M. Fox
President

Acknowledgments

In addition to the contributors, the persons who participated in defining the topics for the chapters and reviewing the first drafts were: Diane Canova, executive director, Therapeutic Communities of America; Patience Drake, fiscal analyst, House Fiscal Agency, Michigan House of Representatives; Bob Galea, Akeela House, Inc.; Henrick J. Harwood, project manager, Lewin-VHI; Mary Jeanne Kreek, associate professor, Rockefeller University; Mary C. Mayhew, deputy chief, Legislative, Government, and Constituent Relations, National Institute on Drug Abuse; Dennis McCarty, Director, Bureau of Substance Abuse Services, Massachusetts Department of Public Health; Douglas H. Morgan, assistant commissioner, Division of AIDS Prevention and Control, New Jersey Department of Health; Charles Palmer, director, Iowa Department of Human Services; Kenneth L. Przybysz, senate chair, Public Health Committee, Connecticut Senate; Ray Rawson, assistant majority leader and chair, Human Resource Committee, Nevada Senate; Pat Rosenman, program analyst, National Institute on Drug Abuse; Peter A. Selwyn, associate director, AIDS Program, Yale–New Haven Hospital; Zili Sloboda, acting director, Division of Epidemiology and Prevention Research, National Institute on Drug Abuse; Frank M. Tims, Chief Services Research Branch, National Institute on Drug Abuse; Leticia Van de Putte, member, Human Resources Committee, Texas House of Representatives; Bailus Walker, professor and dean, College of Public Health, University of Oklahoma; Arthur Y. Webb, chief executive officer, Village Center for Care Fund of New York, Inc.; and Elaine Wilson, chief, Alcohol and Drug Abuse Division, Hawaii State Department of Health.

Other reviewers were: M. Douglas Anglin, director, UCLA Drug Research Center, University of Californa, Los Angeles; Karst Besteman, director, Substance Abuse Center, Institute for Behavior Resources; Kathleen Carroll, assistant professor of psychiatry and director of psychotherapy research, Substance Abuse Center, Connecticut Mental Health Center, Yale University School of Medicine; Richard Catalano, acting director and associate professor, Social Development Research Group, School of Social Work, University of Washington; George De Leon, director, Center for Therapeutic Community Research, National Development and Research Institutes; Richard Frank, professor, Department of Health Care Policy, Harvard Medical School; Mindy Fullilove, associate professor of clinical psychiatry and public health, Community Research Group, New York State Psychiatric Institute and Columbia University; Barbara E. Havassy, professor and director, Treatment Outcome Research, University of California, San Francisco; Jeffery Hoffman, senior vice-president of operations and executive director, Center for Drug Treatment and Research, Koba Associates, Inc.; Harold Holder, director and senior scientist, Prevention Research Center; James A. Inciardi, professor and director, Center for Drug and Alcohol Studies, University of Delaware; Nancy Jainchill, senior principal investigator, Center for Therapeutic Community Research, National Development and Research Institutes; Christine Kasser; Mary Jo Larson, senior research associate, The Heller School, Brandeis University; Richard Lennox, Pacific Institute for Research and Evaluation; Carl G. Leukefeld, professor and director, Multidisciplinary Research Center on Drug and Alcohol Abuse, University of Kentucky; David Lewis, director, Center for Alcohol and Addiction Studies, Brown University; Douglas Lipton, National Development and Research Institutes; Mark Pauly, professor, Department of Health Care Systems, University of Pennsylvania; Jerome J. Platt, professor and director, Division of Addiction Research and Treatment, Department of Mental Health Services, Hahnemann University; Leonard Rubenstein, executive director, Bazelon Center for Mental Health; Louise B. Russell, research professor, Institute of Health, Health Care Policy, and Aging Research, Rutgers University; James L. Sorensen, adjunct professor and chief, San Francisco General Hospital Substance Abuse Services; Donald Steinwachs, director, Health Research and Development Center, Johns Hopkins University; and Stanley Wallack, director, Institute for Health Policy, The Heller School, Brandeis University.

Introduction

Public dollars – federal, state, and local – pay for approximately 70 percent of the costs of treating drug abuse. Yet public policy for treating drug abuse too often is based on unfounded perceptions and entrenched ideologies rather than on the findings of scientific research.

The eleven original articles that comprise this book are the result of a collaboration between researchers and policymakers that was organized by a federal agency and a private foundation. These articles assess research-based knowledge about effective treatment in order to provide guidance to policymakers.

The encouraging results of much recent research on treating drug abuse have been obscured by current debates about related, but separable, issues. Of course it is necessary to reduce demand for drugs by limiting the attractiveness of drug taking and to limit their supply by enforcing laws against drug producers, traffickers, and users. But it is also important to provide treatment interventions that have been proven to assist drug-dependent persons to recover and to become rehabilitated.

Contemporary scientists conceptualize drug addiction as a chronic, relapsing disorder. Using standard methods of research, these scientists have published convincing evidence that treatment works for many people and that there are many effective programs of care. Leading experts on drug-abuse treatment from basic biomedical science, clinical epidemiology, and health services research who participated in the project from which this book was drawn told us that treatment can be made more effective, resulting in better use of public and private funds.

This hopeful view based on science contrasts with the moralism that still drives considerable public expenditure for treating drug abusers. Drug-abuse treatment evolved alongside, and separately from, mainstream health care because abusers have historically been stigmatized. Treatment policy has too often been based on faulty public assumptions that addicts bring their affliction on themselves because they have weak characters and that successful treatment requires them to recognize the error of their ways and abstain from drugs forever. Treatment policy has been judged to have failed by those subscribing to this view because sustained abstinence has not been achieved for sufficient numbers of addicts.

But abstinence is inappropriate as the sole criterion for effective treatment of a chronic disorder. In drug abuse, as in treatment for arthritis or asthma or diabetes, the goal of treatment is ultimately to prevent relapses entirely or to lengthen time between them.

Research on substitution therapy for drug abusers, especially with methadone (a synthetic opiate drug with dependency-producing properties), has demonstrated the usefulness of a chronic illness perspective. When substitution therapy is part of a comprehensive program of drug-abuse treatment, it is an effective intervention, as measured by the prevention of relapses or reduction in their frequency.

The articles commissioned for this book are a result of a project to communicate researchers' current understanding of effective treatment for drug abuse to persons who make policy, mainly for the states. The project was organized by the National Institute on Drug Abuse (NIDA) and the Milbank Memorial Fund. NIDA has conducted or supported more than 80 percent of all drug research in the world. The Fund is an endowed foundation that works with decision makers in the public and private sectors to improve health policy.

Beginning in 1993, the Fund and NIDA convened several meetings of leading researchers on drug treatment and officials of federal, state, and local government. Participants in these meetings formulated topics for articles that would describe current, research-based knowledge about what services for treating drug abuse ought to be provided to whom, by whom, in what setting, at what cost.

Then the Fund and NIDA commissioned articles on these topics from authors who attended the planning meetings and other experts on drug-treatment research. Each author was invited to synthesize research findings in his or her area of expertise and then to apply this knowledge in answering three questions: What treatment programs should policymakers stop financing? What programs should they start to finance? What changes should be made in existing programs?

The resulting articles received extensive review. First, the authors and the policymakers who had participated in the planning meetings met to discuss drafts of all 11 manuscripts. Next, the authors revised their drafts for review by independent experts who had not been associated with the project. Then scientists at NIDA reviewed the authors' final revisions.

The results of the NIDA–Milbank project appear in this book. The first five articles are an overview of the findings of research on treatment for persons who suffer from chronic drug abuse. Thomas McLellan discusses expectations for drug-abuse treatment and provides a model for evaluating it. Dwayne Simpson reviews treatment-outcome studies and arrays evidence to answer questions relating to the motivation, assessment, and retention of patients in treatment and to predicting outcomes. Constance Horgan describes the need and demand for drug-abuse treatment in the context of current barriers to access to care. Barry Brown discusses the history and evolving role of drug-abuse counselors and other practitioners in providing services to meet the multiple needs of persons in treatment, relating changes in staffing patterns to changes in how drug abuse is perceived. Finally, Richard Price analyzes the implementation of treatment practices, particularly the reasons practitioners frequently do not use the best practices.

The next three articles explore the financing of drug-abuse treatment. Allen Goodman offers a conceptual framework for research on the costs of treating drug abuse. Jody Sindelar and Will Manning discuss the importance of distinguishing among outcomes that can be measured by cost-benefit analysis and those that are best evaluated by studies of cost-effectiveness. Margaret Commons and Thomas McGuire assess an innovative approach to state financing of drug-abuse treatment called Performance-Based Contracting.

Each of the articles in the concluding section addresses a special issue in drug-abuse treatment. Scott Henggeler explores treatment for adolescents, emphasizing lessons from interventions with children and adults. David Cole examines the impact of drugs on minority communities and explains how changes in the criminal justice system could address the burgeoning population of addicts cycling in and out of prisons. Finally, Thomas D'Aunno examines research on promoting more effective links between primary health services and treatment for drug abuse.

This book concludes a unique dialogue between scientists and decision makers on important and controversial issues. Dialogues can be enlightening, but they emphasize differences of opinion more often that they resolve them. NIDA and the Fund hope that this book will instruct and stimulate a wide variety of readers. The editors thank the authors, public officials, and expert reviewers whose names are listed in the Acknowledgments.

Joel A. Egertson
Daniel M. Fox
Alan I. Leshner

Part I

Research Findings on Drug-Abuse Treatments

Evaluating the Effectiveness of Addiction Treatments: Reasonable Expectations, Appropriate Comparisons

A. Thomas McLellan, George E. Woody,
David Metzger, Jim McKay, Jack Durell,
Arthur I. Alterman, Charles P. O'Brien

Introduction

Problems of alcohol and drug dependence produce dramatic costs to society in terms of lost productivity, social disorder, and avoidable health-care utilization (National Institute on Drug Abuse 1991; Merrill 1993). Reports from the Robert Wood Johnson Foundation suggest that alcohol abuse costs society approximately $99 billion annually; that abuse of other drugs costs approximately $67 billion annually; and that one-eighth to one-sixth of all deaths here in America are associated in some way with alcohol or drug use (Rice 1990; Robert Wood Johnson Foundation 1994). Perhaps more subtle but no less significant is the fact that more than three-fourths of all foster children in this country are the products of alcohol and/or drug-addicted parents (Children's Defense Fund 1994). While some segments of the public are demanding greater availability and more financing for addiction treatments, there are those in government, insurance, managed care, and the public who question the efficacy of these treatments, and whether they are "worth it" (Saxe et al. 1983; Food and Drug Administration 1980).

There are many issues to be considered in an evaluation of whether and to what extent problems of addiction should be addressed with treatment. First, what results do we expect from an "effective" intervention (regardless of whether it is a treatment intervention); and are conventional treatments for substance-use disorders effective in terms of these expectations? Second, is treatment better and more cost effective than other alternatives such as no treatment at all, self-help groups, community service, jail, etc.? Finally, if treatment is considered an effective solution to the problem, who should deliver treatment, to whom, for how long, and under what circumstances?

Thus, the seemingly simple question of whether treatment for substance-use disorders is "effective," is actually one of the more complex health, social, and financial issues currently facing this nation. The question cannot be answered simply. Rather, it must be re-framed as a series of comparisons that will consider the benefits and liabilities of treatment evaluated against appropriate outcome expectations and against other, plausible alternatives to treatment. In this chapter, we first offer some rationale for what we consider to be reasonable expectations for addiction treatments and, based on these, propose some outcome criteria against which to judge the effectiveness of those treatments. In the second part of the chapter we use these outcome criteria to compare the effectiveness of addiction treatments with several alternatives such as no treatment or incarceration. It should be clear that the purpose of this chapter is not to present an exhaustive review of the now burgeoning literature on treatment outcome in the field of alcohol and drug dependence. Instead, we will compare the results of various addiction treatments with the public's expectations about those treatments and with the results from non-treatment interventions. We believe the data from these comparisons may offer some informative perspectives regarding the issues of the effectiveness and societal "worth" of substance-abuse treatments.

Section I　Reasonable Expectations for "Effective" Interventions

A major issue to be considered in an evaluation of any form of treatment is what we expect an "effective" form of treatment to do? This is not merely an academic or philosophical issue but one that forms the basis for major decisions about the form of treatment, including its goals, patient-admission criteria, staffing patterns, services provided, and treatment duration. Ultimately, the effectiveness of any treatment will be defined in terms of the extent to which that intervention meets these expectations. Most health-care interventions attempt to meet more than one expectation, but the expectations placed upon substance-abuse interventions are particularly diverse and difficult.

Expectations of the Patient

Since the patient is the focus of treatment efforts, his/her expectations must be considered before any others. For many substance-dependent individuals entering treatment there are immediate expectations of relief from the acute and often painful symptoms of withdrawal, craving, and loss of control that they are experiencing. At the same time, there are others who are forced into substance-abuse treatment by the criminal justice system, their employers, or their spouses, and who are not experiencing acute physical or emotional problems and in fact are "unaware" that there is a substance-abuse problem at all. While these patients may not be aware of direct physical or emotional problems, they are often experiencing shame from being "caught" and a mixture of resentment, anger, and worry regarding the recent alcohol or drug-use related situation that led to their treatment admission. These patients typically expect that an "effective" intervention will resolve the social and personal problems that have led to the admission. Still other patients have become aware (typically through failed prior attempts at self-control of their alcohol or drug use) that their substance use has gotten out of control and is preventing them from functioning fully in family, work, and/or social relationships. These patients are often treatment re-admissions seeking a long-term solution to what they have come to see as a chronic and severe problem that has affected most parts of their life.

Thus, the expectations of patients entering substance-abuse

treatment may range from immediate relief from physical symptoms, to short-term resolution of recent addiction-related personal and social crises, to long-term changes in the employment, legal, and family problems that have been brought on by prolonged substance abuse.

Expectations of Others Affected by Substance Abuse

Beyond the patient, there are other constituents who are directly or indirectly affected by the substance-abuse problems of the patient, and who have legitimate expectations of their own regarding the results of addiction treatments. For example, both public and private health insurers and health care delivery organizations (e.g., insurers, HMOs, the Veterans Administration, the Social Security System, etc.) are typically the primary payers for addiction-treatment services. They are anxious for an "effective" treatment in the hope that it will reduce the medical and public health risks associated with substance use. For example, drug use has become a major vector for the spread of serious infectious diseases such as AIDS, hepatitis, and tuberculosis (Metzger et al. 1992). Further, because of the widespread practice of exchanging sex for drugs, substance abuse has become a major risk factor for the spread of sexually-transmitted diseases (Watkins et al. 1992). Finally, from a purely financial perspective, substance-dependent persons use as much as ten times the health care services as non-addicted persons, and their families use as much as five times the health care services as the families of persons without a substance-use disorder (see Saxe et al. 1983). Thus from the perspective of the health insurance and health delivery companies and agencies, a truly "effective" form of treatment for substance abuse would be one that reduced the public health risks of substance abusers and reduced their disproportionate use of expensive health care services.

Employers are often at least partial payers for substance-abuse treatment services. While they realize that uncontrolled substance use is the target problem that must be addressed initially, their primary goal is to have their affected employees returned to an effective level of work performance following treatment and to assure other workers that they will not be put in danger due to substance abuse by co-workers. This is particularly true in the case of employers whose products or services require particular attention and care to ensure safety (e.g., the transportation industry, pharmaceutical industry, nuclear power agencies, etc.). From this perspective, employers consider to be "effective" that substance-abuse treatment which will return employees to safe and effective performance on the job.

Families of substance-dependent individuals are often the major agents of referral into treatment and can be a source of continuing encouragement for the affected individuals during and following treatment. These families typically want an end to the worries, embarrassment, social disruptions, and violence that are so often associated with substance dependence. Thus, for the families of substance abusers, "effectiveness" of addiction treatment will be measured in terms of family peace and safety, and not just reduced substance use.

Police, probation/parole officers, judges, and other agents of the criminal justice system are also major sources of referral to, and payment for, substance-abuse treatments. They are acutely aware of the links between crime and addiction. Current statistics indicate that as many as 75 percent of federal prisoners meet diagnostic criteria for a substance-dependence disorder (Gerstein and Harwood 1990). The statistics on street crime suggest that as much as 50 percent of all property crimes are committed under the influence of alcohol and/or drugs, or with the intent to obtain alcohol and/or drugs with the crime proceeds (Gerstein and Harwood 1990). Finally, and just as importantly to the public, 50 percent of fatal highway accidents are due to the effects of alcohol intoxication (Walsh 1982). Thus, for the criminal justice system and for the public at large, among the more important measures of the "effectiveness" of substance-dependence treatment are reductions in crime, parole/probation violations, and incarceration rates among affected individuals.

In summary, for the patient and particularly for the many treatment stakeholders in society, "effectiveness" of treatment for substance abuse will be measured not just in terms of its effects on alcohol and drug use, but perhaps more importantly, in terms of that treatment's extended effects on the "addiction-related" problems that have limited personal function in the patient, that have become public health and public safety concerns to society, and that have typically been the impetus to treatment admission. These are indeed broad expectations for any type of treatment, and it should be clear that these goals are only imperfectly correlated. That is, the achievement (through treatment or otherwise) of the goal of reduced alcohol and drug use is a necessary, but rarely sufficient requirement for the achievement of the longer-term societal goals of reduced public health and public safety concerns. Regardless, we argue that from both the patient's and society's perspectives, a "truly effective" treatment is one that not only provides reduction of the substance use, but also significantly improves personal and social functioning, particularly in areas of special public health and public safety concern. It is also worth noting that these broad and diverse expectations of treatment are also found in other forms of general medical care. To quote Stewart and Ware in their recent text on outcome evaluation of general medical care (1989):

> Since the 1970s however, the emphasis in America on what patient outcomes to measure to determine health status has been shifting. The focus on the outcomes of medical care is now shifting to the assessment of functioning, or the ability of the patients to perform the daily activities of their lives, how they feel, and their own personal evaluation of their health in general. (Ref. 9, p. 157)

Suggested Outcome Domains for Evaluating the Effectiveness of Treatments for Substance Dependence

Based upon the above discussion from both the patient's and the public's perspectives we have adopted broad "rehabilitation" expectations about the outcomes of substance-dependence treatment – that is, those goals that would make treatment "worth it" both for the patient who undergoes it and for the society that pays for it. We therefore suggest three domains that we feel are relevant to the improved personal function goals of the patient and to the public health and safety goals of society:

1 Reduction of alcohol and drug use;
2 Improvement in personal and social function;
3 Reduction in public health and public safety threats.

In our view, the first two domains are quite consistent with the "primary and secondary measures of effectiveness" typically used by the Food and Drug Administration to evaluate new drug or device applications in controlled clinical trials (Stewart and Ware 1989) and as indicated above, quite consistent with the mainstream of thought regarding the evaluation of other forms of health care (Metzger et al. 1992). We believe the final outcome dimension is more specific to the treatment of substance-use disorders since it acknowledges the significant and possibly unique public health and public safety concerns associated with addiction. Each of these domains and its measurement is discussed in the text that follows.

Reduction of alcohol and drug use

This is the foremost goal of substance-abuse treatments and can be measured accurately and reliably from patient self-report. When information is collected in confidence by independent evaluators and where there is no penalty for accurate reporting, patients' self-reports of alcohol and drug use can be very reliable and accurate measures of this behavior. The validity of patient self-reports has been replicated in many studies over the years (McLellan et al. 1985; Armor, Polich, and Stambul 1976; Ball and Ross 1991; Zanis, McLellan, and Randall 1995; Ehrman and Robbins 1994), but these findings rarely convince the skeptical. For this reason, it has long been the practice of treatment-outcome researchers to also collect laboratory measures of urinalysis for drug screening and breathalyzer readings of blood alcohol content as objective confirmation of at least recent substance use.

Increased personal and social function

As indicated above, improvements in the medical status, psychological health and social function of these patients are important from a societal perspective in that these improvements reduce the problems and thereby the expenses produced by the disorders. In addition, improvements in these personal functional areas are clearly related to the continued maintenance of reduced substance use. There are many ways of measuring improvements in functional status and several specific instruments have been developed (see Food and Drug Administration 1980; McLellan et al. 1980). Measures such as general health status inventories, psychological symptom inventories, family function measures, and simple measures of days worked and dollars earned can be reliably and validly collected either directly from the patient via confidential self-report and/or from medical/psychiatric evaluations and employment records.

Reduction in threats to public health and public safety

The threats to public health and safety from substance-abusing individuals come from behaviors that spread infectious diseases and from behaviors associated with personal and property crimes. It is of course possible to think of these as specific elements of personal health and social function, but we have chosen to separate them into a special criterion domain in recognition of their importance to society. Specifically, the sharing of needles, unprotected sex, and trading sex for drugs are serious addiction-related behaviors that are significant threats to public health. Self-report measures of these behaviors have been developed and validated (Metzger et al. forthcoming). Objective measures of the acquisition of AIDS, STDs, TB, and hepatitis can be obtained by laboratory tests, but these measures underestimate the spread of these diseases to other members of society through contact with substance abusers.

The commission of personal and property crimes for the purpose of obtaining alcohol or drugs and the irresponsible or dangerous use of automobiles or equipment under the influence of alcohol or drugs are major threats to public safety. Objective measures of arrests and incarcerations resulting from these acts can be obtained from public records, although these measures typically underestimate the extent of the criminal and dangerous behaviors actually performed. Thus, treatment-outcome researchers have typically supplemented these public records with confidential self-reports from interviews (Simpson and Savage 1980; Hubbard et al. 1989; Inciardi 1988; Wexler, Falkin, and Lipton 1988; Anglin and Hser 1990).

Suggested Methods for Evaluating the Effectiveness of Substance-Abuse Treatments

Even with basic agreement on the measurement domains to be used in an outcome evaluation, there are still many different methods that can be employed in the evaluation of treatment outcome, all offering particular strengths and limitations. In the interests of enabling direct comparison of effectiveness between substance-abuse treatments and other medical interventions, researchers at the Penn–VA Center have elected to use the designs, methods, and measurement standards recommended by the Food and Drug Administration for the evaluation of new medical devices and pharmacotherapies (Food and Drug Administration 1980). For example, each of the studies to be reported has employed an "*intent to treat*" design, where a random sample of subjects is selected at admission to treatment and fully characterized from that point throughout the course of their treatment and following their discharge. Again, this is a methodological feature that is required by the Food and Drug Administration in their evaluations of new drugs and devices (Food and Drug Administration 1980). This type of evaluation design provides effectiveness estimates that are substantially more conservative than evaluations of samples that have completed the full course of treatment.

A second methodological feature of more rigorous evaluations is the performance of all patient interviews and data collection by _independent evaluators_, not associated with the provision of the intervention. This is critical to the reduction of "demand effects" (i.e., "faking good") that are commonly seen when patients report their levels of improvement directly to the clinical staff who have treated them. In this regard, it is also advisable for subjective reports of post-treatment status to be accompanied by _breathalyzer and/or urine screening tests and/or collateral reports_ to validate patient reports, even when collected by independent evaluators.

Finally, it has been recognized that a high rate of patient follow-up contact is necessary to ensure representative information from the treated sample. Again, the Food and Drug Administration requires _a minimum of 70 percent contact at follow-up_ in their studies (Food and Drug Administration 1980). It has been shown by LaPorte et al. (1981) and by others (Moos 1974) that those patients who are more difficult to find at follow-up typically have worse outcomes. Thus studies reporting contact rates that are less than 70 percent are likely to overestimate the effects of treatment and therefore should be regarded critically. There has been disagreement regarding the appropriate or optimal point at which to evaluate treatment effects, and researchers have used intervals ranging from 1 to 24 months following treatment discharge. In the majority of work to be reported here, we have used a six-month post-treatment follow-up since our work over the past 15 years has suggested that approximately 60 percent to 80 percent of those patients who relapse following treatment, do so within three to four months after discharge (McLellan et al. 1993). Since many of those who relapse return to treatment, later follow-up evaluations of a single treatment episode may become contaminated by the effects of subsequent treatments. We are aware of no single, optimal point at which to evaluate treatment effects, and multiple evaluations are therefore preferable. The six-month evaluations discussed here offer only one, albeit important, indication of treatment effects.

Thus, in the work that follows, we have used the three outcome domains and the most rigorous evaluation methods and measures presently available, to estimate the extent to which the outcomes of substance-abuse treatments actually meet what we believe are the reasonable expectations of the patients and the public at large.

Section II – Appropriate Comparisons to Judge the Effectiveness of Addiction Treatments

---

Do Patients Improve Following Treatment?

Perhaps the most basic question that can be asked of treatment is whether patients who enter care actually show significant reductions in the three outcome domains discussed in Section I of the chapter. Perhaps the most commonly used means of addressing these questions has been a simple comparison of patient status before and after treatment; that is, a standard "Pre–Post" design.

One recent example of a pre- to post-treatment comparison that meets the methodological standards described above is presented in table 1.1 showing the results from a large study of 649 adult alcohol-, cocaine- and opiate-dependent patients admitted to 22 public and private programs (McLellan et al. 1994). All were standard programs that had participated in one of the alcohol and drug rehabilitation-outcome research studies performed by the Penn–VA Center. Twelve of the twenty-two programs were based in several eastern cities, and the remainder were based in suburban settings. Four public and three private outpatient methadone programs were included. Nine private treatment programs (four inpatient, five outpatient) and six public programs (three inpatient, three outpatient) were included. All treatments were in "real world," standard care situations, thus representing a reasonable sample of "treatment as usual."

The admission and follow-up data were collected by independent technicians who were not part of the treatment process or the clinical staff. Follow-up contact rates averaged 92 percent, and urine and breathalyzer reports were collected on randomly selected samples from each program to verify self-reported outcomes. In this study both the admission and follow-up evaluations were performed using the Addiction Severity Index (ASI) (McLellan et al. 1980; 1985; 1992), a standardized, structured, 45-minute clinical research interview, designed to assess problem severity in seven areas commonly affected among substance-abusing individuals: alcohol and drug use, medical, legal, employment, family/social, and psychiatric problems. In each of these areas questions measure the number, frequency, intensity, and duration of problem symptoms in the 30-day periods preceding admission to treatment and preceding the six-month follow-up point. Composite measures of overall status in each problem area were calculated by combining unweighted sets of individual items in each problem area. These composite scores range from 0, indicating no problem in the past 30 days, to 1.0, indicating extremely severe problems.

This total patient population has been divided into the three major drug-preference subgroups in table 1.1. All patients were voluntary participants in the outcome-evaluation study, and a minimum of 75 percent of admissions agreed to participate. There were some demographic differences among the groups as well as severity differences in almost all variables measured, but space constraints do not permit a full discussion of these. In general, the opiate-dependent patients showed more severe problems than either of the other two groups.

Improvements following treatment
Changes in the ASI data from admission to six-month follow-up are presented in table 1.1, divided into the three outcome domains previously discussed. Data are presented for each of the three primary drug-use groups. A within-subjects, multiple analysis of variance (MANOVA) was performed to assess overall improvement from admission to follow-up within each of the three drug-preference groups. As can be seen, the three groups had different patterns of problems at admission, but there was much evidence of significant improvement for all groups, in all three outcome domains at the six-month follow-up. Specifically, the sample of 242 alcohol-dependent patients showed a 76 percent reduction in the number of days of drinking and a 81 percent reduction in the number of days intoxicated from admission to follow-up; 43 percent of alcohol-dependent patients were abstinent from all alcohol for the six-month period. The 212 cocaine-dependent patients showed an 82 percent reduction in days of cocaine use, and the 195 opiate-dependent patients showed a 45 percent reduction in opiate use from admission to follow-up; 51 percent of the cocaine-dependent patients and 39 percent of the opiate-dependent patients were abstinent from all illicit drugs during the six-month period. It can also be seen that these improvements were not confined simply to the alcohol- and drug-use measures, but included significant improvements in the psychiatric, employment, and family status measures, and there were substantial changes in public health and safety measures.

It is important to emphasize that while these results are encouraging it is not possible to attribute these improvements to the direct effects of treatment in the absence of a control group of patients

Table 1.1 Pre- to post-treatment change in three groups of substance-dependent patients.

PROBLEM MEASURE*	OPIATE BASELINE N = 195	OPIATE 6 MONTHS N = 195	t	COCAINE BASELINE N = 212	COCAINE 6 MONTHS N = 212	t	ALCOHOL BASELINE N = 242	t	ALCOHOL 6 MONTHS N = 242
OUTCOME DOMAIN #1 – REDUCTION IN ALCOHOL AND DRUG USE									
Drug Composite Score	.336	.256	***	.228	.081	***	.022	**	.011
Days opiate use	11	6	***	1	2	*	–		–
Days stimulant use	5	3	***	11	2	***	–		–
Days depressant use	6	6		1	1		2	*	1
Alcohol Composite Score	.109	.093		.209	.080	***	.642	***	.158
Days alcohol use	6	5	*	8	3	***	17	***	4
Days drank to intoxication	3	2		6	2	***	16	***	3
OUTCOME DOMAIN #2 – INCREASED HEALTH AND PERSONAL FUNCTION									
Medical Composite Score	.349	.311		.230	.168	*	.229		.223
Days medical problems	8	8		6	4	.08+	7		6
Psychiatric Comp Score	.309	.268	*	.222	.089	***	.220	***	.115
Days psych problems	12	8	***	9	3	***	9	***	4
Employment Comp Score	.675	.641		.621	.571	*	.552		.487
Days worked in past 30	8	10		12	14	*	11	**	14
Employment income	$417	$537	*	$613	$783	*	$697	*	$841
Family Composite Score	.268	.225	*	.250	.136	***	.198	***	.094
Days family conflicts	4	3		3	2		2	**	–
Days social conflicts	2	2		2	1	*	2	*	–
OUTCOME DOMAIN #3 – REDUCTION IN PUBLIC HEALTH AND SAFETY PROBLEMS									
Shared needle/syringe	23%	3%	***	3%	3%		<1%		0%
Had unprotected sex	14%	9%	*	22%	13%	*	19%	**	7%
Legal Composite Score	.133	.102		.064	.024	**	.051	***	.006
Days illegal activity	4	2	*	2	1	**	–		–
Illegal income	$289	$109	**	$105	$83		$26		$1

* All measures derive from ASI interviews covering the 30-day periods prior to baseline and 6-month follow-up.
* = p < .05, ** = p < .01, *** = p < .001 by paired t-test

randomly assigned to receive no treatment (see below). It is possible that these substance-abuse patients would have changed significantly over this same period of time *without treatment*. Of course, random assignment designs including "no-treatment" control groups are not possible in evaluations of ongoing treatments within the real world. Thus, these data are best considered as an indication that substance-abusing patients who receive treatment in these "real world" programs were in much better condition six months after beginning treatment than they were prior to treatment. Further, while these data derive from a series of studies done recently in the Philadelphia region, it should be clear that the nature and amount of changes seen are quite similar to those reported many times over the past decade of evaluation work in this area. Space constraints do not permit a complete discussion of all these studies. The interested reader is referred to studies by Moos, Finney, and their colleagues on the evaluation of alcohol treatments (Moos 1974; McLellan et al. 1980). Large-scale evaluations of drug-abuse treatments have been performed by Simpson and Savage using the DARP data (1980), Hubbard et al. using the TOPS data sets (1989), De Leon studying therapeutic community treatment (1984), and Anglin et al. (1989) and Ball et al. (1988) studying methadone maintenance treatments. While there are of course differences among these studies in the nature of the treatments evaluated and the evaluation paradigms, the results shown in table 1.1 are quite representative of this larger literature showing significant and pervasive changes among substance-dependent patients following standard treatments. In the material that follows, we review efforts designed to determine the causes of these improvements.

Is Treatment More Effective than No Treatment?

While it is ethically not possible to deny available treatment to those whose condition requires it, there are situations where treatments have not been applied to substance-dependent persons and these situations offer some indication of what happens to substance use, personal function and the public health and safety problems of substance-dependent individuals in the absence of treatment. Two recent studies provide information pertinent to this question.

Untreated patients
Metzger et al. (1993) have examined the drug use, needle-sharing

Table 1.2 Drug-related risk behaviors by treatment status.

	In-Tx	Out-Tx
Weekly Injections during prior month:		
Heroin	33% (40)	69% (61)**
Cocaine	22% (27)	61% (54)**
Combined ("Speedball")	32% (39)	45% (40)*
Been to "Shooting Gallery"	33% (41)	55% (48)**
Been to "Crack House"	11% (13)	28% (25)**

* $p < .05$ ** $p < .01$ by Chi-Square

practices, and HIV infection rates of two large samples of opiate-addicted patients in the Philadelphia area. The "In-Treatment" group was composed of 152 patients randomly selected from a large methadone maintenance program. These In-Treatment subjects were asked to refer opiate-using individuals (Out-of-Treatment group – 103 subjects) from their same neighborhoods and social networks but who had been out of all substance-dependence treatments for *at least one year*. Thus, using this chain referral method, the two groups were matched on many relevant demographic, geographic, background, and social factors that are associated with drug use.

Table 1.2 presents an indication of drug use and needle sharing in these two groups, collected from confidential interviews and questionnaires administered at baseline and at subsequent six-monthly intervals, by independent research technicians. As can be seen, despite the fact that the In-Treatment subjects were enrolled in a methadone treatment program, there was some continued opiate and non-opiate drug use and needle sharing. Considered alone, without indication of the prior levels of substance use and public health risk behaviors, these data might lead to a conclusion that treatment was not working. Drug use had not been reduced to zero, and there was still significant public health risk in the form of needle sharing. However, the level of drug use and needle sharing reported by the In-Treatment sample was less than half that seen in the Out-of-Treatment group.

Perhaps the most important data emerging from this study was the differential HIV infection rates between the two samples as seen through prospective follow-up evaluations (including serological examinations) every six months over the next three years, on over

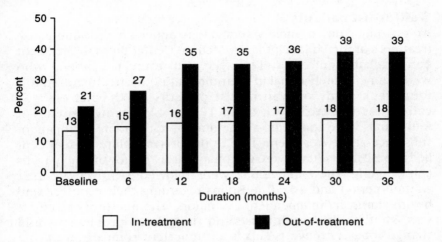

Figure 1.1   Three-year HIV infection rates by treatment status at time of enrollment.

90 percent of the original samples (see figure 1.1). At the initial assessment point, 13 percent of the In-Treatment sample and 21 percent of the Out-of-Treatment sample tested positive for HIV infection. Follow-up testing showed that by the third year, 39 percent of the Out-of-Treatment group, but only 18 percent of the In-Treatment group tested HIV positive. Closer examination of the role of treatment status on HIV conversion revealed that 30 percent of originally HIV-negative subjects *who remained out of treatment*, became infected with the AIDS virus over the three-year period. In comparison, only 8 percent of originally HIV-negative subjects *who remained in the treatment program*, became infected during the same time period.

It bears emphasis that nearly four times as many Out-of Treatment as In-Treatment subjects continued to engage in public health risk behaviors and thereby became infected with the AIDS virus. Though quite remarkable, it must be repeated that even these data do not prove that treatment was the causal agent responsible for these differences in infection rates. It is possible, and even likely, that the "out-of-treatment" subjects may have lacked the motivation for treatment found among the treated subjects, and this lack of desire for personal change, rather than the effects of the treatment itself, may in part explain the status differences seen. In order to make any definitive judgment regarding the causal effects of treatment in reducing AIDS risk behaviors among this group it would have been necessary to somehow find subjects from the two groups who had equal levels of motivation. Obviously this was not possible.

Waiting list patients

An ongoing study of male veterans who applied for cocaine-abuse treatment at the Philadelphia VA Medical Center helps to shed light on the relative outcomes of treated versus untreated patients who were approximately equal in their motivation for treatment. In this four-week study of waiting list patients by Urschel and his colleagues (see McLellan et al. 1992), 42 cocaine-dependent individuals were contacted at the time of application for inpatient substance-abuse treatment. Due to the unavailability of treatment beds, these individuals were put on a waiting list for the next available opening. These individuals were followed each week of their waiting period and asked questions regarding their drug use and health status, by independent evaluators. The question of interest was whether the cocaine use and the related problems would change *without treatment*. This is an important comparison in that these 42 individuals had shown evidence of motivation for change through the act of applying for treatment.

Results indicated that only 16 percent of this group of lower socioeconomic, male veterans received any treatment-related services outside the Veterans Administration during their one-month waiting period. Interestingly, those few patients who did receive some services (typically detoxification and/or temporary housing and food at a community shelter), did show some reductions in their alcohol and drug use, although essentially no improvements in their health and personal functional status. Among the remaining individuals (84 percent) who received no treatment services at all, there were *significant increases in the severity* of medical, psychiatric, social, and drug-abuse problems over the four-week waiting period. Specifically, 53 percent reported *increased* severity of drug problems, 57 percent reported increased severity of medical problems, and 81 percent reported increased employment and support problems.

In summary, this study showed that motivation alone, without treatment, did not result in improved status for these drug-dependent individuals. In fact, there was significant worsening in the overall drug use and health status of the men who did not receive treatment. Again, while these data are by themselves not definitive, they combine with the previous data to suggest an important role for treatment in producing behavioral change and are quite consistent with earlier studies of substance-dependent patients out of treatment (Maddux and Desmond 1986; Gerstein, Judd, and Rovner 1979) and on waiting lists (Rua 1989; Sisk, Hatziandreu, and Hughes 1990).

Is Treatment More Effective than a Criminal Justice Intervention?

While the data presented thus far are quite suggestive that treatment for substance-dependent individuals can produce improvements in substance use, health and personal function, and in public health and safety risks, it remains possible that standard treatment approaches may actually be less effective in producing these favorable outcomes than other kinds of interventions, particularly probation, parole, and incarceration.

A recent study performed at the Federal Probation Department in Philadelphia (see McLellan et al. 1992; Metzger, Cornish, and Woody 1990) evaluated the effects of adding a pharmacological treatment for opiate dependence to standard federal probation/parole as compared with standard probation and with enhanced probation (i.e., twice as many supervision visits). In this study probationers who had committed opiate-related federal crimes and who volunteered for this study were randomly assigned to receive either standard probation plus naltrexone (an opiate antagonist, taken orally) or "double probation." Subjects in the "naltrexone" group met once each week with their probation officer and received a urine screen. In addition, these subjects met once each week with a nurse assigned to the project who provided brief counseling regarding drug problems as well as regular doses of naltrexone, an orally administered opiate antagonist. Subjects in the "double probation" group were required to come to the probation office for a supervision meeting twice weekly and to provide a once-weekly urine screen. The extra probation supervision meeting in this group was included to equate the two groups for the total time and attention. All evaluations were conducted by trained technicians entirely independent of the probation/parole process.

Naltrexone (Trexan ®) is an orally administered, opiate antagonist that has been shown to block the effects of injected opiates for up to 72 hours. There have been few side effects reported among those who have taken the drug, and this medication has been combined with standard counseling to aid opiate addicts in their attempts to combat pressures to relapse following the attainment of drug-free status (Willette and Barnett 1981). In fact, naltrexone has had limited success in the general opiate-abusing population (typically due to poor compliance) but has been useful with those higher socioeconomic strata patients (e.g., addicted doctors, lawyers, etc.) who have been under some externally imposed pressure to take the medication regularly (e.g., loss of license, loss of important job, etc.) (Willette and Barnett 1981). In this study, these voluntary subjects were *not* required to take the medication as part of their probation but when offered the opportunity to take a medication that might reduce their likelihood of incarceration that would be occasioned by a return to opiate use approximately 60 percent of eligible probationers volunteered.

Results of this study were interesting from several perspectives. First, the idea of combining a pharmacological treatment intervention with the standard criminal justice system supervision was well accepted by the probation/parole office, and even the additional work that was required to perform the evaluation was not considered intrusive. Second, the naltrexone was reasonably well accepted by these subjects, and 52 percent continued on the medication for the full six months of the study. This level of participation is more than three times the compliance rate typically seen among samples of opiate addicts who have been prescribed this medication without any legal, employment, or other pressures (Willette and Barnett 1981). Thus, it appears that the legal pressures associated with the threat of incarceration substantially increased treatment participation in this study.

Results of the weekly urine screenings for opiates indicated that 40 percent of the "double probation" subjects, but only 8 percent of the naltrexone subjects tested positive during the course of the study. Of particular importance for the aims of this study, only 23 percent of the naltrexone probation subjects were re-incarcerated during the six months following the study as compared with 55 percent of the subjects in the double probation group. This last result is particularly important when the costs of incarceration are considered. Prison cells are expensive to build and quite expensive to operate. Figures from 1992 suggest that federal, minimum security prison cells cost approximately $42,000 per cell to build and approximately $28,000–$32,000 per inmate to maintain each year. Probation supervision costs range from approximately $9,000 to $14,000 per year and typically result in 40–60 percent incarceration rates due to probation violations (Saxe et al. 1983).

This study illustrates three important points. First, it is possible to combine treatment and correctional approaches to address the problem of substance abuse; these are not mutually exclusive interventions. There are many reports of effective treatments for drug dependence designed for delivery within correctional facilities or in combination with probation and parole. Again, space considerations do not permit a complete review of this literature, but the interested reader is referred to reviews of this work by Inciardi (1988), Wexler et al. (1988) and Anglin et al. (1989). A second and related point

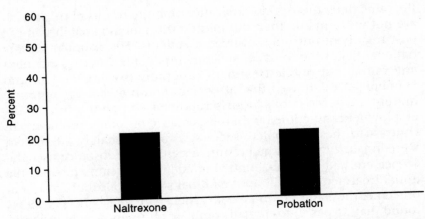

Figure 1.2   Six-month re-incarceration for two groups of opiate-dependent, federal probationers.

has been shown by many other studies within the criminal justice system (Inciardi 1988; Wexler, Falkin, and Lipton 1988; Anglin and Hser 1990), namely, that the addition of substance-abuse treatment to a correctional intervention can result in better outcomes than with the criminal justice system intervention alone. In this case not only did the naltrexone treatment appear to enhance the effects of the probation/parole intervention, but the external pressure applied by the criminal justice system appears to have enhanced compliance with the medication. Third, while this study was focused on a pharmacological treatment for opiate addiction, there is every indication that this paradigm could be applied with other forms of psychological, social, or behavioral treatments (e.g., relapse-prevention training, contingency management) as well as with other pharmacological interventions (e.g., desipramine for cocaine-abusing probationers).

If Treatment is Effective, What Makes it Effective: What are the "Active Ingredients" of Treatment?

The data presented thus far in this chapter combine to indicate that substance-abuse treatments can be effective, not just in reducing alcohol and/or drug use among those treated but also in relieving many of the important personal function and public health and safety problems so often associated with substance dependence. At the same time, there is also indication that the results of treatments are not uniform and there is typically substantial variability in the post-treatment outcomes of treated patients. For example, a large national field study of drug-dependent patients entering inpatient and outpatient public treatment programs (Armor, Polich, and Stambul 1976) showed that at twelve-month follow-up, approximately 12 percent of patients reported complete abstinence, employment, no crime, and no psychiatric or family problems. In contrast to these "complete successes," approximately 18 percent were in jail, 29 percent had resumed significant substance use, and 13 percent had been re-admitted to additional treatment since the initial treatment episode. In a national study of alcohol-treatment outcome, the Rand group (Woody, McLellan, and Luborsky 1984) found that 31 percent reported complete abstinence and no significant social problems at the twelve-month follow-up, while 41 percent had returned to alcohol use, and 19 percent had required additional treatment. Even controlled trials of single treatments in well-specified samples of patients have reported similar levels of variability in outcome (see for example Walsh et al. 1991; Armor, Polich, and Stambul 1976). Given the often extreme variability in outcome status following treatment for substance abuse, researchers have attempted to identify and study those factors that may account for this variability. Several of the most prominent and widely studied factors are discussed briefly below.

Patient factors at treatment admission
The majority of studies attempting to predict outcome have focused on patient variables at the *start* of treatment since these have been considered the most important predictors of patient status *following* treatment. In this regard factors such as greater severity of dependence (Babor et al. 1988), lack of family and social supports (Havassy, Wasserman, and Hall, forthcoming), significant psychiatric symptoms (McLellan et al. 1980; 1983; Rounsaville et al. 1987) and the presence of an antisocial personality diagnosis (Schuckit 1985; Alterman and Cacciola 1991; Hesselbrock, Meyer, and Keener 1985) have been among the more salient and well-replicated patient variables associated with poor post-treatment outcome.

Duration and intensity of treatment
Studies of treated alcoholics have consistently shown that longer stays in treatment and treatment completion are associated with greater reductions in alcohol use and more retention of these

improvements, even after controlling for pre-treatment severity of alcoholism (McKay et al. 1994; Moos, Finney, and Cronkite 1990). Similarly, studies with drug-dependent patients by De Leon (1984), Simpson and Savage (1980), and Hubbard et al. (1989) all support the finding that those patients who stay in treatment longer and who complete a standard course of care ultimately show the best outcomes (regardless of the outcome measure). While these well-replicated findings suggest that a greater "dose" of treatment is responsible for producing these improved outcomes, it is also quite possible that these results merely reflect the outcomes of the most motivated (thus longest staying and most compliant) patients. In this regard, Longabaugh et al. (1995) have shown that patients who were randomly assigned to longer stays in residential programs did *not* have better drinking outcomes than those randomly assigned to shorter stays. This finding suggests that merely longer lengths of time in treatment may not be adequate to produce desired outcomes. Instead, it may be that particular types of treatment "ingredients" are necessary in appropriate intensity and quality to assure patient improvement.

Treatment process measures
While investigations of treatment processes are still relatively new, there is practical clinical value to this type of research. The identification of treatment process and management dimensions that are reliably associated with outcome might enable refinement and enhancement of the "active ingredients" of care and elimination of "inert ingredients." Recently, there have been innovations in the measurement of the treatment environment and the treatment processes that occur during substance-abuse treatments (Ball and Ross 1991). For example, Moos and colleagues have developed and tested measures of the treatment environment in both inpatient and outpatient settings (Moos 1974; Moos, Finney, and Cronkite 1990). Similarly, Ball and his colleagues have demonstrated that it is possible to reliably and validly characterize the leadership qualities, environmental characteristics, number and types of services provided, and other aspects of a drug-dependence treatment program (Ball and Ross 1991). With these additional measures it is now possible to assess potentially relevant dimensions of the treatment as it is delivered.

One clear and tangible result from the availability of these measures coupled with traditional pre–post outcome-evaluation designs is the finding that treatment programs differ in the nature and amount of services provided to clients and that these differences

Table 1.3 Six-month outcome status comparisons among programs.

During the 30 days prior to follow-up, what proportion of patients were:

Treatment Program	Average for All Programs	OPT-1 N=45	Sig. Dif.	OPT-2 N-53	INPT-1 N=54	Sig. Dif.	INPT-2 N=46
Abstinent from alcohol	59%	51%		45%	78%	*	63%
Abstinent from all drugs	84%	80%	*	71%	87%	*	98%
Working >30 hrs/week	77%	80%	*	72%	74%	*	83%
Receiving welfare income	11%	2%	**	28%	9%		4%
Committing crimes	3%	0%	*	7%	4%		0%
Experiencing serious psych symptoms	32%	33%		34%	27%	*	35%
Experiencing serious family conflicts	25%	24%	*	31%	22%		24%

During the 6 months since leaving treatment, what proportion of patients were:

Re-treated for alcohol problems	12%	15%	*	9%	9%	*	15%
Re-treated for drug problems	10%	10%		15%	9%		7%
Hospitalized for medical problems	9%	11%		8%	9%		9%
Hospitalized for psych problems	7%	4%		7%	7%		9%

All figures express as percentage.
* = p < .05, ** = p < .01 by Z test for differences between proportions.

in treatment process correlate with corresponding differences in treatment effectiveness, even after the effects of patient factors are statistically controlled. For example, early studies of alcohol-treatment programs by the Rand Corporation (Armor, Polich, and Stambul 1976), by Emrick (1975), and by Pattison (1969) found marked differences in program organization, intensity of services provided, and in the post-treatment outcomes among inpatient treatment programs. Similarly, studies by Moos, Finney, and Cronkite (1990), evaluating three non-profit and two profit-making residential alcoholism-treatment programs, found substantial differences in the nature of the treatments provided and in the post-treatment outcomes of these five programs. There have been fewer comparative studies of treatment programs for drug-dependent patients, but a multi-site study by Ball and Ross (1991) examined treatment services and outcomes among methadone maintenance programs in three eastern cities. These authors found profound differences in the patterns of services provided to patients and in the outcomes from treatment despite very comparable samples of patients. These authors concluded that differences in program characteristics, such as leadership, organization, staffing patterns, and the amount and range of services provided during treatment, accounted for a significant proportion of the outcome differences seen among these programs.

More recently, McLellan and colleagues compared the during-treatment services and post-treatment outcomes of four private substance-dependence treatment programs (1993). All programs studied were licensed, accredited by the Joint Commission on Accreditation of Hospitals, and had a good reputation in the Philadelphia area. Despite the fact that the goals of treatment, the philosophies of rehabilitation, and the core components of the programs were quite similar (e.g., AA, 12-Steps, Alcohol/Drug Education, group therapy, etc.), there were still substantial differences among the programs in the types and quantities of services actually provided to patients during treatment. The inpatient programs provided significantly more alcohol, drug, and medical services/sessions than the outpatient programs, but services provided in the employment, family, and psychiatric areas were not different between the inpatient and outpatient settings. Although each program employed physicians, nurses, psychologists, and social workers at least part-time, the majority of patients in all programs had very little contact with any of these individuals.

The total group of patients in this study showed statistically significant and clinically impressive improvements by the time of the six-month post-treatment follow-up, both in substance use and in additional measures of personal function and social adjustment. For example, alcohol use was reduced by 74 percent and drug use by 73 percent from admission to follow-up. In fact, 59 percent were abstinent from alcohol and 84 percent were abstinent from all drugs at the follow-up interval. At the same time, there were substantial differences in outcomes among the four programs sampled. For example, drug-use improvement scores ranged from 62 percent to 81 percent across the four programs. Alcohol-use improvements ranged from 53 percent to 84 percent, while abstinence rates ranged from 45 percent to 87 percent. While the results indicated that one of the four programs was particularly inferior, there was still substantial variability among the remaining three programs – even in these licensed, accredited, private programs treating employed, insured middle-class patients. This finding suggests that the variability in treatment outcomes is even greater among less well supported programs treating a more seriously affected segment of the population.

Perhaps most interesting was the finding that these differential outcome results were less accounted for by differences in patient characteristics than by the inter-program differences in the nature and amount of services provided during treatment. Put simply, the program that provided the most services in a particular problem area showed the best outcome in that area, in 9 of 11 criteria measured (McLellan et al. 1993). Thus, consistent with prior findings from public drug-dependence treatment programs as reported by Joe et al. (1992), for residential alcohol-treatment programs as reported by Moos et al. (1990), and for methadone maintenance programs as reported by Ball and Ross (1991), these data suggest that the quantity and range of the treatment services provided within a program (e.g., counseling, physician care, referral for employment, housing, and family therapy, etc.) are important factors in explaining the variability in effectiveness among treatment programs.

While the results of these field evaluations of multiple-treatment programs provide a consistent and face-valid indication that treatment services directed at the multiple problems of substance-dependent patients are important "ingredients" in determining the effectiveness of those treatments, it must be clear that even these results are merely associations. Without proper control groups and random patient assignment, it is impossible to infer causality. However, based upon these field studies, there have now been several controlled clinical trials comparing outcomes of treatments delivered in standard clinical settings, where the "dose" of treatment services has been systematically varied. For example, Woody and his colleagues have evaluated the value of individual psychotherapy when added to paraprofessional counseling services in the course of methadone maintenance treatment (Woody, McLellan, and Luborsky 1984). In that study patients were randomly assigned to receive standard drug counseling alone (DC group) or drug counseling *plus* one of two forms of professional therapy: supportive-expressive psychotherapy (SE) or cognitive-behavioral psychotherapy (CB) over a six-month period. Results showed that patients receiving psychotherapy showed greater reductions in drug use, more improvements in health and personal function, and greater reductions in crime than those receiving counseling alone (Woody, McLellan and Luborsky 1984). These results were found throughout the six months of active treatment and remained signif-icant six months following the end of the interventions (Woody et al. 1987). Stratification of patients according to their levels of psychi-atric symptoms at intake showed that the main psychotherapy effect was seen in those with greater than average levels of psychiatric symptoms. That is, patients with low symptom levels made considerable gains with counseling alone, and there were no differ-ences between treatment groups in this sub-sample. However, patients with more severe psychiatric problems showed few gains with counseling alone but substantial improvements with the addi-tion of the psychotherapy (Woody, McLellan, and Luborsky 1984).

Another controlled study among opiate-dependent subjects extends this observation regarding the potential effectiveness of increased treatment services. McLellan and his colleagues (1993) studied 92 male opiate-dependent patients receiving three "levels" of psychosocial services while in methadone maintenance: (1) minimum methadone services, in which patients received methadone alone with no counseling or other services; (2) standard methadone services, in which patients received regular addictions counseling in addition to methadone; and (3) enhanced methadone services, in which patients received the methadone, addictions counseling, and on-site psychiatric, employment, and family therapy services. It is important to note that patients were randomly assigned to these conditions at the start of their treatment and that the methadone dosage for all groups was 65 mg or higher with no differences in average dosage levels across the three groups. At the end of six months of treatment the minimum services group did show some reductions in opiate use but virtually no other improve-ments. In addition, 69 percent of these patients had to be

32   **A. Thomas McLellan et al.**

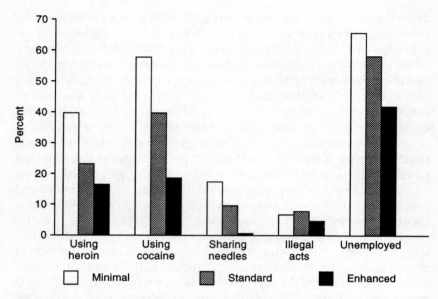

Figure 1.3 Methadone services: target behaviors at six months by level of service.

protectively terminated from the study due to unremitting drug use and/or repeated need for emergency medical care. In contrast, the standard services group showed substantial improvements in both drug and alcohol use as well as employment and crime reduction. The enhanced group showed the greatest number and amount of improvement, particularly in the areas of personal adjustment and public health and safety risk.

Two other studies of outpatient treatments for alcohol and for cocaine dependence also suggest that greater amounts of professional services directed at the "addiction related" problems of substance-dependent individuals during treatment can produce improved outcomes. In a widely cited study of comprehensive services for alcohol-dependent patients Azrin and colleagues developed the "Community Reinforcement Approach" (CRA) and tested it against other "standard" treatment interventions (Azrin 1976). CRA includes conjoint therapy, job-finding training, counseling focused on alcohol-free social and recreational activities, monitored disulfiram, and an alcohol-free social club (Azrin 1976; Hunt and Azrin 1973). In a study in which patients were randomly assigned to CRA or to a standard hospital treatment program, those getting CRA drank less, spent fewer days away from home, worked more days, and were institutionalized less over a 24-month follow-up (Hunt and Azrin 1973). A second controlled study contrasted CRA, a disulfiram (Antabuse®) compliance program, and regular outpatient treatment (Azrin et al. 1982). Once again, those treated with CRA did substantially better on all outcome measures than those in the other treatment conditions.

A more recent set of studies by Higgins et al. (1991; 1993; 1994) has used the CRA approach with cocaine-dependent patients. Here, cocaine-dependent patients seeking outpatient treatment were randomly assigned to receive either standard drug counseling and referral to AA, or a multi-component behavioral treatment integrating contingency-managed counseling, community-based incentives, and family therapy comparable to the CRA model (Higgins et al. 1991). The CRA model retained more patients in treatment, produced more abstinent patients and longer periods of abstinence, and produced greater improvements in personal function than the standard counseling approach. Following the overall findings, this group of investigators systematically "disassembled" the CRA model and examined the individual "ingredients" of family therapy (Higgins et al. 1994), incentives (Higgins et al. 1993), and the contingency-based counseling (Higgins et al. 1991) as compared with groups who received comparable amounts of all components except the target ingredient. In each case, these systematic and controlled examinations indicated that these individual components made a significant contribution to the outcomes observed, thus proving their added value in the rehabilitation effort.

Conclusions

This examination of addiction-treatment effectiveness was begun with a broad discussion of expectations placed upon substance-abuse treatments. In this regard, it was argued that the public stakeholders who are affected by substance abuse and who pay for treatment, and particularly, the patients themselves, expect more from treatment than just reductions in, or even elimination of, substance use. It was argued that the "addiction-related" problems that compromise personal health and that impair social function are important considerations for the patients, their families, and society, and thus should be targeted for improvement as part of "successful" substance-abuse treatment. In this regard, these two domains of outcome expectations for addiction treatment are quite similar to those for many other types of medical treatments. It was also argued that, unlike many forms of medical treatment, those who treat substance dependence and those who evaluate it have a responsibility to consider the special public health and public safety risks produced by addiction (e.g., spread of infectious diseases, drunk driving, drug-related crime) as a third domain of outcome measurement.

Clearly these three outcome expectations – (1) reduction in substance use, (2) improvement in personal health and social function, and (3) reduction in public health and safety risks – represent daunting tasks given the evidence of severe and chronic problems among substance-dependent persons at the start of treatment. Nonetheless, in our review of existing treatment-outcome literature we have purposely maintained this broad, public health and public safety standard for judging treatment effectiveness. Moreover, we have concentrated our review on those studies that have used the most rigorous evaluation methods, including random patient assignment, an intent-to-treat design, and data collection by independent evaluators: the same standards and methods that are typically applied by the FDA in the evaluation of new drugs and medical devices (Food and Drug Administration 1980). Beyond that, we have been careful not to impute causality to treatment unless there was true experimental evidence that the treatment program, therapy, or component under study was clearly the responsible agent of change. Given these broad expectations for the judgment of "effectiveness" and the focus upon methodologically rigorous studies in our review, two findings are quite important from a policy perspective.

First, substance-abuse treatment is "effective" as judged by all three of our criterion measures. Data reviewed indicates that substance-abuse patients show major reductions in their alcohol and drug use following their treatment. These patients also show improved medical and psychological function and often, improved earnings from employment and reductions in utilization of medical and social services. Finally, evaluations of drug-dependent patients following treatment have shown substantial reductions in AIDS-risk behaviors and in drug-related crime. These outcomes have been shown both in controlled clinical trials of experimental interventions and in large-scale evaluations of standard treatments in "real world" settings.

At the same time, it is necessary to point out that this review has also shown substantial variability in effectiveness of substance-abuse treatment across different settings, modalities, and programs. Put simply, not all treatments are effective. The research reviewed has given some clear indications regarding the sources of this variability in outcome. In particular, there is variability across treatments and treatment programs in the types and amount of treatment services provided, and this appears to be clearly associated with outcome variability. Across several types of patients and settings of care, there was consistent and face-valid evidence that patients who receive more services and, particularly, more professional services targeted to the particular profile of problems presented at admission show the best outcomes in all three of the criterion areas.

Second, *substance-abuse treatments can be and have been evaluated in* ②
a scientific manner in the same way that other forms of medical, psychological, and pharmacological interventions are evaluated. This second finding is implicit from the first, but bears emphasis because of the importance of these disorders to the public, because of the dollars expended annually in attempts to treat substance-abusing patients and because there has been so much public skepticism regarding the effectiveness of substance-abuse treatments. The heartening findings reported here suggest that scientific methods that have been proven in other types of intervention evaluations are equally applicable in the evaluation of multi-component treatments for addiction. From a policy perspective, we think this means that substance-abuse treatments *should be evaluated* using public health and public safety criteria that are important to the patients that undergo these treatments and to the society that pays for them.

Note

The Penn–VA Center for Studies of Addiction, 3900 Chestnut St., Phila. Pa., 19104, is supported by grants from NIDA, NIAAA, the Pew Foundation and the Department of Veterans Affairs. Another version of this chapter appeared in the *Milbank Quarterly* 1996 (74: 51–85).

References

Allison, M., and R.L. Hubbard. 1982. *Drug Abuse Treatment Process: A Review of the Literature* (TOPS Research Monograph). Raleigh, N.C.: Research Triangle Press.

Alterman, A.I., and J.S. Cacciola. 1991. The Antisocial Personality Disorder Diagnosis in Substance Abusers: Problems and Issues. *Journal of Nervous and Mental Disorders* 179:401–9.

Alterman, A.I., A.T. McLellan, C.P. O'Brien, et al. 1994. Effectiveness and Costs of Inpatient Versus Day Hospital Cocaine Rehabilitation. *Journal of Nervous and Mental Disorders* 182:157–63.

American Psychiatric Association. 1994. *Diagnostic and Statistical Manual,* 4th edn. Washington.

Anglin, M.D., and Y. Hser. 1990. Legal Coercion and Drug Abuse Treatment. In *Handbook on Drug Control in the United States,* ed. J. Inciardi. Westport, Conn.: Greenwood Press.

Anglin, M.D., G.R. Speckart, and M.W. Booth. 1989. Consequences and Costs of Shutting off Methadone. *Addictive Behaviors* 14(3):307–26.

Armor, D.J., J.M. Polich, and H.B. Stambul. 1976. *Alcoholism and Treatment.* Santa Monica, Calif.: Rand Corporation Press.

Azrin, N.H. 1976. Improvements in the Community Reinforcement Approach to Alcoholism. *Behavior Research and Therapy* 14:339–48.

Azrin, N.H., R.W. Sisson, R. Meyers, and M. Godley. 1982. A Social-Systems Approach to Resocializing Alcoholics in the Community. *Journal of Studies on Alcohol* 43:1115–23.

Babor, T., Z. Dolinsky, B.J. Rounsaville, and J. Jaffe. 1988. Unitary versus Multidimensional Models of Alcoholism Treatment Outcome: An Empirical Study. *Journal of Studies on Alcohol* 49:167–77.

Ball, J.C. and A. Ross. 1991. *The Effectiveness of Methadone Maintenance Treatment.* New York: Springer-Verlag.

Ball, J.C., C.P. Meyers, and S.R. Friedman. 1988. Reducing the Risk of AIDS through Methadone Maintenance Treatment. *Journal of Health and Social Behavior* 29(3):214–26.

Carroll, K.M., M.E. Power, K. Bryant, and B.J. Rounsaville. 1993. One Year Follow-Up Status of Treatment Seeking Cocaine Abusers: Psychopathology and Dependence Severity as Predictors of Outcome. *Journal of Nervous and Mental Disorders* 181(2):71–9.

Children's Defense Fund. 1994. *Children's Defense Fund Report.* Washington.

De Leon, G. 1984. *The Therapeutic Community: Study of Effectiveness.* NIDA Treatment Research Monograph #84-1286. Rockville, Md.: National Institute on Drug Abuse.

Edwards, G., J. Orford, S. Egert, et al. 1977. Alcoholism: A Controlled Trial of Treatment and Advice. *Journal of Studies on Alcoholism* 38:1004–31.

Ehrman, R.N., and S.J. Robbins. 1994. Reliability and Validity of 6-month Timeline Reports of Cocaine and Heroin Use in a Methadone Population. *Journal of Consulting and Clinical Psychology* 62:843–50.

Emrick, C.D. 1975. A Review of Psychologically Oriented Treatments for Alcoholism II. The Relative Effectiveness of Different Treatment Approaches and the Effectiveness of Treatment versus No Treatment. *Journal of Studies on Alcoholism* 36:88–108.

Finney, J.W., R.H. Moos, and D.A. Chan. 1981. Length of Stay and Program Component Effects in the Treatment of Alcoholism: A Comparison of Two Techniques for Process Analyses. *Journal of Consulting and Clinical Psychology* 49:120–31.

Food and Drug Administration. 1980. *Compliance Policy Guidelines* (Associate Committee for Regulatory Affairs, 21 CFR 310). October.

Gerstein, D., and H. Harwood (eds). 1990. *Treating Drug Problems* (vol. 1).

Washington: National Academy Press.

Gerstein, D., L.L. Judd, and S.A. Rovner. 1979. Career Dynamics of Female Heroin Addicts. *American Journal of Drug and Alcohol Abuse* 6(1):1–23.

Havassy, B.E., D. Wasserman, and S.M. Hall. Forthcoming. Social Relationships and Cocaine Use in an American Treatment Sample. *Addiction* (in press).

Hesselbrock, V., R. Meyer, and J. Keener. 1985. Psychopathology in Hospitalized Alcoholics. *Archives of General Psychiatry* 42:1050–5.

Higgins, S.T., A.J. Budney, W.K. Bickel, and G.J. Badger. 1993. Participation of Significant Others in Outpatient Behavioral Treatment Predicts Greater Cocaine Abstinence. *American Journal of Drug and Alcohol Abuse* 20(1):47–56.

Higgins, S.T., A.J. Budney, W.K. Bickel, F. Foerg, R. Donham, and G.J. Badger. 1994. Incentives Improve Treatment Retention Cocaine Abstinence and Psychiatric Symptomatology in Ambulatory Cocaine Dependent Patients. *American Journal of Psychiatry* (in press).

Higgins, S.T., D.D. Delaney, A.J. Budney, et al. 1991. A Behavioral Approach to Achieving Initial Cocaine Abstinence. *American Journal of Psychiatry* 148:1218–24.

Hubbard, R.L., M.E. Marsden, J.V. Rachal, H.J. Harwood, E.R. Cavanaugh, and H.M. Ginzburg. 1989. *Drug Abuse Treatment: A National Study of Effectiveness*. Chapel Hill, N.C.: University of North Carolina Press.

Hunt, G.M. and N.H. Azrin. 1973. A Community Reinforcement Approach to Alcoholism. *Behavior Research and Therapy* 11:91–104.

Inciardi, J.A. 1988. Some Considerations on the Clinical Efficacy of Compulsory Treatment: Reviewing the New York Experience. In *Compulsory Treatment of Drug Abuse: Research and Clinical Practice*. NIDA Research Monograph 86, ed. C.G. Leukefeld and F.M. Tims. Rockville, Md.: National Institute on Drug Abuse.

Joe, G.W., D.D. Simpson, and S.B. Sells. 1992. Treatment Process and Relapse to Opioid Use during Methadone Maintenance. *American Journal of Drug and Alcohol Abuse* 19:124–30.

LaPorte, D., A.T. McLellan, F. Erdlen, and R. Parente. 1981. Alcohol and Drug Abuse Treatment Outcome as a Function of Follow-Up Difficulty. *Journal of Clinical and Consulting Psychology* 49(1):112–19.

Longabaugh, R., M. Beattie, N. Noel, R. Stout, and P. Malloy. 1995. The Effect of Social Investment on Treatment Outcome. *Journal of Studies on Alcohol* 54(4):465–78.

Maddux, J.F., and D.P. Desmond. 1986. Relapse and Recovery in Substance Abuse Careers. In *Relapse and Recovery in Drug Abuse*. NIDA Research Monograph Series 72 (DHHS Pub. No. (ADM) 86–1473), ed. F.M. Tims and C.G. Leukefeld. Rockville, Md.: National Institute on Drug Abuse.

McKay, J.R., A.I. Alterman, A.T. McLellan, and E. Snider. 1994. Treatment Goals, Continuity of Care and Outcomes in a Day Hospital Substance Abuse Rehabilitation Program. *American Journal of Psychiatry* 151(2):254–9.

McKay, J.R., R. Longabaugh, M.C. Beattie, S.A. Maisto, and N. Noel. 1993. Does Adding Conjoint Therapy to Individually-Focused Alcoholism Treatment Lead to Better Family Functioning? *Journal of Substance Abuse* 5(1):44–59.

McLellan, A.T., A.I. Alterman, G.E. Woody, and D. Metzger. 1992. A Quantitative Measure of Substance Abuse Treatments: The Treatment Services Review. *Journal of Nervous and Mental Disorders* 180:101–10.

McLellan, A.T., I.O. Arndt, G.E. Woody, and D. Metzger. 1993. Psychosocial Services in Substance Abuse Treatment?: A Dose-Ranging Study of Psychosocial Services. *Journal of the American Medical Association* 269(15):1953–9.

McLellan, A.T., K.A. Druley, C.P. O'Brien, and R. Kron. 1980. Matching Substance Abuse Patients to Appropriate Treatments. A Conceptual and Methodological Approach. *Drug and Alcohol Dependence* 5(3):189–93

McLellan, A.T., L. Luborsky, J. Cacciola, and J.E. Griffith. 1985. New Data from the Addiction Severity Index: Reliability and Validity in Three Centers. *Journal of Nervous and Mental Disorders* 173:412–23.

McLellan, A.T., L. Luborsky, C.P. O'Brien, and G.E. Woody. 1980. An Improved Evaluation Instrument for Substance Abuse Patients: The Addiction Severity Index. *Journal of Nervous and Mental Disorders* 168:26–33

McLellan, A.T., G. Grissom, A.I. Alterman, P. Brill, and C.P. O'Brien. 1993. Substance Abuse Treatment in the Private Setting: Are Some Programs More Effective Than Others? *Journal of Substance Abuse Treatment* 10:243–54.

McLellan, A.T., L. Luborsky, G.E. Woody, C.P. O'Brien, and K.A. Druley. 1983. Increased Effectiveness of Substance Abuse Treatment: A Prospective Study of Patient-Treatment "Matching." *Journal of Nervous and Mental Disorders* 171(10):597–605.

McLellan, A.T., D. Metzger, A.I. Alterman, J. Cornish, and H. Urschel. 1992. How Effective is Substance Abuse Treatment – Compared to What? In *Advances in Understanding the Addictive States*, ed. C.P. O'Brien and J. Jaffe. New York: Raven Press.

McLellan, A.T., J. Cacciola, H. Kushner, F. Peters, I. Smith, and H. Pettinati. 1992. The Fifth Edition of the Addiction Severity Index: Cautions, Additions and Normative Data. *Journal of Substance Abuse Treatment* 5:312–16.

McLellan, A.T., A.I. Alterman, D.S. Metzger, et al. 1994. Similarity of Outcome Predictors Across Opiate, Cocaine and Alcohol Treatments: Role of Treatment Services. *Journal of Consulting and Clinical Psychology* 62(6):1141–58

Merrill, J. 1993. *The Cost of Substance Abuse to America's Health Care System, Report 1: Medicaid Hospital Costs*. New York: Center on Addiction and Substance Abuse, Columbia University.

Metzger, D., J. Cornish, and G.E. Woody. 1990. Naltrexone in Federal Offenders. In *Problems of Drug Dependence 1989*. NIDA Research Monograph #95. Rockville, Md.: National Institute on Drug Abuse.

Metzger, D.S., G.E. Woody, H. Navilane, and A.T. McLellan. Forthcoming. Risk Assessment Battery: Validity and Reliability of a Brief Questionnaire for the Measurement of AIDS Risk Behaviors. *Journal of the Acquired Immune Deficiency Syndrome* (in press).

Metzger, D., G.E. Woody, D. DePhillipis, A.T. McLellan, C.P. O'Brien, and J. Platt. 1992. Risk Factors for Needle Sharing among Methadone Patients. *American Journal of Psychiatry* 148(5):636–40.

Metzger, D.S., G.E. Woody, A.T. McLellan, et al. 1993. HIV Seroconversion among In and Out of Treatment Intravenous Drug Users: An 18-Month Prospective Follow-Up. *AIDS* 6(9):1049–56.

Miller, W.R. and R.K. Hester. 1986. The Effectiveness of Alcoholism Treatment Methods: What Research Reveals. In *Treating Addictive Behaviors: Process of Change*, ed. W.R. Miller and N. Heather. New York: Plenum Press.

Moos, R.H. 1974. *Evaluating Treatment Environments*. New York: Wiley.

Moos, R.H., J.W. Finney, and R.C. Cronkite. 1990. *Alcoholism Treatment: Context, Process and Outcome*. New York: Oxford University Press.

National Institute on Drug Abuse. 1991. *See How Drug Abuse Takes the Profit Out of Business*. Washington: Department of Health and Human Services.

Pattison, E.M. 1969. Evaluation of Alcoholism Treatment: A Comparison of Three Facilities. *Archives of General Psychiatry* 20:478–83.

Rice, D.P. 1990. Estimates of the Economic Costs of Alcohol, Drug Abuse and Mental Illness. In *Substance Abuse: The Nation's Number One Health Problem*, ed. C. Horgan, M.E. Marsden, and M.J. Larson. Princeton, N.J.: Robert Wood Johnson Press.

Robert Wood Johnson Foundation. 1994. *Costs of Addiction* (Report 14). Princeton, N.J.: Princeton University Press.

Rounsaville, B.J., Z.S. Dolinsky, T.F. Babor, and R.E. Meyer. 1987. Psychopathology as a Predictor of Treatment Outcome in Alcoholics. *Archives of General Psychiatry* 44:505–13.

Rounsaville, B.J., W. Glaser, C.H. Wilber, and H. Kleber. 1983. Short-term Interpersonal Psychotherapy in Methadone Maintained Opiate Addicts. *Archives of General Psychiatry* 40:619–26.

Rua, J. 1989. Treatment Works: The Tragic Cost of Undervaluing Treatment in the Drug War. Paper presented at the "What Works: An International Perspective on Drug Abuse Treatment" Conference, New York. Albany, N.Y.: New York State Division of Substance Abuse Services.

Saxe, L., D. Dougherty, K. Esty, and M. Fine. 1983. *The Effectiveness and Costs of Alcoholism Treatment* (Health Technology Case Study 22). Washington: Office of Technology Assessment.

Schuckit, M.A. 1985. The Clinical Implications of Primary Diagnostic Groups among Alcoholics. *Archives of General Psychiatry* 42:1043–9.

Simpson, D. and L. Savage. 1980. Drug Abuse Treatment Readmissions and Outcomes. *Archives of General Psychiatry* 37:896–901.

Sisk, J.E., E.J. Hatziandreu, and R. Hughes. 1990. *The Effectiveness of Drug Abuse Treatment: Implications for Controlling AIDS/HIV Infection*. Office of

40   A. Thomas McLellan et al.

Technology Assessment, Background Paper No. 6, USGPO No. 052-003-01210. Washington: Office of Technology Assessment.

Stewart, R.G. and L.G. Ware. 1989. *The Medical Outcomes Study.* Santa Monica, Calif.: The Rand Corporation Press

Walsh, D.C. 1982. Employee Assistance Programs. *Milbank Quarterly* 60:492–517.

Walsh, D.C., R.W. Hingson, D.M. Merrigan, et al. 1991. A Randomized Trial of Treatment Options for Alcohol-Abusing Workers. *New England Journal of Medicine* 325:775–82.

Watkins, K.E., D.S. Metzger, G.E. Woody, and A.T. McLellan. 1992. High Risk Sexual Behaviors of Intravenous Drug Users In and Out of Treatment: Implications for the Spread of HIV Infection. *American Journal of Drug and Alcohol Abuse* 18(4):389–98.

Wexler, M.K., G.P. Falkin, and D.S. Lipton. 1988. *A Model Prison Rehabilitation Program. An Evaluation of the Stay'n Out Therapeutic Community.* New York: NDRI Press.

Willette, R.W. and G. Barnett (eds). 1981. *Narcotic Antagonists : Naltrexone.* NIDA Research Monograph 28. Rockville, Md.: National Institute on Drug Abuse.

Woody, G.E., A.T. McLellan, and L. Luborsky. 1984. Psychiatric Severity as a Predictor of Benefits from Psychotherapy. *American Journal of Psychiatry* 141(10):1171–7.

Woody, G.E., A.T. McLellan, L. Luborsky, and C.P. O'Brien. 1987. 12-Month Follow-Up of Psychotherapy for Opiate Dependence. *American Journal of Psychiatry* 144:38–46.

Zanis, D., A.T. McLellan, and M. Randall. 1995. Can You Trust the Self Reports of Drug Users during Treatment? *Drug and Alcohol Dependence.*

2

Effectiveness of Drug-Abuse Treatment: A Review of Research from Field Settings

D. Dwayne Simpson

Historically, treatment evaluation research has relied on outcome or impact studies as the logical first step in efforts to respond to questions about effectiveness. Until the last five years, there has been little emphasis on treatment process research in field settings focusing on patient needs and satisfaction, delivery of services, interactions between patients and counselors, and environmental influences. The first two national, multisite treatment outcome evaluations initiated in the early 1970s and 1980s included exploratory research on organizational and service delivery features in relation to outcomes (Cole and James 1975; Hubbard et al. 1989; James et al. 1976; Joe, Simpson, and Hubbard 1991). In 1988 and 1990, the National Drug Abuse Treatment System Surveys (Price et al. 1991; Price, this volume) provided descriptions of treatment services and procedures at the organizational level, and examination of these measures by Ball and Ross (1991) in relation to patient-level outcomes helped to advance the work in this critical area. More recently, however, several NIDA treatment enhancement and demonstration research projects were funded largely in response to the AIDS epidemic (Magura and Rosenblum 1994; Tims, Inciardi, Fletcher, and Horton, in press). They have linked service delivery process and research efforts based on treatments for cocaine and opioid users and are beginning to fill in some important knowledge gaps.

Policy issues have grown more complex since the late 1960s when public funding for comprehensive community-based mental health and drug-abuse treatment services began (Musto 1987). Concerns at that time focused on whether the new federal strategy for dealing with escalating drug-abuse problems in our society was feasible and effective. The central question – "Does treatment really work?" – emphasized bottom-line outcomes, driven by costs and political implications of this new social policy. Related issues involved the use of "para-professional" versus medically-trained staff (Brown, this volume) and finding appropriate evaluation strategies for treatment research in applied settings (Simpson, Chatham, and Brown 1995). Although suspicions about overall treatment effectiveness persist, today's policy-related queries call for procedural elaborations of the drug-abuse treatment system. For instance, prominent questions include how to identify drug users who are in need of treatment, and how to assess and engage them in the most appropriate types of services for maximizing their chances of recovery.

This chapter addresses these questions with findings from treatment outcome and process research conducted in naturalistic settings, usually based on large and multisite treatment samples. The emphasis is on what works in practice, even though control over treatment assignment, and other evaluation design features for studies conducted in representative community programs, is frequently more limited than in clinical trials or other experimental research settings. Results of early treatment outcome evaluations using national samples are summarized first, followed by a comprehensive overview of the drug-treatment system to provide a context for later sections. Several core questions that serve to organize the body of this chapter are then addressed. These include: "How are drug users who need treatment identified and recruited?"; "What is the role of motivation and readiness for treatment?"; "How are patients inducted into treatment?"; "How are patients assessed and matched to services?"; "How are patients engaged and retained in treatment?"; and "Can one predict which patients are most likely to improve?" Finally, some concluding comments and recommendations are offered.

National Treatment Outcome Evaluations

As indicated by Gerstein and Harwood (1990), global treatment effectiveness questions must be refined and operationalized because of the complexities represented by diverse patient, treatment, and environmental factors. Over the past 25 years, there have been numerous single site and multisite studies of methadone maintenance, therapeutic community, drug-free outpatient, and detoxification programs. National treatment evaluation projects have been central to these efforts, including the Drug Abuse Reporting Program based on 43,943 admissions to 52 programs in the early 1970s (DARP; Sells and colleagues 1975; Simpson and Sells 1990), the Treatment Outcome Prospective Study based on 11,750 admissions to 41 programs in the early 1980s (TOPS; see Hubbard et al. 1989), and the Drug Abuse Treatment Outcome Study, which is currently in progress and based on 10,010 admissions to 100 programs in the early 1990s (DATOS; Fletcher et al. 1993). Each of these national multisite studies included post-treatment follow-up interviews with samples of patients from each modality, and their findings have been central to efforts for maintaining continued federal support of publicly-funded treatment services.

Outcomes of daily opioid users in the first year after leaving major treatment modalities in the DARP were summarized by Simpson and Sells (1982). Overall, roughly one-third had no daily drug use or major criminality, as defined by arrests and incarceration for 30 days or longer, in the year following treatment (and urine testing and official criminal justice records helped confirm the veracity of self-report data). As illustrated in figure 2.1, between-treatment comparisons showed that opioid addicts treated in methadone maintenance, therapeutic-community, and drug-free outpatient programs had significantly better outcomes than those in the detoxification and intake-only comparison groups. It was also found that post-treatment outcomes were directly associated with how long patients remained in treatment; outcomes would therefore appear even more favorable if early program dropouts who never became therapeutically engaged were excluded from figure 2.1. As shown in figure 2.2, 12-year posttreatment longitudinal data from the DARP indicate that these positive outcome trends are long-lasting (Simpson and Sells 1990). Progressive improvements continued throughout the first three years following treatment, influenced in part by readmissions to other post-DARP treatments as well as other

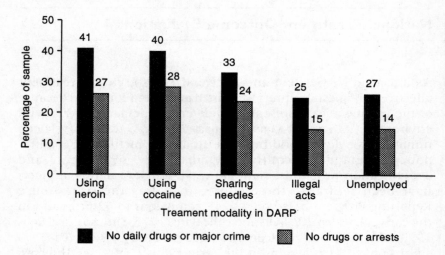

Figure 2.1　Drug-use and crime outcomes for daily opioid users in Year 1 after DARP (from Simpson and Sells 1982).

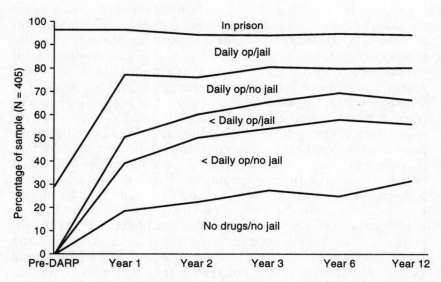

Figure 2.2　Drug-use and crime outcomes over time for daily opioid users treated in DARP (from Simpson and Sells 1990, p. 67).

life events. From years six to twelve, there was a stable rate of about 25 percent who used opioid drugs on a daily basis for all or part of any given year (plus about 8 percent who were incarcerated).

Most other large treatment outcome studies conducted in the last two decades likewise indicate that persons who enter treatment and stay for several months or longer show significant improvements when compared both with their own preadmission baseline drug use and psychosocial functioning, and with comparison groups (Anglin and Hser 1990; De Leon 1989; Gerstein and Harwood 1990; Hubbard et al. 1989; Platt, Husband and Taube 1990–91; Tims and Ludford 1984). The positive relationship between length of time patients spent in treatment and posttreatment outcomes has also

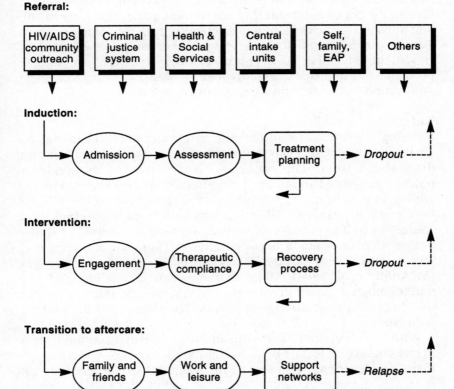

Figure 2.3 Phases of drug-abuse treatment.

been observed consistently within each major modality (De Leon 1984; Hubbard et al. 1989; Simpson 1981; Tims and Ludford 1984), although a minimum engagement period of several months is usually necessary for these improvements to be maintained following treatment.

Phases of Drug-Abuse Treatment

Before further research findings are discussed, several treatment phases are identified to help organize the treatment system into conceptual domains. A four-part model is described below, including Referral, Induction, Intervention, and Transition to Aftercare. As illustrated in figure 2.3, each phase has several steps. It is important to point out that while some patients complete one and move on to the next, others drop out at each step of the process. Therapeutic noncompliance, however, is not unique to drug-abuse treatment. McLellan (this volume) notes that there are similar problems in the medical field involving patients who fail to engage and comply with prescribed treatment regimens.

Referral
Devising effective ways of making drug users and referral agents aware of drug-abuse treatment services is an important task facing drug-abuse treatment agencies. Unfortunately, demand for publicly supported treatment has generally so far exceeded availability that systematic recruiting strategies have seldom been developed or tested. Social indications data from health and legal sources as well as population surveys are sometimes used in statistical models to estimate need for services (Gerstein and Harwood 1990), and recent efforts have focused on telephone surveys (McAuliffe et al. 1994). Major challenges include definitional and methodological variations across time and communities as well as the difficulty of obtaining representative samples of drug-using populations.

With few exceptions, treatment admissions result from some form of crisis involving legal, health, social (family) relations, or employment problems. As represented in figure 2.3, treatment referral strategies and sources vary widely. They include HIV/AIDS community outreach programs, the criminal justice system, community health and social service agencies, centralized treatment intake units, self or family, and employee assistance programs (EAPs).

Homeless shelters, STD clinics, and adolescent runaway programs serve significant numbers of drug users, but they have not become part of the typical referral network. To accommodate community needs for treatment and serve patients effectively, it is important that programs establish and maintain on-going relationships with relevant community agencies. Ideally, this includes descriptions about the types of drug abusers most appropriate for the services offered, periodic updates on availability of services, and agency performance information describing patient retention rates and outcome indicators.

Induction
The major objective of this phase is to help persons who are drug dependent become patients with a commitment to treatment and recovery. Like other types of health-related treatments, it requires a desire for help, acceptance of the role of "patient," and behavioral compliance with therapeutic plans. Due in part to the high demand for services in most communities, however, this treatment phase lacks systematic development and research.

Neither the information about treatment availability nor the fact that a person is in immediate need of treatment ensures a completed admission. Many individuals who are referred never take the first step of inquiring or applying, and there is further attrition between the stages of application and formal admission. Waiting periods and prolonged admission procedures are often assumed to help screen out persons who are not adequately motivated for treatment, but empirical support for this position is lacking. Persons with drug-abuse histories and related problems who come in contact with HIV/AIDS outreach programs and criminal justice systems in many cases have never been in treatment. For many who need treatment, there are several significant barriers which must be overcome involving geographic accessibility, treatment fees, hours of clinic operation, transportation problems, and childcare needs.

Interviews on psychosocial history, functional impairments, treatment readiness, and service needs serve as the basis for planning appropriate intervention strategies. Because licensed psychologists, psychiatrists, and other professionally-trained staff are often in short supply at public treatment programs, admission criteria are sometimes vague and informal in terms of clinical diagnosis for drug dependency and related problems. Routine staff training and supervision for the appropriate application of assessment findings to treatment plans are therefore important. Drug-dependency, legal, medical, mental health, educational, vocational, and social domains are generally evaluated using brief screening instruments, and in some cases more formal assessments of clinical and other problems may be needed. The Addiction Severity Index (ASI, McLellan, Luborsky, O'Brien, and Woody 1980; McLellan, Cacciola et al. 1992) is the most widely used intake and during-treatment progress assessment instrument; however, many programs continue to use open-ended narrative interview schedules that lack the empirical and behavioral coding format of the ASI and other recommended instruments (see Rounsaville, Tims, Horton, and Sowder 1993).

Intervention

This phase has been the central focus of most treatment research. Hoffman and Moolchan (1994) elaborate three procedural steps in reference to methadone treatment – stabilization, commitment, and rehabilitation, which with minor modifications apply to most other drug-treatment strategies as well. The important point is that treatment objectives need to be approached as part of an integrated stage-specific process. The first few weeks focus on detoxification from street drugs and engagement in treatment, followed by compliance and increased commitment as the patient becomes regularly involved in counseling and related therapeutic activities. In time, stages of cognitive and behavioral recovery should begin to emerge (De Leon 1994).

Therapeutic medications have an important role in dealing with acute medical or physical symptoms during addiction withdrawal and to a lesser extent with drug craving. Their value is most clearly established with respect to heroin and other opiates, for which methadone or LAAM can be used effectively on a long-term basis as a maintenance drug (see recent Treatment Improvement Protocols for establishing standard procedural guidelines, CSAT, 1993; 1995 a; 1995 b). Development of effective medications for treatment of cocaine abusers, however, has shown limited success (Campbell, Thomas, Gabrielli, Liskow and Powell 1994; Galloway, Newmeyer, Knapp, Stalcup and Smith 1994; Tims and Leukefeld 1993).

It is important that programs conduct assessments that are relevant to services available, either directly or through referral. This process is fundamental to practical applications of "patient matching" – that is, linking together patient needs and existing program services. Because of the limited resources usually found in public programs, however, matching protocols are seldom elegant. In some instances, it may be limited to assigning patients to a counselor on the basis of language or gender concerns.

Assessments of individual functioning are continued periodically throughout treatment to monitor personal progress. Treatment programs should also track service delivery in each treatment unit – along with patient and counselor attributions and perceptions of the therapeutic process – on a regular basis. In particular, management information systems are needed to monitor overall patient dropout (and retention) rates, session attendance rates, reasons for discharge, and other indicators. If obtained and used systematically, this type of data system can provide the information needed by program managers to document service levels and organizational performance.

Transition to aftercare
In later treatment, increased attention is devoted to preparing patients for independent functioning following discharge. Relationships with family and friends often must be redefined, work and leisure habits established, and support networks (e.g., AA, NA, CA) established and strengthened. Similar to the induction phase of treatment described above, however, development and evaluation of strategies for aftercare have been underemphasized and generally neglected as part of the overall treatment system (Brown 1990–91; Brown and Beschner 1989).

Treatment Research Issues

General questions that span these four phases of treatment are addressed next. Research has not been systematically or evenly divided across these phases, but studies have focused on some of the core issues for each one. Descriptions of findings are organized into the following areas: (1) identifying and recruiting persons in need of treatment, (2) patient motivation and readiness for treatment, (3) induction of drug abusers into treatment, (4) matching patient needs and services, (5) engaging and retaining patients, and (6) predicting improvement following treatment.

Identifying and recruiting persons in need of treatment
Occasional calls for "treatment on demand" – that is, immediate admission and provision of services on request – have neither been subjected to systematic study nor widely implemented. Indeed, its potential impact on publicly-funded programs has been viewed as a moot point given the widespread existence of treatment waiting lists

in many communities. Recent concerns about HIV infection, however, have stimulated an interest in admitting injection drug users in drug-abuse treatment as rapidly as possible. This has led to a congressionally imposed program of interim services in which all injection drug users who can not be inducted into treatment within a two-week period are to be offered, at minimum, HIV prevention counseling and some minimal services including methadone maintenance (or possibly LAAM). Preliminary evidence on the efficacy of interim, or minimum, services of this type has been limited and inconsistent (Calsyn et al. 1994; McLellan, Arndt, Metzger, Wood, and O/'Brien 1993; Yancovitz et al. 1991).

Historically, admissions to community treatment programs frequently report themselves to be self referrals. If the three inter-related categories of self, family, and friends are combined together, they account for one-half to three-fourths of admissions in national multisite treatment studies (for DARP, see Simpson, Savage, Joe, Demaree, and Sells 1976; for TOPS, see Hubbard et al. 1989). The criminal justice system has been the second most common source of referral, accounting for approximately 30 percent of patients admitted to residential and outpatient drug-free programs – but it is only about 5 percent for methadone treatment due to its reluctant use by criminal justice authorities. Other sources (e.g., medical, clergy, employer, community agencies) typically account for no more than 5 percent each. Among more contemporary treatment populations, these traditional patterns of treatment referrals may change as a result of HIV/AIDS and new criminal justice trends toward imposing compulsory treatment.

It is particularly noteworthy that the increase of HIV seroprevalence rates and AIDS among drug users has had an enormous impact on the drug-treatment field, especially in the development of effective community outreach and recruitment strategies (Brown and Beschner 1993). The widespread success of locating drug users by indigenous community workers as part of the pioneering HIV/AIDS outreach studies funded by NIDA has led to implementation of similar programs in virtually every major city in this country. Finding that over 40 percent of the injection drug users recruited for HIV testing and counseling were never in treatment (Liebman, Knezek, Coughey, and Hua 1993) has resulted in greater importance being given to HIV outreach programs as a source of referral to drug-abuse treatment. The never-treated outreach subsample tends to be minority, younger, cocaine users, lower in education, and to have childcare responsibilities. As part of the routine assessment of drug-use history and HIV risk levels, persons who would benefit from drug-abuse treatment are readily identified and given information about local programs. Unfortunately, treatment resources in most communities are not adequate to accommodate the needs identified by these outreach efforts. Treatment referral strategies also vary widely, ranging from merely providing lists of regional treatment programs (but without social networking arrangements), to offering private transportation to a program with openings for immediate admissions.

The other referral source with major implications for treatment demands is the criminal justice system. It employs two general routes leading to compulsory, or coerced, treatment (Leukefeld and Tims 1988), which are being promoted as part of recent crime bills at state and national levels. The first is a diversion program in which nonviolent offenders with drug-related problems are sent to treatment instead of jail or prison (such as TASC and similar programs; see Swartz 1993). Indeed, more communities are beginning to establish drug courts as initiated in Miami to permit referral of drug offenders to treatment programs. This often represents the first contact with formal treatment as evidenced by the fact that Drug Use Forecasting (DUF) data indicate only 4 percent of arrestees are currently in treatment at the time of arrest, and only 22 percent have ever been treated for drug abuse (Lipton 1994). The second route is part of a growing national trend to establish criminal justice facilities devoted to residential drug-abuse treatment, modeled after the successful efforts of Projects REFORM and RECOVERY (Wexler and Lipton 1993). This approach involves designated facilities for providing therapeutic community treatment (or modified approaches) for 6 to 12 months before prison release.

If this trend in social policy continues, it is also expected to have a broader impact on the treatment system through the formal linking of different modalities and creating a continuum of care (from intensive residential in prison to community outpatient support during aftercare). In Texas, for example, legislation was passed in 1991 to create 14,000 beds in state prisons for providing nine months of in-prison drug treatment managed by privately-contracted therapeutic community agencies. Afterwards, inmates are released (as conditions of parole) to a mandatory three months of community-based residential treatment, followed by 12 months of outpatient care (Sellers 1994). There is also a growing number of county residential drug-treatment facilities that treat probationers for several months, as well as short-term jail-based programs. Brief screens for assessing drug-use histories and psychosocial functioning problems related to alcohol and drug use determine who enters these programs, and preliminary findings show that about half have never been in drug treatment before (Simpson, Knight, Chatham, Camacho, and Cloud 1994). Accelerated implementation of these programs in large and multisite applications has been difficult, but evidence concerning their effectiveness promises to have significant policy implications.

Patient motivation and readiness for treatment

Gerstein and Harwood (1990) note that individuals who seek treatment usually share three attributes. First, there is a source of urgency caused by physical or mental health problems (e.g., infections, chronic depression), sharp social pressures (e.g., family problems, legal action), or pending threats or danger (e.g., incarceration, assaults). Second, drug use is recognized as either the direct or indirect cause of problems. And third, there is nervous uncertainty about entering treatment and adapting to a recovery perspective and regimen. These reflect both internal and external pressures to seek treatment. Clearer distinctions between motivational influences and a better understanding of their interactions are needed.

Retrospective accounts of the most important reasons given for entering treatment over the course of a 12-year follow-up study were obtained from male opioid addicts treated in DARP (Simpson and Sells 1990). Collectively, this sample (n = 405) had an average of over six treatment admissions each at the time of follow-up, at which point 62 percent had been abstinent from all opioid drug use for a year or longer (and two-thirds had not used daily in the last 3 years or more). With respect to the reasons they gave for entering treatment programs, nine out of ten reported they decided for themselves and three-fourths felt family pressures were important. Legal influences were cited less frequently, but they were more prevalent than reasons reflecting low availability or quality of drugs, pressure from friends, or medical problems; more specifically, 41 percent and 49 percent cited general legal problems and pressure from parole officer, respectively, as being important.

Work summarized by Prochaska, DiClemente, and Norcross (1992) on stages of change illustrates the importance of cognitive processes and attributions which precede behavioral indicators of recovery. They postulate that modifications of addictive behaviors take place in stages – precontemplation, contemplation, preparation, action, and maintenance – even though progress is not always strictly sequential. Instead, there is frequent recycling through these cognitive and behavioral change stages on the way to long-term recovery. Miller and Rollnick (1991) have developed interview techniques intended to strengthen motivational commitment using supportive exploration of consequences and need for cognitive change, and in their view, there must be a shift in the decisional balance between the benefits and costs associated with drug abuse. Successful induction and engagement in treatment depend on finding ways to enhance and sustain cognitive processes that eventually lead to behavioral change.

Baekeland and Lundwall (1975) reviewed treatment studies showing that poor motivation was a common predictor of dropouts, but observed that measurement and conceptual clarity in these early studies were lacking. Motivation and readiness for drug-abuse treatment have been conceptualized by De Leon and associates (see De Leon and Jainchill 1986; De Leon, Melnick, Kressel, and Jainchill 1994) as composed of four primary dimensions: circumstances, motivation, readiness, and suitability. Related work by Simpson and Joe (1993) identified three dimensions, reflecting self-perceived severity of drug-use problems, desire for help, and treatment readiness. Both of these assessment instruments have predictive validity as indicated by significant associations with treatment retention (in therapeutic community and outpatient methadone treatment settings), and they have begun to identify particular cognitive components that are relevant to therapeutic engagement. More efforts are needed to clarify the comparative roles of internal versus external sources of motivation, however, particularly as they relate to sources and degrees of treatment pressures as perceived by patients. Given the dynamic nature of these cognitive attributions, more study is also needed to monitor changes over time and explore their role in sustaining individual recovery efforts.

Induction of drug abusers into treatment

Persons referred to treatment do not always apply for, or complete, the admission process. Even those who do are not always viewed as being motivated. The social costs resulting from admission failures (from the point of view of crime and health problems) as well as the resources required as part of program intake and assessment lost because of early dropouts suggest that more systematic attention should be given to this phase of treatment. To this end, recent work has focused on program-level factors that represent barriers to entering treatment, as well as patient-level interventions intended to enhance treatment readiness and establish an orientation to the role of patient (Brown and Needle 1994).

With respect to program policy and management influences,

Maddux (in press) found that using rapid intake (for reducing the length of time required for admission) as well as removing financial barriers (by offering no-fee treatment) significantly increased the percentage of opioid addicts retained in methadone treatment. Platt and colleagues (Kirby, Festinger, Lamb, and Platt, forthcoming) report similar benefits of using a rapid intake policy for day treatment of cocaine abusers. Community outreach programs likewise have been found to be more successful in recruiting drug users into treatment through the distribution of coupons or vouchers which guarantee free treatment for a period of time (Bux, Iguchi, Lidz, Baxter, and Platt 1993; Jackson, Rotkiewicz, Quinones, and Passannante 1989; Sorensen, Constantini, Wall, and Gibson 1993). Case management approaches have been shown to help guide and support patient access to health and social service networks (Ashery 1992; Grella, Anglin, Wugalter, and Annon forthcoming; Martin, Inciardi, Scarpitti, and Nelson forthcoming; Mejta, Bokos, Maslar, Mickenberg, and Senay forthcoming; Siegal, Rapp, Fisher, Cole, and Wagner forthcoming). Brady, Besteman, and Greenfield (forthcoming) have demonstrated the efficacy of using a mobile van to provide methadone treatment, thus overcoming problems of community resistance to local fixed-site drug-treatment facilities as well as geographic inaccessibility and transportation costs, factors which inhibit patient enrollment and participation levels.

Patient-level factors believed to increase treatment response include motivational interviewing approaches to enhance internal commitments to treatment (Miller and Rollnick 1991), and external factors such as legal pressures (Anglin and Hser 1990; Leukefeld and Tims 1988). Pretreatment induction efforts have also been developed and tested in which both internal and external influences were merged. For instance, the Weekend Intervention Program (Siegal and Cole 1993) uses three days of marathon counseling sessions based on a cognitive-behavioral approach to supportively assess functional consequences and risks of drug and alcohol use. The program has been effective in improving patient attitudes about treatment activities and reducing early dropout rates.

Matching patient needs and services
It has long been assumed that there is, or should be, an optimal match between clearly defined categories of patients and categories of treatment. Unfortunately, patients and treatments do not fit into convenient categories or types. Instead, there exists a vast array of both patient needs and available services, although few public programs offer a rich mixture of treatment alternatives. Early efforts

to classify patients in community treatment agencies using cluster analytic strategies were abandoned (Joe and Simpson 1975), and it was also found that general categorizations of treatment types used to compare and contrast treatment organization and process across sites (Cole and James 1975) represent an oversimplification of relevant organizational and procedural considerations. For instance, posttreatment outcomes for categories of patients in various DARP treatment modalities and submodalities showed no differences (Simpson and Savage 1981–82); using social and behavioral indicators such as criminal history, legal status at admission, socioeconomic status, and drug-use history for matching patients to treatment in order to improve posttreatment outcomes was unproductive. McLellan and Alterman (1991) have likewise concluded that efforts to find patient–program combinations with clear payoffs in patient recovery rates and therapeutic efficiency have been largely unsuccessful.

The key to a rational approach to matching patients with treatment lies in using assessment techniques that have conceptual and pragmatic linkage to services which realistically can be provided on site or through referral. This is the fundamental mission of treatment, even though it proves in practice to be more difficult than it may sound. Programs would benefit by using the ASI or comparable assessments (rather than relying primarily on narrative accounts of interviews and clinical notes) as a basis for screening and identifying major treatment needs. The ASI is widely used but its value for clinical and evaluation applications is often diminished by nonstandard interpretations of selected items. Price (this volume) found 80–90 percent of outpatient treatment programs report that they conduct some type of mental health assessment for patients, but the level of standardization and utilization of this information is difficult to determine. Indeed, experienced multisite treatment evaluators (personal communications with Doug Anglin, George De Leon, Bob Hubbard, and Tom McLellan) support the concern shown by Price about staff training needs and the "bare bones" treatment approach that exists in many community settings. That is, personnel who are trained to make formal clinical diagnoses are unavailable to most community programs, and the counselors frequently lack the resources, training, or experience to make practical use of them.

Patients vary widely in their needs for services, and these needs change over time. Motivation and treatment readiness levels also waiver. Counseling format, frequency, and focus should be guided by these needs. New patients entering treatment typically have many unresolved crises and related problems, and therefore might benefit from more frequent individualized counseling during the first few months after intake. Later, a shift towards greater reliance on group counseling could be appropriate to take advantage of peer confrontation, support, and bonding. Effective care can be provided within a flexible and supportive environment, sometimes because patients recognize their own needs. For example, Joe, Brown, and Simpson (1994) found that patients in methadone treatment who had higher levels of psychological problems at intake were more likely than other patients to stay 90 days or longer, attend more treatment sessions (especially individual counseling), and discuss psychological issues during sessions. Although they had higher levels of drug use and illegal activity at intake, there were no differences between them and other patients on these measures after 3 months in treatment. In methadone treatment, another option deserving attention for improving long-term care of some patients is "medical maintenance," whereby counseling sessions are tapered off following stabilization with take-home medications of methadone (Novick et al. 1988; Senay, Barthwell, Marks and Bokos 1994; Senay et al. 1993). LAAM may also offer similar possibilities.

More selective attention is needed for underserved groups such as women and minorities in an effort to be more responsive to unique problems of special populations. For instance, a sexuality and assertiveness workshop developed specifically for women addresses topics such as breast health and self-examination, sexual and reproductive anatomy, sexual response, gynecological health, sexually transmitted disease and AIDS/HIV prevention, and communication skills (especially related to AIDS risky behaviors). This module increased women's self-esteem and knowledge, and level of participation was positively associated with length of stay in the treatment program following the workshop (Bartholomew, Rowan-Szal, Chatham and Simpson 1994). Other special needs such as parenting skills for all patients and sexual trauma resolution for women also deserve attention.

Given that HIV seroprevalence rates are higher among minority groups (LaBrie, McAuliffe, Nemeth-Coslett, and Wilberschied 1993) and that they drop out of some types of treatment programs at higher rates than whites (De Leon, Melnick, Schoket, and Jainchill 1993; Kleinman et al. 1992), increased cultural sensitivity should benefit drug-abuse treatment. Culture-related barriers to treatment engagement appear to involve the concept of time, attitudes toward authority figures and health providers, gender roles, spiritual practices, use of leisure time, intergenerational relationships, and most frequently, verbal communication problems (Pérez-Arce, Carr, and

Sorensen 1993; Rowe and Grills 1993; Sue and Sue 1990; Sue and Zane 1987). Misunderstandings caused by different cultural perspectives seem to be compounded by the lack of common language tools, especially because mainstream counseling is largely "talk therapy." Visual representation strategies discussed later in this chapter offer promise as a way of overcoming some of these communication problems (Dansereau, Joe, Dees, and Simpson 1994).

Engaging and retaining patients

Many of the same factors that predict treatment engagement and retention are important for posttreatment outcomes. Those that are reported most commonly fall into three general measurement domains. Patient-specific factors include severity of addiction, criminal involvement, family problems, unemployment, and psychiatric comorbidity (Anglin and Hser 1990). Program-level factors that influence patient decisions about treatment participation include: (1) neighborhood and geographic accessibility, (2) facility attributes and appearance, (3) compatibility with other patients, (4) attitudes of treatment and administrative staff, (5) medication practices, (6) counseling and medical services delivered, (7) treatment philosophies, and (8) administrative procedures and practices (Ball and Ross 1991). Environment and contextual factors include factors such as family relations and social support systems, neighborhood and housing conditions, socioeconomic opportunities and pressures, and local law enforcement practices (Moos, Finney, and Cronkite 1990).

Psychosocial Intervention strategies, however, are central to making improvements in treatment engagement and retention of opiate and cocaine users. Some represent behavioral interventions, while others emphasize cognitive training as a prelude to behavioral change and recovery. The first type are represented by behaviorally-based contingency-management techniques, preferably those that do not lead to discharge from treatment as a result of compliance failures. Positive reinforcement schedules with simple and inexpensive tokens can improve important engagement and compliance behaviors like session attendance and clean urines (Rowan-Szal, Joe, Chatham and Simpson 1994; Stitzer, Grabowski, and Henningfield 1984). Similarly, a reinforcement approach using community-based recreational and leisure activities (e.g., biking, skiing, photography) as incentives appears to be effective in motivating patients to reduce drug use (Sisson and Azrin 1989; Higgins et al. 1991). Family and peer support networks have also been the focus of other behavioral reinforcement strategies for strengthening patient compliance with treatment regimen and recovery efforts (Hunt, Lipton, Goldsmith, and Strug 1984; Sorensen, Gibson, Deitch, and Bernal 1985; Todd 1984).

There is a tendency for drug abusers to be impulsive and lack problem-solving skills (Dansereau, Joe, and Simpson 1993; Husband and Platt 1993). Platt, Prout, and Metzger (1986) have therefore presented a cognitive training module designed to strengthen alternative thinking, consequential thinking, means–end thinking, perspective taking, and social causal thinking. Another cognitive approach that holds promise for dealing with attentional and general problem-solving deficiencies involves "visual representation strategies." Researchers in cognitive psychology have recommended the use of such strategies to clarify problems and potential solutions (Larkin and Simon 1987; Mayer and Gallini 1990; Winn, Li, and Schill 1991). Visual representations tend to help cluster together components that are related, while natural language (spoken or written) tends to string them out. Consequently, language can be less effective for representing parallel lines of thought, feedback loops, and other elements of complex systems. Because counseling involves working with complex systems of interrelated feelings, thoughts, and actions, it should be beneficial to have relevant issues and potential solutions represented visually. Use of special visualization techniques in some applications of family therapy has supported this contention (Liepman, Silvia, and Nirenberg 1989; Van Treuren 1986).

Dansereau and associates assessed the impact of visual representation in drug-abuse counseling using a general purpose node-link mapping system for graphically illustrating personal problems, issues, and plans in group and individual settings. They found mapping-enhanced counseling leads to greater patient commitment to treatment (as measured by attendance at scheduled counseling sessions), more positive counselor perceptions of the patient (e.g., communication effectiveness and motivation), and fewer urinalysis results that are positive for opiates and cocaine during treatment (Dansereau, Joe, and Simpson 1993; forthcoming). The graphic portrayal of addiction and recovery issues provides the patient and counselor with a practical tool that facilitates the interactive course of a session by enhancing communication, focus, and memory for session content.

In response to concerns about counselor training needs and the availability of resources, several non-technical and user-friendly counseling manuals for special issues have been prepared. For example, NIDA has recently printed materials for national distribution on relapse prevention and cue extinction, along with assessment manuals on program evaluation, administration of the ASI, and other diagnostic resources. Some of the materials developed and evaluated under the auspices of NIDA's treatment enhancement and demonstration research projects are also being reprinted for distribution to the field. Platt and colleagues (Kirby, Festinger, Lamb, and Platt, forthcoming) describe their cognitive and behavioral interventions, training in interpersonal problem solving, training in vocational problem solving, and day-treatment modules for anger management, social skills training, and relapse prevention. Other similar comprehensive psychosocial treatment protocols proving to be effective with cocaine/stimulant users include the Matrix Neurobehavioral Model (Shoptaw, Rawson, McCann, and Obert 1994; Magura and Rosenblum 1994), and Living in Balance Program (Hoffman et al. 1994). Simpson and colleagues (summarized in Simpson, Dansereau, and Joe forthcoming) developed and evaluated a series of treatment manuals for HIV/AIDS education, women's assertiveness training, transition to aftercare and support networks, and counselor training in the use of visual representation techniques. And Sacks, De Leon, Bernhardt, and Sacks (1994) are developing a manual-driven protocol for use in modified therapeutic-community treatment programs for homeless, mentally ill substance abusers.

Predicting improvements following treatment

The most consistent predictor of favorable posttreatment outcomes is length of time spent in treatment. Few would argue, however, that this effect is due simply to the elapsed time between admission and discharge. Indeed, recent studies by Hoffman et al. (1994), McLellan, Arndt et al. (1993), Shoptaw et al. (1994), and Simpson, Joe, Rowan-Szal, and Greener (1995) support expectations that frequency and intensity of services are directly related to patients' cognitive and behavioral improvements. In addition to patient-level engagement effects, other findings consistently show that program-level indicators of quality and quantity of services are likewise associated with more positive outcomes when examined in publicly-funded methadone maintenance programs (Ball and Ross 1991; Joe, Simpson and Hubbard 1991; Joe, Simpson, and Sells 1994), private chemical dependency programs (McLellan, Grissom et al. 1993), and alcohol treatment programs (Moos, Finney, and Cronkite 1990).

Patient background and related characteristics generally account for a much smaller share of outcome variance than do treatment-related variables (Anglin and Hser 1990). In effect, this suggests there are no patient types who should be considered untreatable. Nevertheless, findings from the DARP indicated that heavy criminal involvement is a predictor of poor posttreatment recovery in most outcome domains, which tends to merge with a general set of predictors reflecting general social dysfunction (Simpson and Sells 1982). Anglin and Hser (1990) likewise conclude that more stability in family background, intact marriage, employment, low criminality, less severe drug use, and less severe psychiatric disorders predict better outcomes. Psychiatric comorbidity, involving drug dependency and psychiatric disorders, generally complicates treatment; this is especially true for patients diagnosed as having antisocial personality disorders (Woody, McLellan, O'Brien, and Luborsky1991).

Finally, it should be added that alcohol abuse has often been given too little attention in the treatment of illicit drug use. Studies have found heavy alcohol consumption to be associated with a variety of behavioral and psychosocial problems and linked to different responses to treatment. Among these are higher rates of medical illness (Baden 1970; Force and Miller 1974; Stimmel, Vernance, and Tobias 1972), higher death rates (Cherubin, McCusker, and Baden 1972), greater criminal activity (Roszell, Calsyn, and Chaney 1986), greater use of illicit drugs during treatment (Maddux and Elliot 1975), and poorer social functioning (Chatham, Rowan-Szal, Joe, Brown and Simpson 1995; Rounsaville, Weissman, and Kleber 1982). Associated psychological problems include depression, obsessive-compulsive behavior, somatization, phobic anxiety, and psychosis (El Bassel, Schilling, Turnbull, and Su 1993). Nevertheless, the relationship to treatment outcome is unclear. It has been associated with higher rates of treatment failure by some (Gearing 1970; Joseph and Appel 1985; Perkins and Bloch 1970), but unrelated to outcome by others (Rounsaville, Weissman and Kleber 1982; Stimmel 1981). Because of the multiple problems presented by these patients, however, they usually are described as difficult to treat.

Concluding Comments

Outcome evaluations in the past 25 years have consistently supported the effectiveness of drug-abuse treatment. However, failure to maintain stable federal funding during this time for a progressive research program that addresses therapeutic and methodological needs of the field has been costly in regard to our scientific knowledge base. In particular, we need better understanding of treatment dynamics and influences on complex drug-abuse recovery processes for making health care reform and policy recommendations. New work funded by NIDA in the last five years, especially under the auspices of treatment enhancement demonstration research grants, has helped.

National treatment evaluation studies, treatment evaluation research centers, and treatment enhancement demonstration projects working closely with community-based treatment agencies provide valuable information about existing services and needs in the field. Most patients (especially in outpatient treatment) receive only brief drug-abuse counseling, but there are needs for a wide variety of other problems that intersect with drug use and addiction. Unfortunately, resources and access to corollary services in the national infrastructure for publicly-funded drug-abuse treatment have diminished markedly since the early 1980s (Etheridge, Craddock, Dunteman and Hubbard 1995; Gustafson 1991; Price, this volume). Unmet are many requests for vocational training and job placement, public health care (for HIV/AIDS, TB, sexually transmitted diseases), preventive medical services for adults and their children, and mental health services. Although there is considerable diversity across programs (both within and between states) in staff training and financial resources, there are widespread needs in the areas of resource development and management, patient-needs assessments, and applied counseling skills.

Because of the shortage of treatment services in most communities, recruitment of new drug-abuse patients is not usually feasible or viewed as a priority. In addition, special efforts needed to engage and retain difficult patients seem unnecessary. Why expend significant time and energy on those who are unwilling to participate if others are waiting for treatment? However, programs have always owned the responsibility for creating sufficient motivation for treatment participation and behavior change rather than demanding that the patient appear before them "ready for treatment." Drug abusers are apt to be ambivalent about adopting the role of patient and pursuing a life course which is largely alien to them and likely to lead to isolation from many of the people with whom they have associated. Treatment programs must have resources to meet their responsibility for recognizing and, in so far as possible, resolving these issues as a part of the work of treatment.

To a significant degree, AIDS and the threat of HIV infection are changing public thinking about both treatment recruitment and retention issues. Citing concerns about AIDS, the Congress and the Secretary of Health have mandated both outreach and interim services (including interim methadone) to target injection drug users with a view toward providing an intervention sufficient to reduce risk of AIDS in this population. While comprehensive treatment is not contemplated in either the outreach or interim services mandated, it is apparent that some behavior-change strategies must be derived from drug-abuse treatment. Responsibility for providing services to this population fall primarily on the local treatment community.

The high prevalence of drug-abuse problems among criminal justice populations has caused renewed interest in compulsory treatment. Several options seem reasonable to pursue, but widespread implementation of these programs without an on-going evaluation plan threaten their political endurance. An integrated network of community-based treatments (including self-help groups) will also be needed to provide continuing care during social reentry from correctional settings. The function of existing community programs which currently provide primary treatment is expected to be expanded, in some instances, to meet continuing-care needs of prison-based treatments as well. As a result, existing needs for more staff, resources, and training in drug-abuse treatment programs are anticipated to become even more acute.

Persons who participate actively and stay in drug-abuse treatment longer have more favorable outcomes, so it is therefore important to identify factors that promote motivation, satisfaction, engagement, and retention. This is a major objective of process research in which service delivery, patient characteristics, counseling strategies, and the interactions between these elements are examined (see Ball and Ross 1991; Joe, Simpson, and Sells 1994; and Moos, Finney, and Cronkite 1990). But treatment is a dynamic and transitional process only partially influenced by patient interactions within the treatment environment. Many other contextual and environmental factors exert direct as well as indirect effects on persons trying to recover from addiction.

Compared with impact assessments focusing on posttreatment outcomes, process studies require a sophisticated set of measurement and analytical approaches. For instance, measures representing internal operations in the treatment system and patient responses are necessary, which are then examined as sequential and interactive events that influence later outcomes. Cognitive attributions of patient and counselor (the basis of therapeutic alliance and stages-of-change concepts) are fundamental. Within this framework, specific treatment activities – including new or alternative approaches and how well they are delivered – need to be examined and related to indicators of engagement. Data systems for this work are complex and require carefully coordinated and collaborative efforts of service providers and evaluation groups.

In conclusion, all four phases of the treatment continuum – referral, induction, intervention, and transition to aftercare – are critical elements of an integrated system for responding to drug-abuse problems in our society. Personal and public health concerns argue for effective procedures for recruiting drug abusers into treatment, securing their participation, and retaining them long enough to establish foundations for recovery. Several general observations and recommendations for improving treatment are summarized below.

Referral. Drug users who are identified by social service agencies and community outreach programs (e.g., HIV/AIDS) as being in need of treatment – especially for low-fee or no-fee treatment – are not being served adequately by existing publicly-funded drug-abuse treatment programs. Better integration of HIV/AIDS outreach services with treatment providers, and more efficient coordination of treatment resources in community-based and criminal justice settings, along with guidelines for allocating limited treatment services, are needed.

Induction. There are barriers to treatment entry and participation, especially in low-income indigent populations who cannot pay for treatment fees, transportation, and childcare. Motivation and commitment for change are also low among many drug abusers, especially youth with comparatively short addiction histories and antisocial peer reference groups. Treatment fees and related barriers to care should be removed or reduced by programs, and improved strategies are needed for inducting drug users into treatment as well as motivating those who are not ready for change.

Intervention. Structured evaluations of patient needs required for treatment assignment and for monitoring progress over time are not well developed or implemented. Integrated intake and in-treatment data systems which track patient and program management objectives are often lacking. For too many patients, attendance rates for counseling sessions are low, individual sessions are crisis-oriented, and group sessions (which can capitalize on positive peer involvement) are underutilized. Treatment plans that are not behaviorally oriented fail to help guide progress in defining and reaching personal goals. Counseling staff have large caseloads (frequently exceeding 35 patients) and operate with limited resources and training opportunities. As a result there has been a major decline in the quantity of services delivered at public programs during the past decade. Patient assessments and improved staff training to guide practical decisions about matching available services to patient needs are required, and management information systems on patient flow and services are needed to improve delivery and public accountability of program services. Reductions in patient caseloads, routine supervision and training, user-friendly counseling manuals and materials, and better access to community services are needed by counselors.

Aftercare. Patients leaving treatment return to social environments with low employment rates, high crime, and easily accessible drugs. Vocational training and job placement assistance, and access to community-based recovery support networks (e.g., AA/NA/CA) are needed.

References

Anglin, M.D., and Y.I. Hser. 1990. Treatment of Drug Abuse. In *Drugs and Crime,* ed. M. Tonry and J.Q. Wilson, 393–460. Chicago: University of Chicago Press.

Ashery, R.S. (ed.) 1992. *Progress and Issues in Case Management* (NIDA Research Monograph 127, DHHS pub. no. (ADM) 92-1946). Rockville, Md.: National Institute on Drug Abuse.

Baden, M. 1970. Methadone-Related Deaths in New York City. *International Journal of the Addictions* 5:489–98.

Baekeland, F., and L. Lundwall. 1975. Dropping out of Treatment: A Critical Review. *Psychological Bulletin* 82(5):738–83.

Ball, J.C., and A. Ross. 1991. *The Effectiveness of Methadone Maintenance Treatment: Patients, Programs, Services, and Outcome.* New York: Springer-Verlag.

Bartholomew, N.G., G.A. Rowan-Szal, L.R. Chatham, and D.D. Simpson. 1994. Effectiveness of a Specialized Intervention for Women in a Methadone Program. *Journal of Psychoactive Drugs* 26:249–55.

Brady, J., K. Besteman, and L. Greenfield. Forthcoming. Evaluating the Effectiveness of Mobile Drug Abuse Treatment. In *The Effectiveness of Innovative Strategies in the Treatment of Drug Abuse,* ed. F.M. Tims, B.W. Fletcher, J.A. Inciardi, and A.M. Horton, Jr. (in press). Westport, Conn.: Greenwood Press.

Brown, B.S. 1990–91. AIDS and the Provision of Drug User Treatment. *International Journal of the Addictions* 25(12A):1503–14.

Brown, B.S., and G.M. Beschner. 1989. AIDS and HIV Infection – Implications for Drug Abuse Treatment. *Journal of Drug Issues* 19(1):141–62.

Brown, B.S., G.M. Beschner, and National AIDS Research Consortium (eds). 1993. *Handbook on Risk of AIDS: Injection Drug Users and Sexual Partners.* Westport, Conn.: Greenwood Press.

Brown, B.S., and R.H. Needle. 1994. Modifying the Process of Treatment to Meet the Threat of AIDS. *International Journal of the Addictions* 29(13):1739–52.

Bux, D.A., M.Y. Iguchi, V. Lidz, R.C. Baxter, and J.J. Platt. 1993. Participation in an Outreach-Based Coupon Distribution Program for Free Methadone Detoxification. *Hospital and Community Psychiatry* 44:1066–72.

Calsyn, D.A., E.A. Wells, A.J. Saxon, T.R. Jackson, A.F. Wrede, V. Stanton, and C. Fleming. 1994. Contingency Management of Urinalysis Results and Intensity of Counseling Services Have an Interactive Impact on Methadone Maintenance Treatment Outcome. *Journal of Addictive Diseases* 13(3):47–63.

Campbell, J.L., H.M. Thomas, W. Gabrielli, B.I. Liskow, and B.J. Powell. 1994. Impact of Desipramine or Carbamazepine on Patient Retention in Outpatient Cocaine Treatment: Prelimary Findings. *Journal of Addictive Diseases* 13(4):191–9.

Center for Substance Abuse Treatment. 1995a. *Matching Treatment to Patient Needs in Opioid Substitution Therapy* (Treatment Improvement Protocol Series #20 DHHS pub. no. (SMA) 95–3049). Rockville, Md.

———. 1995b. *LAAM in the Treatment of Opiate Addiction* (Treatment Improvement Protocol Series). Rockville, Md.

———. 1993. *State Methadone Treatment Guidelines* (Treatment Improvement Protocol Series, DHHS pub. no. (SMA) 93-1991). Rockville, Md.

Chatham, L.R., G. Rowan-Szal, G.W. Joe, B.S. Brown, and D.D. Simpson. 1995. Heavy Drinking in a Population of Methadone Maintained Clients. *Journal of Studies on Alcohol* 56(4):417–22.

Cherubin, C., J. McCusker, and M. Baden. 1972. The Epidemiology of Death in Narcotic Addicts. *American Journal of Epidemiology* 96:11–22.

Cole, S.G., and L.R. James. 1975. A Revised Treatment Typology Based on the DARP. *American Journal of Drug and Alcohol Abuse* 2(1):37–49.

Dansereau, D.F., G.W. Joe, S.M. Dees, and D.D. Simpson. 1996. Ethnicity and the Effects of Mapping-Enhanced Drug Abuse Counseling. *Addictive Behaviors* 21:363–76.

Dansereau, D.F., G.W. Joe, and D.D. Simpson. 1993. Node-Link Mapping: A Visual Representation Strategy for Enhancing Drug Abuse Counseling. *Journal of Counseling Psychology* 40(4):385–95.

De Leon, G. 1984. Program-Based Evaluation Research in Therapeutic Communities. In *Drug Abuse Treatment Evaluation: Strategies, Progress, and Prospects*, ed. F.M. Tims and J.P. Ludford (NIDA Research Monograph Series no. 51, DHHS pub. no. (ADM) 84-1329), 69–87. Rockville, Md.: National Institute on Drug Abuse.

———. 1989. Psychopathology and Substance Abuse: What is Being Learned from Research in Therapeutic Communities. *Journal of Psychoactive Drugs* 21:177–88.

——. 1994. A Recovery Stage Paradigm and Therapeutic Communities. In *Proceedings of the Therapeutic Communities of America 1992 Planning Conference, Chantilly, VA.* Providence, R.I.: Manisses Communications Group.

De Leon, G., G. Melnick, D. Kressel, and N. Jainchill. 1994. Circumstances, Motivation, Readiness and Suitability (the CMRS scales): Predicting Retention in Therapeutic Community Treatment. *American Journal of Drug and Alcohol Abuse* 2(4):495–515.

De Leon, G., G. Melnick, D. Schoket, and N. Jainchill. 1993. Is the Therapeutic Community Culturally Relevant? Findings on Race/Ethnic Differences in Retention in Treatment. *Journal of Psychoactive Drugs* 25(1):77–86.

De Leon, G., and Jainchill, N. 1986. Circumstance, Motivation, Readiness, and Suitability as Correlates of Treatment Tenure. *Journal of Psychoactive Drugs* 18(3):203–8.

El Bassel, N., R.F. Schilling, J.E. Turnbull, and K. Su. 1993. Correlates of Alcohol Use among Methadone Patients. *Alcoholism: Clinical and Experimental Research* 17(3):681–6.

Etheridge, R., S. Craddock, G. Dunteman, and R. Hubbard. 1995. Treatment Services in Two National Studies of Community-Based Drug Abuse Treatment Programs. *Journal of Substance Abuse* 7(1):9–26.

Fletcher, B.W., R.L. Hubbard, P.M. Flynn, R.M. Etheridge, and J.W. Luckey. 1993. DATOS Research Program: A Coordinated Interactive Alliance of Research and Practice. Symposium at NIDA Second National Conference on Drug Abuse Research and Practice, Washington. July.

Force, E., and J. Miller. 1974. Liver Diseases in Fatal Narcotism: Role of Chronic Disease and Alcohol Consumption. *Archives of Pathology* 97:166–9.

Galloway, G.P., J. Newmeyer, T. Knapp, S.A. Stalcup, and D. Smith. 1994. Imipramine for the Treatment of Cocaine and Methamphetamine Dependence. *Journal of Addictive Diseases* 13(4):201–16.

Gearing, F.R. 1970. Evaluation of Methadone Maintenance Treatment Program. *International Journal of the Addictions* 5(3):517–45.

Gerstein, D.R. and H.J. Harwood (eds). 1990. *Treating Drug Problems: Vol. 1. A Study of the Evolution, Effectiveness, and Financing of Public and Private Drug Treatment Systems* (Committee for the Substance Abuse Coverage Study Division of Health Care Services, Institute of Medicine). Washington: National Academy Press.

Grella, C.E., M.D. Anglin, S.E. Wugalter, and J.J. Annon. Forthcoming. The Effectiveness of the Los Angeles Enhanced Methadone Maintenance Project: Reducing HIV Risk among Injection Drug Users. In *The Effectiveness of Innovative Strategies in the Treatment of Drug Abuse*, ed. F.M. Tims, J.A. Inciardi, B.W. Fletcher, P. Delaney, and A.M. Horton, Jr. (in press). Westport, Conn.: Greenwood Press.

Gustafson, J.S. 1991. Do More . . . and Do It Better: Staff-Related Issues in the Drug Treatment Field that Affect the Quality and Effectiveness of

Services. In *Improving Drug Abuse Treatment* (NIDA Research Monograph 106, DHHS pub. no. (ADM) 91-1754), ed. R.W. Pickens, C.G. Leukefeld, C.R. Schuster, 53–67. Rockville, Md.: National Institute on Drug Abuse.

Higgins, S., D. Delaney, A. Budney et al. 1991. A Behavioral Approach to Achieving Initial Cocaine Abstinence. *American Journal of Psychiatry* 148:1218–24.

Hoffman, J.A., B.D. Caudill, J.J. Koman III, J.W. Luckey, P.M. Flynn, and R.L. Hubbard. 1994. Comparative Cocaine Abuse Treatment Strategies: Enhancing Client Retention and Treatment Exposure. *Journal of Addictive Diseases* 13(4):115–28.

Hoffman, J.A., and E.T. Moolchan. 1994. The Phases-of-Treatment Model for Methadone Maintenance: Implementation and Evaluation. *Journal of Psychoactive Drugs* 26(2):181–97.

Hubbard, R.L., M.E. Marsden, J.V. Rachal, H.J. Harwood, E.R. Cavanaugh, and H.M. Ginzburg. 1989. *Drug Abuse Treatment: A National Study of Effectiveness.* Chapel Hill: University of North Carolina Press.

Hunt, D.E., D.E. Lipton, D.S. Goldsmith, and D.L. Strug. 1984. Problems in Methadone Treatment: The Influence of Reference Groups. In *Behavioral Intervention Techniques in Drug Abuse Treatment* (NIDA Research Monograph 46, DHHS pub. no. (ADM) 89-1578), ed. J. Grabowski, M. Stitzer, and J. Henningfield. Washington: U.S. Government Printing Office.

Husband, S.D., and J.J. Platt. 1993. The Cognitive Skills Component in Substance Abuse Treatment in Correctional Settings: A Brief Review. *Journal of Drug Issues* 23:31–42.

Jackson, J.F., L.G. Rotkiewicz, M.A. Quinones, and M.R. Passannante. 1989. A Coupon Program, Drug Treatment, and AIDS Education. *International Journal of the Addictions* 24:1035–51.

James, L.R., O. Watterson, J.R. Bruni, and S.G. Cole. 1976. Validation of Drug Abuse Treatment Classification Checklists. In *The Effectiveness of Drug Abuse Treatment. Vol. V: Evaluation of Treatment Outcomes for 1972–1973 DARP Admission Cohort,* ed. S.B. Sells and D.D. Simpson, 407–52. Cambridge: Ballinger Publishing Company.

Joe, G.W., B.S. Brown, and D.D. Simpson. 1994. Psychological Problems and Client Engagement in Methadone Treatment. (Manuscript submitted for publication.)

Joe, G.W., and D.D. Simpson. 1975. Research on Patient Classification for Drug Users in the DARP. *American Journal of Drug and Alcohol Abuse* 2(1):29–35.

Joe, G.W., D.D. Simpson, and R.L. Hubbard. 1991. Treatment Predictors of Tenure in Methadone Maintenance. *Journal of Substance Abuse* 3:73–84.

Joe, G.W., D.D. Simpson, and S.B. Sells. 1994. Treatment Process and Relapse to Opioid Use during Methadone Maintenance. *American Journal of Drug and Alcohol Abuse* 20(2):173–97.

Joseph, H., and P. Appel. 1985. Alcoholism and Methadone Treatment: Consequences for the Patient and Program. *American Journal of Drug and Alcohol Abuse* 11(1&2):37–53.

Kirby, K.C., D.S. Festinger, R.J. Lamb, and J.J. Platt. Forthcoming. Improving Retention and Outcome in the Treatment of Cocaine Addiction. In *The Effectiveness of Innovative Strategies in the Treatment of Drug Abuse*, ed. F.M. Tims, J.A. Inciardi, B.W. Fletcher, and A.M. Horton, Jr. (in press). Westport, Conn.: Greenwood Press.

Kleinman, P.H., S. Karg, D.S. Lipton, G.E. Woody, J. Kemps, and R.B. Millman. 1992. Retention of Cocaine Abusers in Outpatient Psychotherapy. *American Journal of Drug and Alcohol Abuse* 18:29–43.

LaBrie, R.A., W.E. McAuliffe, R. Nemeth-Coslett, and L. Wilberschied. 1993. The Prevalence of HIV Infection in a National Sample of Injection Drug Users. In *Handbook on Risk of AIDS: Injection Drug Users and Sexual Partners*, ed. B.S. Brown, G.M. Beschner, and National AIDS Research Consortium, 16–37. Westport, Conn.: Greenwood Press.

Larkin, J.H., and H.A. Simon. 1987. Why a Diagram is (Sometimes) Worth Ten Thousand Words. *Cognitive Science* 11:65–99.

Leukefeld, C.G., and F.M. Tims (eds). 1988. *Compulsory Treatment of Drug Abuse: Research and Clinical Practice* (NIDA Research Monograph 86, DHHS pub. no. (ADM) 88-1578). Washington: U.S. Government Printing Office.

Liebman, J., L.D. Knezek, K. Coughey, and S. Hua. 1993. Injection Drug Users, Drug Treatment, and HIV Risk Behavior. In *Handbook on Risk of AIDS: Injection Drug Users and Sexual Partners*, ed. B.S. Brown, G.M. Beschner, and National AIDS Research Consortium, 355–73. Westport, Conn.: Greenwood Press.

Liepman, M.R., L.Y. Silvia, and T.D. Nirenberg. 1989. The Use of Family Behavior Loop Mapping for Substance Abuse. *Family Relations* 38:282–7.

Lipton, D.S. 1994. The Correctional Opportunity: Pathways to Drug Treatment for Offenders. *Journal of Drug Issues* 24(2):331–48.

Maddux, J.F. Forthcoming. Outcomes of Innovations to Improve Retention on Methadone. In *The Effectiveness of Innovative Strategies in the Treatment of Drug Abuse*, ed. F.M. Tims, J.A. Inciardi, B.W. Fletcher, and A.M. Horton, Jr. (in press). Westport, Conn.: Greenwood Press.

Maddux, J.F., and B. Elliot III. 1975. Problem Drinkers among Patients on Methadone. *American Journal of Drug and Alcohol Abuse* 2(2):245–54.

Magura, S., and A. Rosenblum (eds). 1994. *Experimental Therapeutics in Addiction Medicine*. Binghamton, N.Y.: The Haworth Press, Inc.

Martin, S.M., J.A. Inciardi, F.R. Scarpitti, and A.L. Nielsen. Forthcoming. Case Management for Drug Involved Parolees: A Hard Act to Follow. In *The Effectiveness of Innovative Strategies in the Treatment of Drug Abuse*, ed. F.M. Tims, J.A. Inciardi, B.W. Fletcher, and A.M. Horton, Jr. (in press). Westport, Conn.: Greenwood Press.

Mayer, R.E., and J.K. Gallini. 1990. When Is an Illustration Worth Ten Thousand Words? *Journal of Educational Psychology* 82:715–26.

McAuliffe, W.E., R. LaBrie, N. Mulvaney et al. 1994. *Assessment of Substance Dependence Treatment Needs: A Telephone Survey Manual and Questionnaire* (revised edition). Cambridge: National Technical Center for Substance Abuse Needs Assessment.

McLellan, A.T., and A.I. Alterman. 1991. Patient Treatment Matching: A Conceptual and Methodological Review with Suggestions for Future Research. In *Improving Drug Abuse Treatment* (NIDA Research Monograph 106, DHHS pub. no. (ADM) 91-1754), ed. R.W. Pickens, C.G. Leukefeld, and C.R. Schuster, 114–35. Rockville, Md.: National Institute on Drug Abuse.

McLellan, A.T., I.O. Arndt, D.S. Metzger, G.E. Wood, and C.P. O'Brien. 1993. The Effects of Psychosocial Services in Substance Abuse Treatment. *Journal of American Medical Association* 269(15):1953–96.

McLellan, A.T., J. Cacciola, H. Kushner, F. Peters, I. Smith, and H. Pettinati. 1992. The Fifth Edition of the Addiction Severity Index: Cautions, Additions, and Normative Data. *Journal of Substance Abuse Treatment* 5:312–16.

McLellan, A.T., G.R. Grissom, P. Brill, J. Durell, D.S. Metzger, and C.P. O'Brien. 1993. Private Substance Abuse Treatments: Are Some Programs More Effective than Others? *Journal of Substance Abuse Treatment* 10:243–54.

McLellan, A.T., L. Luborsky, C.P. O'Brien, and G.E. Woody. 1980. An Improved Evaluation Instrument for Substance Abuse Patients: The Addiction Severity Index. *Journal of Nervous Mental Disease* 168:26–33.

Mejta, C.L., P. Bokos, E.M. Maslar, J. Mickenberg, and E. Senay. Forthcoming. The Effectiveness of Case Management in Working with Intravenous Drug Users. In *The Effectiveness of Innovative Strategies in the Treatment of Drug Abuse*, ed. F.M. Tims, J.A. Inciardi, B.W. Fletcher, and A.M. Horton, Jr. (in press). Westport, Conn.: Greenwood Press.

Miller, W.R. and S. Rollnick. 1991. *Motivational Interviewing: Preparing People to Change Addictive Behavior*. New York: Guilford Press.

Moos, R.H., J.W. Finney, and R.C. Cronkite. 1990. *Alcoholism Treatment: Context, Process, and Outcome*. New York: Oxford University Press.

Musto, D.F. 1987. *The American Disease: Origins of Narcotic Control* (expanded edition). New York: Oxford University Press.

Novick, D.M., E.F. Pascarelli, H. Joseph et al. 1988. Methadone Maintenance Patients in General Medical Practice. *Journal of American Medical Association* 22:3299–3302.

Pérez-Arce, P., K.D. Carr, and J.L. Sorensen. 1993. Cultural Issues in an Outpatient Program for Stimulant Abusers. *Journal of Psychoactive Drugs* 25(1):35–44.

Perkins, M.E., and H.I. Bloch. 1970. Survey of a Methadone Treatment Program. *American Journal of Psychiatry* 126:33–40.

Platt, J.J., S.D. Husband, and D. Taube. 1990-91. Major Psychotherapeutic Modalities for Heroin Addiction: A Brief Overview. *International Journal of the Addictions* 25(12A):1453–77.

Platt, J.J., M.F. Prout, and D.S. Metzger. 1986. Interpersonal Cognitive Problem-Solving Therapy (ICPS). In *Cognitive-Behavior Approaches to Psychology*, ed. W. Dryden and W. Golden, 261–89. New York: Harper & Row.

Price, R.H., A.C. Burke, and T.A. D'Aunno, et al. 1991. Outpatient Drug Abuse Treatment Services, 1988: Results of a National Survey. In *Improving Drug Abuse Treatment* (NIDA Research Monograph 106, DHHS pub. no. (ADM) 91-1754), ed. R.W. Pickens, C.G. Leukefeld, C.R. Schuster, 63–92. Rockville, Md.: National Institute on Drug Abuse.

Prochaska, J.O., C.C. DiClemente, and J.C. Norcross. 1992. In Search of How People Change: Applications to Addictive Behaviors. *American Psychologist* 47(9):1102–14.

Rounsaville, B.J., F.M. Tims, A.M. Horton, and B.J. Sowder (eds). 1993. *Diagnostic Source Book on Drug Abuse Research and Treatment* (NIDA Research Monograph, NIH pub. no. 93-3508). Rockville, Md.: National Institute on Drug Abuse.

Rounsaville, B.J., M.M. Weissman, and H.D. Kleber. 1982. The Significance of Alcoholism in Treated Opiate Addicts. *Journal of Nervous and Mental Disease* 170(8):479–88.

Roszell, D.K., D.A. Calsyn, and E.F. Chaney. 1986. Alcohol Use and Psychopathology in Opioid Addicts on Methadone Maintenance. *American Journal of Drug and Alcohol Abuse* 12(3):269–78.

Rowan-Szal, G.A., G.W. Joe, L.R. Chatham, and D.D. Simpson. 1994. A Simple Reinforcement System for Methadone Clients in a Community-Based Treatment Program. *Journal of Substance Abuse Treatment* 11(3):217–23.

Rowe, D., and C. Grills. 1993. African-Centered Drug Treatment: An Alternative Conceptual Paradigm for Drug Counseling withAfrican American Clients. *Journal of Psychoactive Drugs* 25(1):21–33.

Sacks, S., G. De Leon, A. Bernhardt, and J. Sacks. 1994. Modified Therapeutic Community for Homeless People with Mental Illness and Chemical Abuse Disorders: A Treatment Manual. (Unpublished manuscript.)

Sellers, T. 1994. Texas Criminal Justice System Chemical Dependency Treatment Initiatives. Presented at the Fourth National Conference on Drugs and Crime, Dallas, Texas. February.

Sells, S.B., and Associates. 1975. The DARP Research Program and Data System. *American Journal of Drug and Alcohol Abuse* 2(1):1–136.

Senay, E.C., A. Barthwell, R. Marks, and P.J. Bokos. 1994. Medical Maintenance: An Interim Report. *Journal of Addictive Diseases* 13(3):65–9.

Senay, E.C., A.G. Barthwell, R. Marks, P. Bokos, D. Gillman, and R. White. 1993. Medical Maintenance: A Pilot Study. *Journal of Addictive Diseases* 12(4):59–76.

Shoptaw, S., R.A. Rawson, M.J. McCann, and J.L. Obert. 1994. The Matrix Model of Outpatient Stimulant Abuse Treatment: Evidence of Efficacy. *Journal of Addictive Diseases* 13(4):129–41.

Siegal, H.A., R.C. Rapp, J.H. Fisher, P.A. Cole, and J.H. Wagner. Forthcoming. Treatment Induction and Case Management: Two Promising Drug Treatment Enhancements. In *The Effectiveness of Innovative Strategies in the Treatment of Drug Abuse*, ed. F.M. Tims, J.A.

Inciardi, B.W. Fletcher, and A.M. Horton, Jr. (in press). Westport, Conn.: Greenwood Press.

Siegal, H.A., and P.A. Cole. 1993. Enhancing Criminal Justice Based Treatment through the Application of the Intervention Approach. *Journal of Drug Issues* 23(1):131–42.

Simpson, D.D. 1981. Treatment for Drug Abuse: Follow-up Outcomes and Length of Time Spent. *Archives of General Psychiatry* 38(8):875–80.

Simpson, D.D., L.R. Chatham, and B.S. Brown. 1995 The Role of Evaluation Research in Drug Abuse Policy. *Current Directions in Psychological Science* 4(4):123–6

Simpson, D.D., D.F. Dansereau, and G.W. Joe. Forthcoming. The DATAR Project: Cognitive and Behavioral Enhancements to Community-Based Treatments. In *The Effectiveness of Innovative Strategies in the Treatment of Drug Abuse*, ed. F.M. Tims, J.A. Inciardi, B.W. Fletcher, and A.M. Horton, Jr. (in press). Westport, Conn.: Greenwood Press.

Simpson, D.D., and G.W. Joe. 1993. Motivation as a Predictor of Early Dropout from Drug Abuse Treatment. *Psychotherapy* 30(2):357–68.

Simpson, D.D., G.W. Joe, G. Rowan-Szal, and J. Greener. 1995. Client Engagement and Change during Drug Abuse Treatment. *Journal of Substance Abuse* 7(1):117–34.

Simpson, D.D., K. Knight, L.R. Chatham, L.M. Camacho, and M. Cloud. 1994. *Prison-Based Treatment Assessment (PTA): Interim Report on Kyle ITC Evaluation*. Fort Worth: Texas Christian University, Institute of Behavioral Research.

Simpson, D.D., and L.J. Savage. 1981–82. Client Types in Different Drug Abuse Treatments: Comparisons of Follow-Up Outcomes. *American Journal of Drug and Alcohol Abuse* 8(4):401–18.

Simpson, D.D., L.J. Savage, G.W. Joe, R.G. Demaree, and S.B. Sells. 1976. *DARP Data Book: Statistics on Characteristics of Drug Users in Treatment During 1969-1974*. Fort Worth: Texas Christian University, Institute of Behavioral Research.

Simpson, D.D., and S.B. Sells. 1982. Effectiveness of Treatment for Drug Abuse: An Overview of the DARP Research Program. *Advances in Alcohol and Substance Abuse* 2:7–29.

—— (eds). 1990. *Opioid Addiction and Treatment: A 12-Year Follow-Up.* Malabar, Fla.: Krieger Publishing Co.

Sisson, R.W., and N.H. Azrin. 1989. The Community Reinforcement Approach. In *Handbook of Alcoholism Treatment Approaches: Effective Alternatives*, ed. R.K. Hester and W.R. Miller, 242–58. New York: Pergamon Press.

Sorensen, J.L., M.F. Constantini, T.L. Wall, and D.R. Gibson. 1993. Coupons Attract High-Risk Untreated Heroin Users Into Detoxification. *Drug and Alcohol Dependence* 31:247–52.

Sorensen, J.L., D. Gibson, D. Deitch, and G. Bernal. 1985. Methadone Applicant Dropouts: Impact of Requiring Involvement of Friends or Family in Treatment. *International Journal of the Addictions* 20:1273–80.

Stimmel, B. 1981. Methadone Maintenance and Alcohol Use. In *Drug and Alcohol Abuse: Implications for Treatment* (NIDA Research Monograph, DHHS pub. no. (ADM) 80-958), ed. S.E. Gardner, 57–74. Rockville, Md.: National Institute on Drug Abuse.

Stimmel, B., S. Vernance, and H. Tobias. 1972. Hepatic Dysfunction in Heroin Addicts: The Role of Alcohol. *Journal of American Medical Association* 222:811–2.

Stitzer, M., J. Grabowski, and J. Henningfield. 1984. Behavioral Intervention Techniques in Drug Abuse Treatment: Summary of Discussion. In *Behavioral Intervention Techniques in Drug Abuse Treatment* (NIDA Research Monograph 46, DHHS pub. no. (ADM) 89-1578), ed. J. Grabowski, M. Stitzer, and J. Henningfield, 147–56. Washington: U.S. Government Printing Office.

Sue, D.W., and D. Sue. 1990. *Counseling the Culturally Different*. New York: John Wiley & Sons.

Sue, D. W., and N. Zane. 1987. The Role of Culture and Cultural Techniques in Psychotherapy. *American Psychologist* 42(1):37–45.

Swartz, J. 1993. TASC – The Next 20 Years: Extending, Refining, and Assessing the Model. In *Drug Treatment and Criminal Justice* (Sage Criminal Justice System Annuals, vol. 27). ed. J.A. Inciardi, 127–48. Newbury Park, Calif.: Sage Publications.

Tims, F.M., J.A. Inciardi, B.W. Fletcher, and A.M. Horton, Jr. (eds) Forthcoming. *The Effectiveness of Innovative Strategies in the Treatment of Drug Abuse* (in press). Westport, Conn.: Greenwood Press.

Tims, F.M. and C.G. Leukefeld (eds). 1993. *Cocaine Treatment: Research and Clinical Perspectives* (NIDA Research Monograph 135, NIH pub. no. 93-3639). Rockville, Md.: National Institute on Drug Abuse.

Tims, F.M., and J.P. Ludford (eds). 1984. *Drug Abuse Treatment Evaluation: Strategies, Progress, and Prospects* (NIDA Research Monograph No. 51, DHHS pub. no. 84-1329). Washington: U.S. Government Printing Office.

Todd, T.C. 1984. A Contingency Analysis of Family Treatment and Drug Abuse. In *Behavioral Intervention Techniques in Drug Abuse Treatment* (NIDA Research Monograph 46, DHHS pub. no. (ADM) 89-1578), ed. J. Grabowski, M. Stitzer, and J. Henningfield. Washington: U.S. Government Printing Office.

Van Treuren, R.R. 1986. Self-Perception in Family Systems: A Diagrammatic Technique. *Social Casework: Journal of Contemporary Social Work* 67(5):299–305.

Wexler, H.K., and D.S. Lipton. 1993. From Reform to Recovery: Advances in Prison Drug Treatment. In *Drug Treatment and Criminal Justice* (Sage Criminal Justice System Annuals, vol. 27), ed. J.A. Inciardi, 209–27. Newbury Park, Calif.: Sage Publications.

Winn, W., T-Z, Li, and D. Schill. 1991. Diagrams as Aids to Problem Solving: Their Role in Facilitating Search and Computation. *Educational Technology Research and Development* 39(1):17–29.

Woody, G.E., A.T. McLellan, C.P. O'Brien, and L. Luborsky. 1991.

Addressing Psychiatric Comorbidity. In *Improving Drug Abuse Treatment* (NIDA Research Monograph 106, DHHS pub. no. (ADM) 91-1754), ed. R.W. Pickens, C.G. Leukefeld, and C.R. Schuster, 152–66. Washington: U.S. Government Printing Office.

Yancovitz, S.R., D.C. Des Jarlais, N.P. Peyser, et al. 1991. A Randomized Trial of an Interim Methadone Maintenance Clinic. *American Journal of Public Health* 81:1185–90.

3

Need and Access to Drug-Abuse Treatment

Constance M. Horgan

Drug abuse imposes enormous burdens both on those who abuse drugs and on those who do not. Need for and access to treatment may be viewed from the viewpoint of both individual well-being of the drug user and broader societal concerns. The large social costs associated with issues such as drug-related crime and consequences of drugs in the workplace point up societal interest in ensuring access to drug-abuse treatment for those in need.

The purpose of this chapter is to describe what we know about need for and access to drug-abuse treatment. First, the context of need and access is examined in terms of historical changes in the patterns of drug use and it is placed in a broad social perspective. Next, a series of questions are explored: who needs treatment, who receives treatment, and where is treatment provided? Finally, the policy implications of need for and access to treatment are examined in the light of a rapidly changing health-care delivery system. To the extent possible, the data presented refer to illicit drugs and do not include abuse of alcohol and nicotine. When treatment data are presented that include both alcohol and illicit drugs, the more comprehensive term, substance abuse, is used.

I   Need and Access in Context

1.1   Changing attitudes and patterns of drug use

The use of illicit drugs in the United States has fluctuated with shifting public attitudes and types of governmental responses, resulting in changing levels of need for and access to treatment (Musto 1991). Laissez-faire approaches to drug use during the late 1800s gave way to increased regulation of cocaine and opiates as the addictive properties of these drugs became better understood. Cocaine and opiate use declined during the first half of the 1900s, only for heroin to emerge again as a problem in the 1950s and 1960s. A more tolerant attitude toward drugs emerged in the 1970s, as overall use of a variety of illicit drugs increased, peaking in the late 1970s for most drugs. However, cocaine use became more common in the 1980s, particularly the use of crack, its cheaper derivative. Although overall use of cocaine has declined since the mid-1980s, the number of heavy users has remained relatively stable (Gfroerer and Brodsky 1993). The role of these heavy users is reflected in the increasing number of cocaine- and heroin-related emergency room visits reported in the Drug Abuse Warning Network in recent years (SAMHSA 1993).

Examination of long-term trends in drug use, show that patterns of drug use are cyclical (Musto 1991). Recent epidemiological data indicate that the significant declines in the prevalence of illicit drug use that occurred throughout the 1980s did not continue into 1993 (SAMHSA 1994). These data may reflect a short-term interruption of the declining trend, a leveling off, or perhaps the start of an increase in illicit drug use.

1.2   Current use of drugs

A substantial portion of the US population have used or currently use illicit drugs, including marijuana, cocaine, heroin, inhalants, hallucinogens, and the non-medical use of psychotherapeutic drugs. In 1993, 37 percent had used illicit drugs at some point during their lives, 12 percent had used these substances within the last year, and almost 6 percent were current users, defined as any use of these substances within the past month (SAMHSA 1994). These estimates are based on the 1993 National Household Survey on Drug Abuse (NHSDA), which provides a comprehensive estimate of substance use in the civilian, non-institutionalized population over twelve years of age. It is the primary source for national prevalence data on

Drug abuse occurs within the broader sociocultural context of American society. Since the 1960s, multiple social crises, such as declining employment opportunities for low-income individuals, shortage and rising costs of housing, less stable families, high school drop-out rates, etc. have contributed to a drug-abusing population who may also have multiple social problems (Johnson and Muffler 1992). Drug abusers often require housing, social services, family services, vocational counseling, and other non-medical services.

1.4 Policies to control drug use

The two major strategies to control illegal drug use are: reducing the illicit drug supply and reducing Americans' demand for drugs (Reuter 1992). Supply-reduction strategies seek to curtail the supply of drugs through intercepting and seizing illegal drug shipments, source country control of production, and domestic law enforcement, such as arrest and imprisonment of drug dealers. Demand-reduction strategies aim to decrease the number of people who want to use illicit drugs, primarily through prevention, early intervention, and treatment services. More money and effort traditionally have gone into supply reduction than demand reduction; however, disentangling the effects of various policies on drug use is difficult.

Rydell and Everingham (1994) examined the relative effectiveness of four types of cocaine control programs through an economic model predicting how much would have to be spent annually to reduce cocaine consumption by one percent. Three of the programs were supply-side in orientation: source country control, interdiction, and domestic enforcement. The fourth program focused on treatment of heavy users, and thus was a demand-side intervention. The supply-side interventions discourage consumption by raising the retail price of the drug because the cost to dealers of supplying cocaine increases. Treatment reduces consumption by discouraging use while in treatment and after treatment for many consumers. The analysis by Rydell and Everingham (1994) showed that treatment of heavy users was by far the most cost-effective form of drug control. An expenditure of $34 million on treatment of heavy users could reduce cocaine consumption by as much as an expenditure of $250 million on domestic enforcement, the least expensive of the three supply-side interventions.

Drug-use patterns also have implications for which demand-side strategies are implemented. The patterns of declining light use and unabated heavy use, described ab⌐   ⌐ important implications for assessing treatment needs. ⌐   ⌐dell (1994) examined the relative contributions of light and heavy cocaine users to total cocaine consumption. They found the relative contribution of heavy cocaine users to total consumption is so great, that even if the number of new users per year continues to decline at the current rate, total consumption will hardly be affected. From a policy perspective, these findings indicate that cocaine-related problems can be reduced by a combined approach which both prevents initiation (prevention) and also reduces consumption by heavy users. Indeed, expanding the treatment system for chronic, heavy users is a high priority in the 1994 National Drug Control Strategy (White House 1994).

1.5 Societal cost perspective

While the health consequences to drug abusers in terms of illness, injuries, disability, and premature death are substantial, there are very large costs to the rest of society, including family, employers, and victims of abuse-related crime and accidents. The total economic cost of drug abuse was estimated to be $67 billion in 1990 (unpublished data from Rice as reported in Horgan et al. 1993). Crime plays the major role in drug-related costs, with almost 70 percent of total costs primarily linked to criminal activity. The costs of crime include the cost of persons incarcerated in prison as a result of a conviction for a drug-related crime, the cost of victims of crime, and the cost of crime careers (Rice et al. 1991). Lost productivity related to illness and premature death accounted for 17 percent of total cost in 1990. The direct medical costs of drug abuse represented only 5 percent of the total economic cost, and another 10 percent of total cost was associated with AIDS related to injecting drug use. Although specific cost estimates vary across studies because of differences in underlying assumptions and definitions, all show substantial economic costs.

The large "externalities" or costs to others place drug abuse squarely in the public health arena. The public health implications of the higher incidence of many infections, including HIV/AIDS, tuberculosis, and other infections such as viral hepatitis and endocarditis among drug users are well documented (Des Jarlais and Friedman 1988; Haverkos and Lange 1990). Pregnant women who use drugs are at risk of experiencing health problems themselves, as well as of giving birth to infants who may experience withdrawal and various other problems, such as low birth weight and neurobehavioral deficiencies. This has large implications for both the health care system, in terms of high neonatal costs and other health costs, as well as other systems, including the education and social service systems (Horgan et al. 1991). The safety and public health benefits of drug-abuse treatment derive both from reductions in actual use and from reductions in the consequences of drug abuse, such as crime, workplace, and family burden.

2   Who Needs Treatment?

2.1   Dimensions of need

Cleary (1989) has pointed out that in the psychiatric area, need for treatment is a relative concept that is a function of the person using the term, with epidemiologists, providers, and individuals in the community having different ideas about what constitutes need. For example, epidemiologists are likely to define need in terms of definitions of disease that can be operationalized in a consistent manner, whereas providers will tend to define need in terms of whether the patient can be effectively treated. Perceived need for drug-abuse treatment by individuals in the community may relate to the symptoms of distress that are observed in the drug user. Cleary (1989) emphasizes that methodological refinements in measuring need do not solve the problem of the term need having different meanings depending on the perspective of the person defining need.

Difficulties in estimating need for drug treatment relate both to lack of agreement in how to measure need and to inadequacies in data sources in covering key populations that need treatment, such as arrestees and the homeless (Epstein and Gfroerer 1994; Harwood and Zenzola 1993). Use of drugs is not, in and of itself, an indication of need for treatment. Consumption of drugs can be viewed conceptually as ranging along a continuum: abstinence, use, abuse, and dependence. The level and pattern of consumption for illicit drugs, and the seriousness of associated consequences, including physical, emotional, and social problems, vary across individuals and determine need for treatment. Stages of drug history are defined in Gerstein and Harwood (1990) as:

- Use – low or infrequent doses: experimental, occasional. Damaging consequences are rare or minor.
- Abuse – higher doses and/or frequencies: sporadically heavy, intensive. Effects are unpredictable, sometimes severe.
- Dependence – high, frequent doses: compulsion, craving, withdrawal. Severe consequences are very likely.

Transition to higher stages of addiction are determined by the specific pattern of consumption and the existence of other factors which are biological, psychological and social in nature. The need for treatment results from a combination of these factors. Need for treatment may begin to appear for some individuals in the abuse stage. Individuals new to the abuse stage or showing little impairment generally do not need treatment, but may benefit from other interventions such as preventive counseling or education. Treatment is usually viewed as needed when progression to chronic abuse or dependence has occurred.

Measurement of problem levels of use indicative of need for treatment is more complex than simple consumption patterns, and involves assessment of physiological and psychological symptoms of dependence and abuse, psychosocial problems, and consequences of consumption. Several studies, many unpublished, have used alternative methods and data sets to develop need estimates and are reviewed in Epstein and Gfroerer (1994) and Harwood and Zenzola (1993). The Epidemiological Catchment Area (ECA) study sponsored by the National Institute of Mental Health has been used to apply clinical criteria, for mental disorders, including drug dependence, to a general population. Most other estimates rely on data from the National Household Survey on Drug Abuse (NHSDA) and use a variety of algorithms to estimate need. Additionally, some studies use supplementary data to estimate need in populations underreported in household surveys, e.g., the criminal justice and the homeless populations.

The 1980–84 Epidemiological Catchment Area study used the Diagnostic Interview Schedule in household interviews in five communities to provide mental health assessments based on the American Psychiatric Association's Diagnostic and Statistical Manual of Disorders (DSM-III) (Robbins and Regier 1991). Problems with using ECA data to estimate drug-treatment need include the fact that the ECA was conducted prior to the widespread use of crack cocaine, and that it may underrepresent those in high drug-using populations, such as the criminal justice and homeless populations. Its major strength is that it was the first survey to apply clinical criteria to determine the existstence of a diagnosable drug-abuse disorder.

Gerstein and Harwood (1990) used an algorithm to create four categories of need: unlikely, possible, probable, and clear. Three factors were used to create the categories: (1) frequency of consumption; (2) physiological and psychological symptoms of dependence and abuse; and (3) psychosocial problems and other consequences of consumption. Symptoms included such measures as needing larger amounts to get the same effect or feeling sick because of use. Problems included measures such as having trouble at school or work or finding it harder to handle problems. Using this technique and 1991 NHSDA data, Harwood and Zenzola (1993) found that for current drug users, defined as users within the last 30 days, 11 percent had clear need, 21 percent had probable need, 18 percent had possible need, and 50 percent were unlikely to need treatment.

Epstein and Gfroerer (1994) use an algorithm that approximates the criteria from the *Diagnostic and Statistical Manual of Mental Disorders*, Third Edition, Revised (DSM-III-R) for illicit drug dependence, which defines a person as dependent for a substance if they meet three out of nine criteria pertaining to that substance. The NHSDA includes items on symptoms and problems that are combined to approximate five of the nine DSM-III-R criteria for dependence: (1) tolerance; (2) withdrawal; (3) inability to stop or control use of the substance; (4) giving up or reducing social, occupational or recreational activities; or (5) physical problem due to use. Epstein and Gfroerer (1994) define a person as dependent and thus needing treatment if they have two out of these five criteria.

2.2 Population in need

Given the different methodologies in developing national need estimates, it is not surprising that there is a range of estimates. Irrespective of the method of determining need, the consensus is that a large number of individuals are in need of treatment.

Using ECA data and projecting estimates to 1990, Regier et al. (1993) found that 5.7 million individuals or 3.1 percent of the US adult population had a diagnosable drug disorder. This analysis did not explicitly address the issue of whether all individuals with a diagnosable drug disorder need treatment or whether some individuals without a diagnosable disorder were in need of treatment, although the presumption is equivalence with need for treatment.

Using the NHSDA, supplemented by other sources, Harwood and Zenzola (1993) estimated that in 1991 there were 4.9 million individuals in need of treatment for drug problems, based on the clear and probable need criteria. This includes 3.67 million in the general population; 723,000 individuals on probation or parole, 424,000 persons incarcerated in prisons or jails, and 110,000 homeless individuals. Also using the 1991 NHSDA, Epstein and Gfroerer (1994) estimated that in the population aged 12 and older, the prevalence of individuals needing drug-abuse treatment was 1.28 percent, representing 2.59 million persons in the civilian non-institutionalized population. The comparable numbers using the Harwood and Zenzola methodology were 1.93 percent of the population, accounting for 3.91 million persons. It appears that the Harwood and Zenzola estimates include a broader group of drug abusers, while the Epstein and Gfroerer estimates define a smaller, more severely impaired group of drug abusers needing treatment. Both of these estimates are lower than the ECA estimates, which indicate the size of the population with a diagnosable drug disorder.

Level of need, no matter how defined, varies in different subsets of the population (Cleary 1989; Gerstein and Harwood 1990). Knowledge of how need for treatment varies for population subgroups is important in planning the allocation of drug-treatment resources. Most of the national need estimates have focused on overall drug-treatment need estimates, with little emphasis on variation by demographic or other characteristics.

Gerstein and Harwood (1990) used their methodology to estimate need in 1988. Of those in need of drug treatment in the household population, 51 percent were less than 25 years of age, 68 percent were male, and 24 percent of adults were either unemployed or not participating in the labor force. Of individuals involved with the criminal justice system, 35 percent of those in prisons and jails and 28 percent of those on probation and parole were estimated to be in need of treatment (Gerstein and Harwood 1990).

Although use of drugs is not necessarily an indication of need for treatment, frequency and level of consumption is commonly used as a proxy for need for treatment in the absence of data which incorporate information on symptoms and problems related to drug abuse. An examination of frequent cocaine users indicates that they are more likely than non-users to be male (62 versus 48 percent), to be unemployed (32 versus 7 percent), and to engage in heavy alcohol use (32 versus 3 percent) (Gfroerer and Brodsky 1993). Those who are uninsured are also more likely to frequently use illicit substances (Larson et al. 1993).

Particular groups of drug users are sometimes identified as special populations, having special needs or special access problems, and often are targeted for special categorical funding to improve service access and delivery. These groups include the homeless, the criminally involved, dually diagnosed with mental and substance disorders, injecting drug users, pregnant women, adolescents, and minorities. These special populations are usually treated within regular treatment programs, but sometimes specialized separate programs have been developed. The effectiveness of such specialized programs has not been addressed, nor is there evidence that specialized programs do in fact increase access to treatment (Weisner and Schmidt 1994). More research is needed about whether separate special-population programs have increased access or improved outcomes.

3 Who Gets Treatment?

3.1 Demand for treatment

It is important to distinguish between need for treatment and demand for treatment. Demand for treatment is most commonly assessed in terms of service utilization. Most persons who are in need of drug-abuse treatment do not actually receive it. Data from the Epidemiological Catchment Area study indicate that only 30 percent of those with drug-abuse disorders received any services in the de facto treatment system, broadly defined to include the specialty treatment sector, the general medical sector, the human service sector, and the voluntary sector, which includes mutual help groups (Regier et al. 1993).

Demand for medical treatment is related to wanting and seeking treatment. In the drug-abuse area, not all persons who are in treatment may want treatment. Indeed, it is more common that drug abusers will resist treatment rather than seek it out (Steinberg 1992). Many drug abusers may deny the need for treatment and may eventually be coerced into treatment in some fashion, either through court orders or by threats from family or employers (Leukefield and Tims 1988). The fact that drug abuse involves criminal behavior, e.g., purchasing illegal substances, may also contribute to denial because of the stigma attached to this behavior (Steinberg 1992). Once in treatment, criminal justice clients who have been coerced into treatment stay longer and fare no worse than those who have not been referred by the criminal justice system (Hubbard et al. 1989).

The demand for drug-abuse services is determined by a complex array of factors. Service utilization is typically described as being influenced by three broad categories of factors: individual or person level; organizational or system level; and environmental influences (Weisner and Schmidt 1994). Individual-level variables, including sociodemographic characteristics such as age and marital status, cultural beliefs and attitudes about treatment efficacy, perceptions of symptom severity, and social networks, appear to influence the treatment-seeking process. Organizational variables, such as managed care and interorganizational linkages, and environmental factors, such as insurance mandates and criminalization philosophy, also clearly influence access and utilization.

3.2 Population in specialty treatment

This section describes users of services in the specialty substance-abuse sector and describes other factors influencing use of services as an indication of access to specialized treatment services. In 1992, 63 percent of clients in specialty substance-abuse treatment had a problem with drug abuse; 25 percent had a drug-only problem, 38 percent had both drug and alcohol problems, and 37 percent had an alcohol-only problem (SAMHSA 1995). In order to focus more clearly on the drug-abuse problem, national estimates of the demographic characteristics for clients treated in drug-only and combined drug and alcohol treatment facilities are presented below and are based on data from the Drug Services Research Survey, a nationally representative survey of drug-abuse treatment providers in 1990 (Batten et al. 1993).

Age. About 27 percent of clients in specialty drug/alcohol treatment were under 25 years of age; 35 percent were between 25 and 34; 27 percent were between 35 and 44 years; and 12 percent were 45 or older. This age distribution points up the preponderance of young adults in the treatment system. The percentage of 25 to 34 year-olds in drug treatment is almost twice their proportion in the national population. Only 9 percent of those in treatment are younger than 18 years old and about one-fourth of these (2 percent of total) are less than 15 years of age.

Race/ethnicity. White clients constitute 63 percent of all clients in treatment in drug/alcohol facilities, black clients make up 24 percent, and Americans of Hispanic origin comprise 11 percent of clients in treatment.

Employment status and insurance. Half of those in treatment were employed at admission to treatment. Only 30 percent of clients had private or public insurance as the expected source of payment for treatment.

Primary drug of abuse. Two-thirds of those in treatment for drug abuse were admitted to treatment for either cocaine (including crack) or heroin/other opiates as their principal drug of abuse. Cocaine (including crack) accounts for 40 percent of admissions; heroin or other opiates represent 27 percent; marijuana/hashish for 20 percent; and other drugs, including benzodiazepenes and amphetamines, for the remainder.

Financial. Demand for treatment is also related to the ability and willingness of someone to pay for treatment. Contrary to much of medical care, most clients in drug-abuse treatment do not have insurance as the expected source of payment. For example, nationally in 1990 only 16 percent of clients in drug and combined drug and alcohol treatment facilities had private insurance as the expected source of payment, and another 14 percent had the public insurance programs of Medicaid and Medicare as primary sources of payment. Thus in the drug-abuse treatment area, there is a tremendous reliance on public, non-insurance-based financing, such as the federal ADM block grant and state and local funding.

Supply. Other factors influence entry into treatment, such as the availability of space in a treatment program. Almost 88 percent of all treatment capacity in drug and combined drug and alcohol facilities was estimated to have been used on a given date in 1990. This national system-wide utilization rate is very high, and in fact many facilities were functioning at an exceptionally high service-utilization level as shown by waiting-list information. About 42 percent of all facilities reported that they usually had more applicants than capacity for treatment, with an average wait of about 14 days to enter treatment; however, this was especially true for facilities that were primarily publicly funded.

4 Where is Treatment Provided?

4.1 Overview of treatment system

The US substance-abuse treatment system consists of several distinct sectors, which together have been described as the de facto services system (Regier et al. 1993). The major sectors are: specialty substance abuse; non-specialty medical; and other, which includes services outside of the health care system.

Specialty sector – history. Treatment for substance abuse encompasses a continuum of services provided in a variety of settings. A specialized treatment system currently exists which provides a wide range of services, including detoxification and rehabilitation services in both ambulatory and residential settings. In the early 1960s, formal treatment was largely provided in prisons. The 1960s and 1970s saw the development of modern treatment modalities, including methadone maintenance and therapeutic communities. In the early 1970s, treatment also moved to a community-based model involving outpatient care. In the early 1980s, there was a shift to a medicalized model focusing on hospital-based treatment (Besteman 1992). In recent years, an increasing emphasis on managed care has resulted in a shift from inpatient to outpatient settings (Larson et al. 1993; Callahan et al. 1994). During the 1980s, there was a major organizational change within the specialty substance-abuse system as drug and alcohol treatment merged into combined treatment both at the individual program level and at the state and local administrative level. Between 1982 and 1990, the proportion of combined drug and alcohol treatment units tripled, accounting in 1990 for 76 percent of all treatment units, while the proportion of alcohol-only units declined from 51 to 13 percent and the number of drug-only units declined from 26 to 11 percent (Schmidt and Weisner 1993). Thus, many different types of specialized treatment co-exist in this broad-based treatment system, which has developed over the last three decades as a fragmented system with separate tracks for publicly and privately financed clients (Schlesinger et al. 1991; Gerstein and Harwood 1990).

Specialty sector – setting. The specialty treatment system encompasses a continuum of services provided in a variety of settings. Specialty substance-abuse treatment may take place either in the ambulatory setting, which includes outpatient and intensive outpatient services, or in the residential setting, which includes hospital inpatient, short-term residential and long-term residential services, including therapeutic communities. Most clients are treated in the ambulatory setting. Across the nation in 1992, on a given day, about 945,000 clients received substance-abuse treatment in the specialized sector (SAMHSA 1995). Approximately 87 percent of clients were treated on an outpatient basis, including 7 percent receiving treatment through an intensive outpatient program. Only about 11 percent of clients were in an inpatient or residential facility for rehabilitation services. This includes 8 percent who were in long-term residential care where the length of stay was typically over 30 days. Less than 2 percent of clients were involved in detoxification in any type of setting, and about 12 percent of clients received methadone in conjunction with their treatment (SAMHSA 1995). Not reflected in these numbers are the specialized services provided in private practice by psychiatrists, psychologists, and social workers.

There are variations in the type of care utilized by substance-abuse clients treated in drug-only and combined drug and alcohol facilities by demographic characteristics of clients, as reflected in national survey data from 1990 (Batten et al. 1993). Outpatient drug maintenance programs have the oldest clients, with more than three-fifths over 34 years of age and only 7 percent less than 25 years of age. Outpatient drug-free programs treat the youngest population, with almost one-third of their clients younger than 25 years of age. About one-third of clients in residential treatment settings are black, a significantly higher proportion than in the treatment population at large. Blacks and Hispanics are disproportionately represented in outpatient maintenance programs, while whites predominate in outpatient drug-free settings.

Non-specialty medical sector. Substance-abuse treatment services are also provided in the non-specialty sector. Non-specialty treatment may be provided in private settings by general medical practitioners and in facilities that are not exclusively used for substance abuse. Schlesinger et al. (1991) estimate that including these types of providers would increase the estimates of those in treatment for a substance-abuse problem by 40 percent for an inpatient setting and 20 percent for outpatient care. Frequently, the services provided in this nonspecialty setting involve the treatment of other medical conditions concurrently with the substance-abuse problem. Treatment for substance abuse may be delivered under another diagnosis, particularly when substance abuse is seen as a secondary condition.

The primary care setting is increasingly recognized as an important setting for substance-abuse problems from a screening and early intervention perspective and for referral to specialized services. Many individuals who have a drug-abuse problem are encountered in the primary care and/or other medical settings. Emergency rooms, psychiatric care settings, and medical specialties such as infectious diseases, have a significant portion of patients whose medical problems are related to drug abuse (Babor 1990).

Other sectors. Early drug-abuse treatment in the United States was viewed as a criminal justice system issue. Although now most of specialty substance-abuse treatment takes place in the community, the criminal justice system still plays a role in the provision of treatment in this country (Besteman 1992). In 1989, it was estimated that about 5 percent of convicted offenders in local jails were receiving treatment while incarcerated (Harlow 1991). Additionally, a substantial proportion of substance-abuse treatment in non-correctional specialty settings occurs as a condition imposed by the court or criminal justice system, including arrests for driving under the influence of drugs, alcohol, or both substances.

Although not part of the formal treatment system, mutual help groups play an important role in the recovery process for many individuals with substance-abuse problems. Mutual help groups may be used in different ways: as the only form of external help, concurrently with formal treatment, or sequential with the treatment system. Mutual help groups include Alcoholics Anonymous, Cocaine Anonymous, and Narcotics Anonymous. These groups are typically based on the 12-step model to personal change with abstinence as the goal. Due partially to the groups' philosophy of maintaining anonymity, accurate counts of current or former members are not available.

Relative importance of sectors. As noted previously, there is a large gap between the prevalence of a diagnosable drug-abuse problem and the proportion of these individuals who receive treatment in any component of the de facto treatment system. Less than 30 percent of persons with a diagnosable disorder received any treatment in any sector. Some people received service in more than one sector. About 14 percent received treatment in the specialty sector, and almost 12 percent were treated in the non-specialty sector. About 6 percent received services in some other component of the human-services sector, and 9 percent received services in the voluntary sector, including mutual help groups, clergy, etc. (Regier et al. 1993; Narrow et al. 1993). These numbers substantiate the very significant role that sectors other than the specialty sector play in the delivery of drug-abuse services. This emphasizes the need for appropriate recognition and treatment of disorders in the non-specialty sectors, and appropriate referral to the specialty sector when needed.

4.2   Two-tiered specialty system
The current specialty system can be viewed as having two distinct tiers, distinguished primarily by source of funding (Gerstein and Harwood 1990). The public tier treats clients whose treatment is paid for by government. The private tier treats clients whose treatment is largely paid through private insurance and patient fees. The two tiers also differ with respect to client characteristics, treatment settings, and capacity.

Public. The public tier providers are largely publicly owned or private non-profits with the bulk of their funding from public sources. On any given day, over three-fourths of clients in drug-only and combined drug and alcohol treatment facilities are treated in the public tier (Batten et al. 1993). The public tier encompasses a range of facility types, including both outpatient drug-free and outpatient methadone and residential facilities. In 1990, over 65 percent of drug and combined drug and alcohol treatment facilities were in the public tier (Batten et al. 1993). The public tier developed in the 1960s and the 1970s with a strong federal role, which has since shifted to the states.

Private. The private tier consists primarily of private for-profit facilities that receive the bulk of funding from private sources, such as private insurance. The private tier also encompasses a range of facility types; however, the strong link of this tier with the hospital setting is apparent. In 1990, about 34 percent of drug and combined drug and alcohol treatment facilities were in the private tier (Batten et al. 1993). This tier evolved in response to the expansion of substance-abuse benefits within private health insurance and grew rapidly during the 1980s. It is characterized by higher levels of reimbursement and a greater chance that a client can gain immediate access to treatment than the public tier (Gerstein and Harwood 1990).

4.3   Special issues for the delivery system

Growth of managed care. Managed care has grown rapidly in recent years, as public and private decision-makers are turning to it as a means of controlling costs. Private health insurance that does not incorporate some form of managed care is becoming rare. In 1990, only 5 percent of employees were enrolled in traditional insurance plans that did not rely on utilization-management techniques. Approximately 57 percent of employees were in conventional plans with utilization management, and another 38 percent were in some type of network plan, including HMOs (Hoy et al. 1991). By 1993, network-type managed-care plans, including HMOs, covered 51 percent of privately insured individuals (Gabel et al. 1994). The trend is similar in the public sector with 36 state Medicaid programs using some form of managed care for at least some beneficiaries (Bachman and Batten 1993). Numbers on the use of managed-care strategies for substance abuse, either as part of the overall health-insurance package or as a separate benefit, were not available; however, it is clear that use of managed-care strategies for substance-abuse services, particularly utilization review and selective contracting, is widespread and has led to drastic change in practice (England and Vaccaro 1991), particularly the reduction in the use of inpatient substance-abuse treatment. A unique aspect of managed care for substance abuse and mental health has been the growth of specialty carve-out arrangements for managing these services (Freeman and Trabin 1994).

Changes in insurance coverage. Changes in the insurance market are affecting access to private insurance. Many employers have been dropping health insurance or groups from health insurance over the last few years (Larson et al. 1993). Access to insurance benefits is reduced by employers shifting to part-time or contract workers, dropping coverage for certain groups, such as dependants or retirees, dropping certain health plan options, or excluding "pre-existing conditions," which may include substance abuse (GAO 1990). Benefit changes are also contributing to an erosion of substance-abuse coverage which may be inadequate for chronic substance-abuse conditions (Larson et al. 1993). Separate benefit limits on substance-abuse services are almost always more restrictive than on other medical services, and use of increased copayments for inpatient and outpatient substance-abuse services is widespread (Foster Higgins 1990).

5   Policy Implications

The American health care system is in the process of rapid transformation. Key to its evolution has been the explosive growth of managed care, resulting in substantial change in the way providers deliver services and relate to payers and insurers. As these changes proceed, we should remain cognizant of several aspects of the drug-abusing population if we are to ensure that the population in need of treatment has access to the most appropriate services.

5.1   Meeting multiple needs
Substance abusers often require supplementary services beyond drug-abuse treatment. These may include medical needs, or other needs such as psychosocial counseling, financial counseling, housing, parenting training, child care, etc. Provision of these services has been shown to improve treatment outcomes (McLellan et al. 1993). These multiple needs can be met either directly in the treatment program or through appropriate linkages to other sectors. In particular, links to the acute health care system are critical, in light of the health care needs of the drug-abusing population, especially the growing HIV/AIDS epidemic.

5.2   Expanding the covered population
Much of the focus of state health reform efforts is moving toward the goal of universal access, especially through expanding existing employment-based insurance. It should be recalled that the substance-abusing population is disproportionately unemployed. To the extent that health reform efforts are employment linked, particular concern must be paid to handling the drug-abuse population without an employment link.

5.3 Adequacy of the benefit package

Drug abuse has been described as a chronic, recurring condition. Over the lifetime of a person with a drug-abuse problem, there may be several relapses into dependency and need for treatment. To the extent that reform initiatives include a limited private insurance-like benefit, care must be taken that, once the limits are reached, there are provisions that the client has access to further services.

5.4 Evolution and integration of the treatment system

The majority of substance-abuse clients are now treated in the publicly-funded treatment tier. This is largely a system with little experience of private insurance and one that routinely provides wrap-around services, such as social services, vocational training, etc., as components of treatment, which enhance treatment retention and effectiveness, yet are not typically covered under private insurance. While eliminating a two-tiered system may be a desirable social goal, retention of certain non-medical aspects of the public system is desirable for sub-groups who need these kinds of services for successful outcomes.

The drug-abusing population and the drug-abuse treatment system have distinctive characteristics and shortcomings that should be taken into account as the American health care system continues to undergo transformation. While there is considerable room for improving access for those in need of treatment, there is the danger that things could become worse if special issues are not adequately addressed.

Note

This chapter was commissioned by the Milbank Memorial Fund in collaboration with the National Institute on Drug Abuse. The author gratefully acknowledges suggestions received from John Capitman, David Lewis, Mary Ellen Marsden, and one anonymous reviewer. The research assistance of Julie Buckley is also appreciated. Helpful comments were also received from participants at a meeting, "The Use of Research for Drug Abuse Treatment Policy," held on 19 July 1994 in Arlington, Virginia.

References

Babor, T.F. 1990. Alcohol and Substance Abuse in Primary Care Settings. In *Conference Proceedings: Primary Care Research, An Agenda for the 90s*. DHHS pub. no. (PHS)90-3460, ed. J. Mayfield and M.L. Grady Washington.

Bachman, S., and H.L. Batten. 1993. Medicaid Managed Care for the SSI Disabled: Capitated and Fee-for-Service Programs. Office of

Management and Budget, Health Care Financing Administration Briefing (HCFA Contract No: 18-C-90096/1-01). Institute for Health Policy, Brandeis University, Center for Vulnerable Populations, Waltham, Mass., January 25.

Barthwell, A.G., and Gibert, C.L. 1993. Screening for Infectious Diseases Among Substance Abusers. Treatment Improvement Series. DHHS Pub. No. (SMA) 93-2048. Washington.

Batten, H.L., C.M. Horgan, J.M. Prottas, et al. 1993. Drug Services Research Survey Phase I Final Report: Non-Correctional Facilities. Report submitted by Institute for Health Policy. Brandeis University, Waltham, Mass., February 22.

Besteman, K.J. 1992. Federal Leadership in Building the National Drug Treatment System. In *Treating Drug Problems, Volume II*, ed. D.R. Gerstein and H.J. Harwood. Washington: National Academy Press.

Burt, M.R., and B.E. Cohen. 1989. *America's Homeless: Numbers, Characteristics, and Programs that Serve Them.* Urban Institute Report 89-3. Washington: The Urban Institute Press.

Callahan, J.J., D.S. Shepard. R.H. Beinecke, M.J. Larson, and D. Cavanaugh. 1994. Evaluation of the Massachusetts Medicaid Mental Health/Substance Abuse Program. Report prepared for the Mental Health/Substance Abuse Program, Massachusetts Division of Medical Assistance. Prepared by Heller School, Brandeis University, Waltham, Mass., January 24.

Cleary, P. 1989. The Need and Demand for Mental Health Services. In *The Future of Mental Health Services Research.* DHHS pub. no. (ADM) 89-1600, ed. C. Taube, D. Mechanic, and A. Hohmann. Rockville, Md.: National Institute on Drug Abuse.

Des Jarlais, D.C., and S.R. Friedman. 1988. HIV Infection among Persons Who Inject Illicit Drugs: Problems and Prospects. *Journal of Acquired Immune Deficiency Syndromes* 1:267–73.

England, M.J., and V.A. Vaccaro. 1991. New Systems to Manage Mental Health Care. *Health Affairs* 10(4):129–37.

Epstein, J.F., and J.C. Gfroerer. 1994. Estimating Substance Abuse Treatment Need from the NHSDA. In *Proceedings of the Section on Survey Research Methods of the American Statistical Association* (in press).

Everingham, S.S., and Rydell, C.P. 1994. *Modeling the Demand for Cocaine.* Rand Report no. MR-332-ONDCP/A/DPRC. Santa Monica, Calif.: Rand Corporation.

Foster Higgins. 1990. *Health Benefits Survey: Mental Health Abuse Benefits, 1989.* Report 5: Mental Health and Substance Abuse Benefits. Princeton, N.J.

Freeman, M.A., and T. Trabin. 1994. Managed Behavioral Healthcare: History, Models, Key Issues, and Future Course. Report prepared by Behavioral Health Alliance for Center on Mental Health Services, Substance Abuse and Mental Health Services Administration, Department of Health and Human Services. October 5.

Gabel, J., D. Liston, G. Jensen, and Marsteller. 1994. The Health Insurance Picture 1993: Some Rare Good News. *Health Affairs* 13(1):327–36.

Gerstein, D.R., and H.J. Harwood. 1990. *Treating Drug Problems.* Institute of Medicine, vol.1. Washington: National Academy Press.

Gfroerer, J.C. and M.D. Brodsky. 1993. Frequent Cocaine Users and Their Use of Treatment. *American Journal of Public Health* 83(8):1149–54.

Harlow, C.W. 1991. *Drugs and Jail Inmates, 1989.* Bureau of Justice Statistics Special Report. U.S. Department of Justice, Office of Justice Programs. Washington

Haverkos, H.W., and R.L. Lange. 1990. Serious Infections Other than Human Immunodeficiency Virus among Intravenous Drug Abusers. *Journal of Infectious Diseases* 161:894–902.

Harwood, H.J., and T. Zenzola. 1993. How Many People Are in Need of Treatment. Paper prepared by Lewin-VHI for Office of National Drug Control Policy (Task No.93H), Washington, July 14.

Horgan, C., M.E. Marsden, M.J. Larson, et al. 1993. Substance Abuse: the Nation's Number One Health Problem, Key Indicators for Policy. Report prepared by the Institute for Health Policy, Brandeis University for the Robert Wood Johnson Foundation, Waltham, Mass., October.

Horgan, C., M. Rosenbach, E. Ostby, and B. Butrica. 1991. Targeting Special Populations with Drug Abuse Problems: Pregnant Women. *NIDA Drug Abuse Services Research Series: Background Papers on Drug Abuse Financing and Services Research* (1):123–44.

Hoy, E.W., R.E. Curtis, and T. Rice. 1991. Change and Growth in Managed Care. *Health Affairs* 10(4):18–36.

Hubbard, R.L., M.E. Marsden, J.V. Rachal, H.J. Harwood, E.R. Cavanaugh, and H.M. Ginzburg. 1989. *Drug Abuse Treatment: A National Survey of Effectiveness.* Chapel Hill, N.C.: The University of North Carolina Press.

Johnson, B.D. and J. Muffler. 1992. Sociocultural Aspects of Drug Use and Abuse in the 1990s. In *Substance Abuse – A Comprehensive Textbook,* ed. J.H. Lowinson, P. Ruiz, R.B. Millman, and J.G. Langrod. Baltimore: Williams and Wilkins.

Johnston, L.D., P.M. O'Malley, and J.G. Bachman. 1993. *Secondary School Students.* National Survey Results on Drug Use from Monitoring the Future Study, 1975–1992, vol. 1, NIH pub. no. 93-3597. Bethesda, Md.: National Institutes of Health

Keer, D.W., J.D. Colliver, A.N. Kopstein, et al. 1994. *Restricted Activity Days and Other Problems Associated with Use of Marijuana or Cocaine Among Persons 18–44 Years of Age: United States, 1991.* Advance Data from Vital and Health Statistics no. 246. Hyattsville, Md.: National Center for Health Statistics.

Kessler, R.C., K.A. McGonagle, S. Zhao, et al. 1994. Lifetime and 12-Month Prevalence of DSM-III-R Psychiatric Disorders in the United States. Results from the National Comorbidity Survey. *Archives of General Psychiatry* 51(1):8–19.

Larson, M.J., and C.M. Horgan. 1994. *Variations in State Medicaid Program Expenditures for Substance Abuse Units and Facilities.* NIDA Services

Research Monograph no. 1: Financing Drug Treatment through State Programs. Rockville, Md.: National Institute on Drug Abuse.

Larson, M.J., C. Horgan, M.E. Marsden, C. Tomkins, S. Wallack and A. Hendricks. 1993. *Health Insurance Coverage for Substance Abuse Services.* Rockville, Md.: Substance Abuse and Mental Health Services Administration.

Leukefeld, C.G., and F.M. Tims. 1988. Compulsory Treatment: A Review of Findings. In *Compulsory Treatment of Drug Abuse: Research and Clinical Practice.* NIDA Research Monograph 86. DHHS Pub. No. (ADM) 88-1578, ed. C.G. Leukefeld and F.M. Tims,. Rockville, Md.: National Institute on Drug Abuse.

Leukefeld, C., R.W. Pickens, and C.R. Schuster. 1992. Recommendations for Improving Treatment. *International Journal of Addictions* 27(10):1223–39.

McLellan, A.T., I.O. Arndt, D.S. Metzger, G.E. Woody, and C.P. O'Brien. 1993. The Effects of Psychosocial Services in Substance Abuse Treatment. *Journal of the American Medical Association* 269(15):1953–9.

Musto, D.F. 1991. Opium, Cocaine and Marijuana in American History. *Scientific American* 265(1).

———. 1992. Historical Perspectives on Alcohol and Drug Abuse. In *Substance Abuse – A Comprehensive Textbook*, ed. J.H. Lowinson, P. Ruiz, R.B. Millman, and J.G. Langrod. Baltimore: Williams and Wilkins.

Narrow, W.E., D.A. Regier, D.S. Rae, R.W. Manderscheid, and B.Z. Locke. 1993. Use of Services by Persons with Mental and Addictive Disorders: Findings from the NIMH ECA Program. *Archives of General Psychiatry* 50(2):95–107.

Regier, D.A., W.E. Narrow, and D.S. Rae. 1993. The de facto US Mental and Addictive Disorders Service System: Epidemiologic Catchment Area Prospective 1-Year Prevalence Rates of Disorders and Services. *Archives of General Psychiatry* 50(2):85–94.

Reuter, P. 1992. Hawks Ascendant: The Punitive Trend of American Drug Policy. *Daedalus* 121(3):15–22.

Rice, D.P. 1993. Unpublished Preliminary Data. San Francisco: Institute for Health and Aging, University of California, San Francisco.

Rice, D.P., S. Kelman, and L. Miller. 1991. Estimates of Economic Costs of Alcohol and Drug Abuse and Mental Illness, 1985 and 1988. *Public Health Reports* 106(3):280–92.

Robbins, L.N., and D.A. Regier (eds). 1991. *Psychiatric Disorders in America.* New York: Free Press.

Russo, R. 1991. Primary Care and Intravenous Drug Abuse Treatment. In Improving Drug Abuse Treatment. NIDA Research Monograph 106; DHHS pub. no. (ADM)91-1754, ed. R.W. Pickens, C.G. Leukefeld, C.R. Schuster. Rockville, Md.: National Institute on Drug Abuse.

Rydell, C.P., and S.S. Everingham. 1994. *Controlling Cocaine: Supply versus Demand Programs.* Rand Report no. MR-331-ONDCP/A/DPRC. Santa Monica, Calif.: Rand Corporation.

Schlesinger, M., R. Dorwart, and R. Clark. 1991. Public Policy in a Fragmented Service System. NIDA Drug Abuse Services Research Series: Background Papers on Drug Abuse Financing and Services Research. 1:16–57.

Schmidt, L., and C. Weisner. 1993. Developments in Alcoholism Treatment. In *Recent Developments in Alcoholism*, ed. M. Galanter. New York: Plenum.

Steinberg, R. 1992. The Market for Drug Treatment. In *Treating Drug Problems*, Volume II, ed. D.R. Gerstein and H.J. Harwood. Washington: National Academy Press.

Substance Abuse and Mental Health Services Administration. 1993. Estimates from the Drug Abuse Warning Network – 1992 Estimates of Drug-Related Emergency Room Episodes. Advance Report Number 4 (September). Washington: U.S. Department of Health and Human Services.

———. 1994. Preliminary Estimates from the 1993 National Household Survey on Drug Abuse. Advance Report Number 7 (July). Washington: U.S. Department of Health and Human Services.

———. 1995. Overview of the National Drug and Alcoholism Treatment Unit Survey (NDATUS): 1992 and 1980-1992. Advance Report Number 9 (January). Washington: U.S. Department of Health and Human Services.

U.S. General Accounting Office. 1990. Health Insurance: Cost Increases Lead to Coverage Limitations and Cost Shifting. GAO/HRD-90-68 (May). Washington.

U.S. Office of Management and Budget. 1993. Federal Drug Controls Programs: Budget Summary Fiscal Year 1994 (April 23). Washington: Executive Office of the President.

Weisner, C., and L.A. Schmidt. 1994. A Framework for Evaluating Research on Access and Utilization of Drug Abuse Services. Prepared for NIDA Health Services Research Program (January 24). Washington.

The White House. 1994. National Drug Control Strategy: Reclaiming Our Communities from Drugs and Violence. Washington: Office of National Drug Control Policy, Executive Office of the President.

4

Staffing Patterns and Services for the War on Drugs

Barry S. Brown

The declaration of a War on Drugs was made without benefit of either a standing army or a ready reserve. The Drug Abuse Office and Treatment Act of 1972 provided funds for a national program of community-based drug-abuse treatment (SAODAP 1972). In so doing, the President, together with a unanimous Congress, redefined drug abuse as a health rather than a criminal justice issue, and made access to treatment available to clients voluntarily seeking treatment in their own communities (Jaffe 1979). Prior to that time, two major facilities, one in Lexington, Kentucky, and one in Fort Worth, Texas, provided the great bulk of publicly funded drug-abuse treatment. These were oriented to the criminal justice system, with 80 percent of their clientele initially coming from correctional settings (Pescor 1938). By 1977, only 20 percent of clients being treated in publicly funded settings were coming from the criminal justice system (NIDA 1981). Indeed, the Treatment Alternatives to Street Crime program (TASC), funded through the Drug Abuse Office and Treatment Act of 1972, went so far as to permit adjudicated drug users to volunteer for drug-abuse treatment in lieu of further criminal processing (Weinman 1990). During this period, the number of community-based treatment programs grew from less than 600 prior to 1970 to more than 3000 by 1975 and came to

include at least one program in every state and in each of three terri-
tories (NIDA 1976).

The Paraprofessional Movement

A major health-care program had been initiated. A behavior
disorder found to afflict tens of thousands was earmarked for treatment and, to a considerable degree, the mental health community
was otherwise engaged. On the one hand, character disorders – as
drug users were likely to be described at the time – were generally
regarded as unattractive clients (Brown 1996). They were both more
intractable and less cooperative than other, readily available, mental
health clients. In addition, they were also largely unknown to all but
those few mental health professionals who had experience in
correctional settings or in the Lexington and Fort Worth public
health settings. Drug use translated into heroin use in the early
1970s, with over 80 percent of a sample of more than 40,000 clients
entering treatment from 1969 to 1972 reporting heroin as their
primary drug (Simpson et al. 1978). And the shadowy world of
"ripping and running," of "copping" and of such related activities as
"boosting, pimping, tricking" or "hustling" was foreign in both form
and language. Fortunately for the mental health professional – and
for the drug-abuse client – both guide and translator were available
in the person of the paraprofessional, and typically ex-addict, drug-
abuse counselor.

In 1958, Synanon was founded on the premise that recovering
addicts could work with active addicts to help the latter graduate to
recovering status and to allow the former to remain drug free.
Synanon begat Phoenix House, Daytop Village, Gateway, and nearly
200 other therapeutic-community programs. It also spawned an
interest and a confidence in the paraprofessional drug-abuse counselor that came to extend well beyond the therapeutic-community
movement. Indeed, while proponents of the therapeutic community and of methadone maintenance treatment found themselves
locked in ideological conflict over several important issues of service
delivery, both agreed on the desirability of paraprofessional, and
typically ex-addict, counselors, although not always with equal
enthusiasm (Lowinsohn and Millman 1979). Nonetheless, of all
human-service delivery programs, drug-abuse treatment has probably become the most frequent employer of its own graduates. Thus,
drug-abuse treatment has provided its graduates continuing support

to their rehabilitation efforts, and has provided its clients visible evidence of reward for their rehabilitation efforts.

The ex-addict paraprofessional not only provided a vitally needed personnel source, the ex-addict paraprofessional also offered critical strengths that complemented the skills provided by their academically trained colleagues – who were also, typically, their supervisors. The professional could describe and measure human behavior and could design a comprehensive course of therapeutic action. The paraprofessionals could relate to addict-clients in a manner that took advantage of experience they shared with their clients. The paraprofessional could deal empathically with the client's efforts to modify the role-demands and expectations of others in the community, and deal confrontively with efforts at self-denial or manipulation. Moreover, the ex-addict paraprofessional counselor could act as role model. S/he was not voicing an abstract notion of rehabilitation, s/he had made the journey. In the parlance of the times, the ex-addict counselor, "had walked the walk, and could talk the talk."

Little wonder that the ranks of counseling were filled with significant numbers of ex-addict paraprofessionals while the ranks of administrators/directors were filled with more traditionally trained staff. And while the disparity in status – often complicated by co-occurring ethnic differences – sometimes led to difficulty, in general the status differences appear to have been seen as the expected corollary of educational differences (Brown and Needle 1994). Nor was the lack of education necessarily a barrier to advancement. Administrators of therapeutic-community programs were sometimes drawn from the ranks of ex-addicts. Far less frequently paraprofessionals could become administrators of methadone programs. However, clinical supervisors and chief counselors were frequently individuals who had distinguished themselves through their work in the treatment setting rather than their work in the classroom.

Two other factors are also worth noting as having probably fueled the interest in using paraprofessionals. On the one hand, the development of community-based drug-abuse treatment occurred not long after the establishment of the paraprofessional counseling movement in mental health. That field had discovered, albeit somewhat belatedly, that psychiatric aides – hired to be custodial staff – not only spent a significant period of time with their psychiatric patients but interacted with those patients in ways that were different from those of mental health professionals, but which appeared nonetheless positive, e.g., holding or hugging patients to lend emotional support (Reissman and Popper 1968; Sobey 1970).

In addition, aspects of the Civil Rights Movement and the War on Poverty – particularly the Community Action and Model Cities Programs in the latter – involved empowering community members to act on behalf of themselves and their communities. In those programs an emphasis was placed on recruiting from the community, then using those indigenous nonprofessionals to help guide the change process within their communities. It seems likely that these movements lent an ideology and, in at least some instances, the War on Poverty lent resources and personnel to the War on Drugs.

By 1976, 35 percent of full-time drug-abuse treatment program staff were nonprofessional counselors. (Data were not collected on the number who were recovering addicts, but it is reasonable to assume they constituted a substantial proportion of nonprofessional counseling staff.) In comparison, there were only 2 percent who were physicians, 10 percent who were nursing staff, 3 percent psychologists, and 6 percent social workers (NIDA 1976).

The thrust of drug-abuse treatment in the early and mid-70s reflected a view of the addict-client as showing social, not psychological, deficit (Robins 1979). The typical addict-client was a minority-group male, living in the inner city, with a limited educational and job history and an extensive history of criminal activity. As described by Dole and his colleagues (1968), "the slum-born, minority group, criminal addict needed help to become a productive member of society. Many of these individuals came to us from jail with no vocational skills, no family and no financial resources. They were further handicapped by racial discrimination and by their police records."

In the face of that social deficit, the emphasis of drug-abuse treatment was on the creation of prosocial skills and encouraging an acceptance of personal and social responsibility. The first and prototypic methadone program, organized by Dole and Nyswander and as described by Gearing (1968), provided vocational rehabilitation/job development, legal counseling, assistance in obtaining financial entitlements as well as counseling designed to develop skills in coping with the demands of community living. In drug-free outpatient programs, as reported by Kleber and Slobetz (1979), "counseling programs tend, on the whole, to focus on the 'here and now'. . . . The therapeutic goals of counseling will most often focus on questions of social adjustment with peers, family, school, job, etc." Therapeutic communities emphasized the graduated assumption of responsibility by addict-clients seen to be immature and irresponsible at program entry. Given these emphases on providing opportunities/demands for prosocial functioning, and the apparent absence of psychological impairment, the dearth of traditional mental health staff was not a significant concern.

At the same time the drug-abuse treatment field was significantly involved in guaranteeing appropriate training opportunities to drug-abuse treatment staff generally, and to paraprofessional counselors particularly. In 1973, the National Training System was organized under federal auspices. The System was composed of regional centers at which brief courses were provided on a variety of subjects, although counseling practices were the major emphasis of the courses offered (Dendy 1979). Thousands of program staff were exposed to those courses, and it is likely that many more were influenced by the course work provided. The National Training System complemented the on-the-job training being provided at local programs. These initiatives to upgrade counseling skills were to lead ultimately to a credentialing of drug-abuse counselors in an effort to provide quality control to a service delivery field heavily invested in hiring key staff on the basis of personal attributes and history, rather than academic qualifications alone.

Nonetheless, concerns about the quality of care provided by ex-addict paraprofessional counselors were sufficient to stimulate a number of studies through the mid and late 1970s comparing the functioning and effectiveness of ex-addict and non-addict counselors. The several studies found no, or few, differences in the ways in which counselors viewed their roles and undertook their jobs (Kozel and Brown 1973; LoSciuto et al. 1984; Aiken et al. 1984a), or in their effectiveness in producing positive behavioral change (Longwell et al. 1978; Brown and Thompson 1976; Aiken et al. 1984b). Beyond these overall results several individual findings are worth noting.

Longwell and his colleagues found greater reductions in opiate use among those clients who had counselors assigned to them consistently throughout the study period than among those who did not. Also, while none of the studies contrasted the performance of paraprofessional counselors with that of traditional mental health professionals, the studies by LoSciuto et al. (1984) and Aiken et al. (1984a; 1984b) did make use of a sample of non-addict counselors who had, at minimum, completed college, 42 percent having also obtained masters' degrees and an additional 29 percent some graduate training. By comparison, 84 percent of the ex-addict counselors had high school degrees only. In light of these educational differences, the absence of differences in client outcomes is striking. Moreover, LoSciuto and colleagues (1984) found that clients of ex-addict counselors were more likely than other clients to report themselves as deriving benefit from counseling sessions, and to report both wanting their counselors to help them with personal problems and expecting that their counselors would help them, while Aiken et al. (1984a) found that ex-addict counselors were significantly more likely to engage the client in his or her own community.

Consistent with these findings regarding counselor effectiveness, Durlak (1979), in a review of studies across the fields of mental health and substance abuse, reported no differences in outcomes for clients of professionals and paraprofessionals in 29 of the 42 studies reviewed, reported more positive outcomes for clients of paraprofessionals in 12 of the 42 studies and more favorable outcomes for professionals in only one study. A more recent review of the literature by Christensen and Jacobson (1994) comes to the same conclusion as that reached by Durlak. Counselors are found equally effective whether their expertise is based on experience only or a combination of academic credentials and experience. For these reasons "paraprofessionals" have sometimes been described as professionals of experience, and traditional mental health "professionals" as professionals of education (Brown 1993).

Treatment was not the only area of drug-abuse programming importantly influenced by the efforts of nonprofessionals. In the late 1970s a body of parents, concerned about the extent of drug use in their communities and the government's seeming unwillingness to act on their behalf, organized themselves to promote drug-abuse prevention through a combination of community organization and political action. However, the two groups of paraprofessionals neither found or ever sought common ground although both can be characterized as professionals of experience committed to containing the drug abuse in their communities. Indeed, it seems likely that the two groups, the parents' movement and the ex-addict counselors, never saw themselves as sharing common interests and were, in fact, probably only vaguely aware of each other. Whereas the ex-addict counselors were inner-city, male-dominated, primarily paid staff concerned with "hard drugs," the parents' movement was composed of suburban, female-dominated, primarily volunteer staff concerned with "soft drugs." More importantly, where the ex-addict counselors extolled (and personified) triumph over drug use with governmental intercession, the parents' movement extolled the avoidance of drug use and independence from government. Nonetheless, both groups championed the contributions of persons who traded on experience and hard work to make a difference in the drug-abuse field.

The Mental Health Movement

By the start of the second decade of the War on Drugs, a new phenomenon was being noted which was destined to bring a traditional mental health perspective more forcefully into play in drug-abuse treatment. The drug-abuse client was no longer seen as showing evidence of social deficit alone. A substantial number of clients now showed evidence of psychological deficit as well. Several investigators reported higher levels of psychological disorder among clients being admitted to treatment in the late 1970s and early 1980s than had been been found earlier (McLellan et al. 1983; Rounsaville et al. 1982a; De Leon et al. 1985; Nurco 1985). Of particular significance were reports of current or historic depression, other mood disorders and, less frequently, anxiety disorder (Rounsaville and Kleber 1985). Moreover, psychological disorder was viewed as having substantial prognostic importance (McLellan et al. 1983; Rounsaville and Kleber 1985).

To meet the needs of those drug users showing symptoms of psychological disorder, later to be christened the dually diagnosed client, there appeared to many to be a need for traditional mental health workers. It may have been hoped that a decade of drug-abuse treatment – with considerable national attention and reasonable funding – would have lent an air of respectability, if not glamor, to the field of drug-abuse treatment, allowing for easier recruitment of mental health professionals than was the case when war was first declared.

The reports of significant psychological dysfunction accompanying clients' drug use also prompted concerns about refining both the psychiatric nosology and psychodiagnostic strategies in drug abuse. A team of experts was commissioned to develop criteria appropriate to the drug-abuse client and to update the Diagnostic and Statistical Manual of Mental Disorders (DSM III) accordingly. Plans were made to update the International Classification of Diseases (ICD-8) as well (Jaffe 1993). The DSM-III was revised in 1987 (DSM-IIIR) and the ICD (ICD-10) shortly thereafter. Intake forms were expanded to include a broader array of questions about psychological functioning and history. In addition, paper and pencil tests regarding psychological functioning and standard psycho-diagnostic interviews came into wider use.

In drug-abuse treatment, the use of psychotherapeutic drugs, in particular anti-depressants, became increasingly common, extending even to therapeutic-community regimens. However, it was the increasing influence of the mental health community on the conduct of drug-abuse counseling that was most notable. A study by Woody and his colleagues (1983) lent considerable weight to the argument favoring an infusion of mental health professionals into the drug-abuse field. In that study it was found that a core of drug-abuse clients showed greater positive behavioral change and reduction in psychological symptoms consequent to the combined efforts of traditional drug-abuse counseling and psychotherapies than was shown consequent to the efforts of traditional drug-abuse counseling alone. That study and subsequent analyses clarified that those clients with higher levels of psychopathology – other than sociopathy – were most likely to derive benefit from the addition of psychotherapy (Woody et al. 1984; Woody et al. 1985). In this well-designed clinical trial there appeared clear evidence of the importance of psychotherapy for some number of drug-abuse clients. However, several issues are worth noting.

First, as the authors themselves made clear, the vast majority of drug-abuse clients in their study showed dramatic and equivalent rehabilitative gain, no matter whether they were seen by drug-abuse counselors only or by drug-abuse counselors in conjunction with therapists providing supportive-expressive or cognitive-behavioral psychotherapies. Moreover, studies are far from uniform in suggesting a need for mental health professionals to achieve reductions in the psychological problems of drug-abuse clients. De Leon (1985) reported reductions in psychological dysfunction associated with length of time in the therapeutic community. Similarly, Rounsaville et al. (1982b) reported a reduction in depressive symptoms consequent to treatment making use of traditional drug-abuse counseling staff. Other studies have found that psychologically disturbed clients could be retained in treatment as long as those without disturbance, could show equivalent compliance with program requirements, and could achieve equal behavioral improvement (Hubbard et al. 1989; Agosti et al. 1991; Joe et al. 1995).

It has been speculated that the achievement of change in behaviors may lead to change in psychological functioning. In this thinking, change in behavior is seen as leading to change in self-perception and the perceptions of others, which together can lead to reductions in psychological symptoms. Indeed, Vaillant and

Milofsky (1982), reporting the results of follow-up studies of alcohol clients, found reductions in psychological symptoms occurring consequent to abstinence from alcohol.

For whatever reasons, as shown in table 4.1, it does not appear from data collected through federal reporting systems that concerns about increasing numbers of the dually diagnosed, although voiced by service providers and state drug-abuse administrators (Greenberg and Brown 1984), stimulated a significant increase in the representation of traditional mental health workers in drug-abuse treatment settings (NIDA 1976; SAMHSA 1993). It should be noted, however, that findings from a comparison between the National Drug Abuse Treatment Utilization Survey (NDATUS) and the National Drug and Alcoholism Treatment Unit Survey (NDATUS) must be regarded as suggestive only as the change in name (while retaining the initials) implies important changes in the reporting system.

In the 15-year period between 1976 and 1991, the percentage of full-time psychiatrists relative to all staff has gone from 1.0 percent to 1.1 percent, the number of full-time physicians other than psychiatrists has gone from 1.0 percent to 1.1 percent, nursing staff has gone from 10.0 percent to 8.7 percent (RNs only are included in the 1991 reporting), social workers from 5.8 percent to 6.3 percent, psychologists from 3.1 percent to 3.5 percent, while counselors

Table 4.1 Comparisons of 1976 and 1991 percentages of full-time staff positions.*

Staff	1976 (N=31,100) %	1991 (N=101,534) %
Psychiatrists	1.0	1.1
Other physicians	1.0	1.1
Nurses**	10.0	8.7
Psychologists	3.1	3.5
Social Workers	5.8	6.3
Counselors***	35.0	35.8
Other direct care	22.5	17.6
Administrative	21.6	26.0

* Based on data from the National Drug Abuse Treatment Utilization Survey (1976) and the National Drug and Alcoholism Treatment Unit Survey (1991).

** Nursing staff in 1991 were RNs only.

*** Counselors in 1991 included both credentialed and non-credentialed staff.

(credentialed and other) have gone from 35.0 percent to 35.8 percent. An additional 22.5 percent of staff in 1976 and 17.6 percent in 1991 were involved in other direct care efforts, while 21.6 percent in 1976 and 26.0 percent in 1991 provided administrative services.

Although the data suggest a remarkable stability in employment categories it is necessary, again, to point to several cautions in interpreting that data. As noted, the data for 1976 reflect drug-abuse treatment programs, the data for 1991 reflect both alcohol and drug-abuse treatment programs. The total number of staff available to clients in the years compared is very different, in part of course, due to the absence of alcohol treatment staff in the earlier survey. Nonetheless, client:staff ratios are also remarkably similar between the two years. The ratio of clients to all direct care staff was 9.8:1 in 1976, 10.77:1 in 1991; the ratio of clients to all nonprofessional counselors was 22.16:1 in 1976; 22.26:1 in 1991.

Part-time staff are not included in the data reported because of the absence of full-time equivalency data for 1976. It should be noted that degreed staff are more likely to be part-time staff than are non-degreed counselors. However, the representation of the different types of staff change little when full-time equivalents are considered for the 1991 data. Psychiatrists and other physicians come to constitute 1.6 percent and 1.8 percent of all staff, respectively, nursing 10.7 percent, while social workers remain constant at 6.3 percent and psychologists grow only to 3.8 percent. Counselors, credentialed and not, drop slightly to 34.3 percent. Moreover, part-time staff constituted 33 percent of all service staff in 1976 and a roughly equivalent 30 percent in 1991.

It should be noted also that volunteer staff are not calculated in this reporting; however, in 1991 they constituted only 3.7 percent of direct care FTEs (SAMHSA 1993).

Finally, and perhaps most importantly for this comparison, there appears to be a greater percentage of private programs (18.5 percent), as reflected by the designation "private for profit," in the 1991 sample, than was found in the 1976 sample in which 6 percent of programs report receiving only private funding.

It is apparent that whatever the belief about the utility of mental health staff, or of traditionally degreed staff generally, the weight of treatment falls on the shoulders of the counseling staffs who have born that weight since the establishment of community-based treatment. Whatever the reasons, the representation of mental health professionals would not appear to have increased in concert with increasing evidence of psychological difficulty. Calls for increased use of psychotherapy with drug-abuse clients (Woody et al. 1991), however well intentioned, appear destined to go unanswered.

Indeed, Hubbard (1994) reports a dramatic diminution in the percentage of clients reporting receipt of psychological services between 1979–81 admissions and 1991–93 admissions. During that approximate 10-year period reports of receipt of psychological services went from 16.1 percent to 4.2 percent for methadone programs, 71.3 percent to 8.5 percent for outpatient drug-free programs, and from 53.1 percent to 7.7 percent for residential programs. In national surveys of outpatient treatment programs, Price and D'Aunno (1992b) found that programs reported 36 percent of clients receiving mental health services in 1988, with that figure dropping below 30 percent by 1990.

While questions can be raised about the extent of need for psychotherapy, it is reasonable to posit that some number of clients can benefit from a psychologically oriented counseling. In this regard, it is noteworthy that Rounsaville and Kleber (1985), in their review of the drug-abuse and psychotherapy literature, report that drug-treatment programs are unlikely to reject clients on the basis of psychological difficulty.

In recognition of the limited resources available to most programs, efforts can be made to forge relationships with community mental health facilities to provide training and consultation to counseling staff as well as services to a limited number of clients, or a staff member or members may be recruited on a full- or part-time basis to provide these same services on behalf of the program.

Educational Status of Treatment Staff

Although mental health staff remain in short supply, there is reason to believe that the drug-abuse counselor of the 1990s is somewhat better educated than the drug-abuse counselor of the 1970s. Hubbard et al. (1989) report a majority of counselors in outpatient drug-free programs (11 of 19 "who provided information") as having graduate degrees, and a distinct minority (5 of 19) with high school diplomas only. Mulligan et al. (1989) found a comparable 21 percent of alcohol and drug-abuse counselors in Massachusetts (N = 1328) lacking college degrees and 45 percent with masters' or doctoral degrees. However, educational credentials varied widely by modality, with zero percent of community mental health center staff lacking college degrees compared with 53 percent of drug detoxification staff. Working with a sample of 588 outpatient treatment programs, Price and D'Aunno (1992a) conclude that the master's degree is the most frequent educational achievement among outpatient treatment staff (34 percent), with the bachelor's degree next (23 percent) and only 21 percent with less than a bachelor's degree.

Similarly, Winick (1991) reports an increasing emphasis on academic accomplishment in an effort to achieve professionalization in the therapeutic community. Indeed, Winick (1991) details reductions in the representation of ex-addict counselors in therapeutic-community programs to permit the greater representation of non-using professional staff.

Not surprisingly, the proportion of ex-addict staff to all treatment staff nonetheless appears greater in therapeutic communities (approximately 40 percent over all New York programs – Winick, 1991) than among outpatient programs (27 percent ex-addict or recovering alcoholic – Price et al. 1991). Price and D'Aunno (1992a) also report large differences in percentages of recovering staff between outpatient methadone and outpatient drug-free programs. Less than 10 percent of methadone treatment staff are recovering addicts or alcoholics compared with 27 percent to 37 percent of outpatient drug-free staff depending on type of setting. As might be expected, outpatient drug-free staff were more likely to value the ability to overcome addiction as a useful job qualification than were methadone staff (Price and D'Aunno 1992b). Thus, in lieu of an ability to attract mental health professionals – or perhaps with a view toward melding drug-abuse and mental health concerns – staffing initiatives have focused on upgrading the quality of counseling staff through a demand for greater academic achievement and/or certification of counseling knowledge and skills.

Vocational Services

While considerable attention and concern have focused on psychological problems, other client needs continue to demand the attention of drug-abuse treatment staffs. The most recent and comprehensive description of client characteristics and reported needs is available from the Drug Abuse Treatment Outcome Study (DATOS). Preliminary data from that study report findings for 6000 clients admitted during the period 1991–1993 to 50 programs nationwide as compared with 10,000 admissions, in the period 1979–1981, to the 37 programs included in the Treatment Outcome Prospective Study (TOPS – Hubbard 1993; 1994). Hubbard found that today's clients are significantly older (a majority of clients being above 30), more likely to be female (more than a third overall), and somewhat more likely to be living in stable partner relationships (more than 25 percent overall). Perhaps more significantly for our purposes is the finding that, in spite of increases in the proportion of clients with high school degrees or GEDs across all modalities, rates of full-time employment have declined across all modalities. Less than 20 percent of 1991–3 admissions reported full-time employment in the period prior to treatment entry.

Employment, or engagement in productive activity, has long been regarded as a criterion of program effectiveness and cited as an essential element of client rehabilitation (Hall 1983). Nonetheless, findings from DATOS suggest that little attention is devoted to employment issues in contemporary drug-abuse treatment. A high of 8.9 percent of residential drug-free clients report receipt of employment services during treatment compared with 5.4 percent in outpatient drug-free treatment and 2.3 percent in methadone treatment programs (Hubbard 1994).

Findings that comparatively few clients receive vocational services are not new. Hubbard and Harwood (1981) reported that only about two-thirds of a sample of 194 outpatient and residential clinics provided any vocational services to clients, although another study has indicated that vocational assistance is a particularly strong client interest (Hargreaves 1980). What is a concern is that the provision of vocational services was found to be substantially lower today than was the case a decade earlier in spite of the increased need (Hubbard 1994). Similarly, data from the national survey of outpatient programs found only a third of clients reported to be receiving vocational services in 1988 (Price and D'Aunno 1992c) and that figure had dropped to 22 percent by 1990 (Price and D'Aunno 1992b). Not surprisingly, there has been a call for greater use of trained vocational specialists to meet client need (Deren and Randall 1990; Livingston et al. 1990).

Different models exist for making use of vocational specialists. In a study involving the random assignment of treatment programs to conditions of (a) the addition of vocational specialists to work with clients directly, (b) the addition of vocational specialists to work as consultants to counseling staffs through consortia of programs, and (c) a control condition involving no addition of vocational specialists, it was found that the addition of vocational specialists led to significantly greater retention and lesser drug use in the vocational specialist groups than in the control. No differences were found between the use of vocational specialists to provide direct services or to provide consultation only to counseling staffs; however, no differences were found between the vocational specialist and control groups with regard to employment rate among the clinic's clients (NIDA 1982).

Studies of specific models of vocational rehabilitation have included several supported work programs (Friedman 1978; Dickinson and Maynard 1981; Manpower Demonstration Research Corporation 1980), and behavioral skills training (Hall et al. 1981a; 1981b; Platt and Metzger 1987; Platt et al. 1988; Platt et al. 1993). Although these projects were not uniform in their effects, in general they impacted significantly on one or more of the standard outcome criteria of illicit drug use, employment, and/or arrest.

Programs of vocational assistance are important on two counts. On the one hand, employment/productive activity is one of the three treatment goals programs developed with and for clients (and is consequently one of the three outcome criteria by which we judge program efficacy), and it has been found to be linked to success with regard to reductions in drug use and criminality – the other two outcome criteria goals (Fisher and Anglin 1987; Anglin and Fisher 1987; Platt and Labate 1976).

While this points to the utility of employment specialists, and to the obvious wisdom of making use of models which have been found effective, fiscal realities suggest a difficulty in obtaining the level of participation that might be wished from the vocational rehabilitation community. On the other hand, research also suggests that the use of vocational specialist consultants working with counseling staffs can be effective in implementing new and effective programs. This was the model for use with the Job Seeker's Workshop program developed by Hall and her colleagues (Loeb et al. 1982); it later formed the core of a successful training program to implement that program in a national sample of methadone programs (Sorensen et al. 1988; Hall et al. 1988). These findings suggest a use of specialized staff as program consultants to counseling staffs, providing services only in selected instances.

Two issues should be kept in mind in this emphasis on counseling staff efforts. On the one hand, counselors too are finite. Indeed, Gustafson (1991) reports that poor pay and inadequate fringe benefits, work with "undesirable" clients in undesirable areas, and fear of AIDS is already hampering the State of New York in hiring and retaining both professional and paraprofessional counselors. Moreover, the report of the Institute of Medicine (IOM – Gerstein and Harwood 1990) expresses concern about escalating caseloads experienced by a number of programs consequent to the reductions in real dollar funding for drug-abuse treatment experienced since 1976. Staff burnout is frequently raised as a problem in association with this issue, and while it remains a somewhat obscure concept, staff burnout is nonetheless a real concern for program administrators.

A second issue involves the need to provide effective training to counseling staffs in the interventions in which they are to become invested. Counselors do not accept automatically the innovations discovered by others (Bigelow et al. 1984), but have been found accepting of training intended to make themselves and their programs more effective (Gustafson 1991; Sorensen et al. 1988).

Counselors, credentialed or not, are the linch pin of drug-abuse treatment. To stint on the availability, retention, or effective functioning of competent staff by virtue of inadequate pay or haphazard training is poor economic and social policy. Since the system of drug-abuse treatment is constructed around their efforts, it behooves us to take steps to shore up still further their capacities to provide effective treatment services.

Medical Services

In contrast to reports regarding mental health and vocational counseling services, data from both DATOS (Hubbard 1994) and the National Survey of Drug Abuse Treatment Services (Price and D'Aunno 1992a; Price and D'Aunno 1992b) suggest that medical services are being provided to substantial numbers of clients. Findings from DATOS (1991–3 admissions) indicate that nearly half (45.5 percent) of all methadone clients report receipt of medical services and nearly a quarter (23.3 percent) of drug-free clients report receiving medical services. This accords with National Survey findings that 38 percent of outpatient clients received medical services in 1988 (Price and D'Aunno 1992c) although this figure drops to 26 percent by 1990 (Price and D'Aunno 1992b). A majority (58.6 percent) of DATOS residential clients reported receiving medical services, although this is down significantly from the 74.7 percent reporting receipt of medical services a decade earlier (Hubbard 1994).

Supportive Services

Rates of receipt of non-medical services that may be seen as significant to developing and maintaining drug-free living are far lower. Although financial problems were reported by 44–62 percent of TOPS clients, outpatient programs in the National Survey reported that only 27 percent of clients received financial counseling in 1988 (Price and D'Aunno 1992c), and only 16 percent by 1990 (Price and D'Aunno 1992b). More pointedly, less than 2 percent of DATOS clients reported receiving financial services (Hubbard 1994).

Moreover, while 43.1 percent of outpatient drug-free DATOS clients are referred through the criminal justice system, only 3.5 percent of those clients reported the receipt of legal services. Similarly, although 41.9 percent of clients are referred to residential programs through the criminal justice system, only 12.4 percent reported the receipt of legal services (Hubbard 1994). And while approximately 20 percent of outpatient clients were reported to have received legal counseling in 1988, that figure had nearly halved by 1990 (Price and D'Aunno 1992b).

Family-related services are little in evidence across all modalities, and are significantly reduced from the level of services available a decade earlier. Only 2.7 percent of 1991–3 methadone clients reported receiving family services compared with 10.2 percent of 1979–81 methadone clients; 9.8 percent of 1991–3 outpatient drug-free clients reported receiving family services compared with 45.9 percent of 1979–81 outpatient drug-free clients. A somewhat higher proportion of 1991–3 residential clients (22.2 percent) reported the receipt of family services, down only slightly from 1979–81 rates (26.3 percent) (Hubbard 1994).

To the extent one sees financial, legal, and/or family issues as associated with community stabilization, the absence of services to deal with those issues must be viewed with concern. Certainly, the absence of those services may, in part, explain the relatively high rates of relapse experienced with drug-abuse treatment. Strategies of relapse prevention/aftercare, which provide a mix of behavioral skills training, counseling, case management, and peer-based mutual support have proven successful in dealing with these and other issues of community stabilization (McAuliffe and Chien 1986; Nurco et al. 1991; Hawkins et al. 1986; Catalano et al. 1991; Mackay and Marlatt 1991). To make use of those strategies, and of the further advances likely to grow from continuing research in relapse prevention/aftercare, it will be necessary to have available appropriate staff to implement those strategies. Similarly, there will be a need to make available appropriate staff to undertake narrower tasks of establishing linkages with community agencies appropriate to permit the client's effective reentry into the community, i.e., to conduct case management functions.

While counseling staffs, if they exist in sufficient numbers, can assume some portion of these responsibilities, specialists should be employed to organize and direct relapse prevention/aftercare initiatives and, in the instance of case management, to establish the initial ties to community agencies and organizations relevant to clients' needs as well as to monitor the treatment program's continuing relationship with those community agencies and organizations.

The reduction in availability of family services has particular relevance when joined to reports of an increasing number of women being admitted to drug programs. Female clients are far more likely to have responsibility for dependent children than are male clients (Eldred and Washington 1975). Colten (1982) reported that 49 percent of female clients had children living with them. Moreover, female clients who did not have their children living with them were likely to be making use of their mothers to provide necessary child care (Tucker 1979). It is apparent that in defining family services to include services on behalf of the client to provide supports to drug-free living, and services to provide supports to effective child care, e.g., through parenting-skills training efforts and through linkages with appropriate community service agencies, we may effect both the reintegration of the client into society and the prevention of a second generation of dysfunctional behaviors. To date, most treatment programs have lacked the resources to embrace these larger responsibilities.

AIDS and Drug-Abuse Treatment

Perhaps the greatest challenge to the treatment community, and to the time and skills of service providers, is posed by the threat of lethal disease that now endangers the clients of drug-abuse treatment programs. The challenge of AIDS has stimulated a call on the part of some to increase the availability of comprehensive programs of methadone treatment (Brown 1991) and a call on the part of others to develop interim methadone clinics, devoid of counseling or significant social support, in recognition of our inability to make comprehensive care available for all in need and at risk of infection (Dole 1991).

While that debate continues, many treatment programs have initiated AIDS prevention programming, although only a few provide HIV testing as a part of those efforts. As found in the survey of outpatient treatment programs (Price and D'Aunno 1992a), 53 percent of programs in 1988 were conducting HIV counseling to a "great" or "very great" extent; however, only 6 percent provided HIV testing to more than half their clients. Moreover, only 17 percent of programs were able to make special staff available for HIV prevention efforts to a "great" or "very great" extent (Price and D'Aunno 1992c; D'Aunno and Mohr 1993). Thus, we can conclude that to the extent HIV prevention efforts are offered, those efforts rely on existing medical and counseling staffs or other community agencies.

At the same time several observers have reported difficulty in recruiting and retaining staff in the wake of AIDS concerns (Winick 1991; Gustafson 1991; Brown 1991). The impact of AIDS concerns on the hiring and retention of staff is unclear. What impact there is may be experienced in only narrow areas of the country, e.g., the Northeast – at least for the present. That impact may also be greater for staff with more marketable skills. And that impact may be greater in terms of the quality rather than the quantity of staff who make themselves available. In any event, to the extent that AIDS exists as a meaningful threat to a community, it is unlikely to be a drawing card to employment in drug-abuse treatment.

Moreover, it seems likely that program responsibilities will grow rather than diminish in association with the AIDS pandemic. Many programs are already called upon to extend or to initiate linkages with community medical care facilities (Selwyn et al. 1989) – now including hospices. To a limited extent, programs have become involved in the provision of outreach services for purposes of HIV prevention (Price and D'Aunno 1992c). In general, outreach has been undertaken by community-based organizations other than treatment providers, often resulting in the creation of an expanded pool of treatment applicants (Liebman et al. 1993). Indeed, the relationship of treatment programs both to outreach and to syringe exchange programs will need to be explored since both appear to create new clients for drug-abuse treatment (Lurie and Rheingold 1993). Treatment programs are also likely to be called upon to determine their responsibility to spouses and sexual partners of injection drug-abuse clients, that is, to determine whether and to whom to provide HIV prevention information and counseling, or to make provision to see that those services are provided (Brown and Beschner 1989). In short, the already difficult and challenging job of rehabilitation has now been made immeasureably more difficult by the new responsibilities for client survival and community protection that drug treatment programs are increasingly called upon to provide.

Conclusion

Two decades of study have established the importance of several components for the effective treatment of drug-abuse clients. Vocational programming, an attention to mental health issues, and relapse prevention/aftercare initiatives have all been found to be associated with client rehabilitation. All must be mediated through drug-abuse treatment counseling staffs.

In spite of some suggestion of a relative stability in client:staff ratios over time, there is ample evidence of a deterioration in service availability in the face of an increasingly complex client population. Throughout this period the central service provider has been, and remains, the drug-abuse counselor. That provider, however, appears to have greater education and training than his/her counterpart of 15 to 20 years ago, although Price et al. (1991) find that even today nearly half (44 percent) of treatment staff have bachelors' degrees or less. Moreover, it is likely that those with more advanced degrees are disproportionately represented among program supervisors and administrators, i.e., have little or no direct care responsibilities. In short, making treatment more effective means, in large part, increasing the capability of largely non-professional drug-abuse counselors.

A first effort is simply to increase the numbers of counseling staff to serve clients. Programs with lower client to staff ratios are more effective than programs with higher ratios (McCaughrin and Price 1992). If we have reason to believe that treatment is largely effective, i.e., typically leads to positive behavior changes, then one strategy for increasing program effectiveness is to guarantee that we can bring to bear the level of services required to produce change.

Moreover, the number of counseling staff, and of treatment staff generally, needs to be increased to contend with the greater array of client issues that are to be addressed. In the view of this writer all clients admitted to drug-abuse treatment should receive HIV prevention counseling and have access to HIV testing with appropriate pre- and post-test counseling as a part of each program's initial health screening for clients. This calls for the availability of adequate medical and counseling staffs. Staffing should also be adequate to link clients with health service facilities in the community and to provide, or arrange to have provided, counseling for sexual partners or family members.

Moreover, rehabilitation services in terms of job training and job finding will probably require the services of a vocational specialist (full- or part-time depending on the size of program) to provide support and assistance to counseling staffs, to assume a caseload of particularly complex cases, and to establish and maintain ties with appropriate community agencies and potential employers.

Mental health services can be made available in a similar manner in which the limited resources typically available to programs can be used to employ a specialist or specialists to provide consultation and guidance for counseling staff, assume a small caseload, and effect liaison with appropriate community agencies.

The need to effect the transition from treatment to the community suggests the need for an additional staff member. A case manager/aftercare coordinator will be appropriate to develop linkages with community agencies that can provide needed services for clients while in treatment and when exiting from treatment. Those services may include housing, legal assistance, financial benefits, family assistance, child care, and contacts with church or other organizations that have the potential to provide ongoing social support for clients. It would be expected that counseling staff would follow up on the leads generated by the coordinator.

Finally, the need to ensure service delivery consistent with findings regarding treatment efficacy requires an increase in counseling staffs. More specifically, to permit counseling staffs the ability to provide the level of services needed to achieve rehabilitative and survival goals will require appropriately small caseloads to allow a concentrated effort with clients assigned, and to guarantee time for training, consultation, and supervision. Support for counseling staffs should extend, as well, to the provision of salaries and benefits commensurate with the requirements and responsibilities of their jobs.

References

Agosti, V., E. Nunes, J.W. Stewart, and F.M. Quitkin. 1991. Patient Factors Related to Early Attrition from an Outpatient Research Clinic: A Preliminary Report. *International Journal of the Addictions* 26:327–34.

Aiken, L.S., L.A. LoSciuto, M.A. Ausetts, and B.S. Brown. 1984a.

Paraprofessional versus Professional Drug Counselors: Diverse Routes to the Same Role. *International Journal of the Addictions* 19:153–73.

——. 1984b. Paraprofessional versus Professional Drug Counselors: The Progress of Clients in Treatment. *International Journal of the Addictions* 19:383–401.

Anglin, M.D., and D.G. Fisher. 1987. Survival Analysis in Drug Program Evaluation: II. Partitioning Treatment Effects. *International Journal of the Addictions* 22:377–87.

Bigelow, G.E., M.L. Stitzer, and I.A. Liebson. 1984. The Role of Behavioral Contingency Management in Drug Abuse Treatment. In *Behavioral Intervention Techniques in Drug Abuse Treatment*, ed. J. Grabowski, M.L. Stitzer, and J.E. Henningfield (36–52). Rockville, Md.: National Institute on Drug Abuse.

Brown, B.S. Forthcoming. Policy Issues and Policy Development in Drug Abuse. In *Mental Health Services: A Public Health Perspective*, ed. B.L. Levin, and T. Petrilla (in press). New York: Oxford University Press.

——. 1993. Observations on the Recent History of Drug User Counseling. *International Journal of the Addictions* 28:1243–55.

Brown, B.S., and G.M. Beschner. 1989. AIDS and HIV Infection – Implications for Drug Abuse Treatment. *Journal of Drug Issues* 19:141–62.

Brown, B.S., and R.H. Needle, 1994. Modifiying the Process of Treatment to Meet the Threat of AIDS. *International Journal of the Addictions* 29:1739–52.

Brown, B.S., and R.F. Thompson. 1976. The Effectiveness of Formerly Addicted and Nonaddicted Counselors on Client Functioning. *Drug Forum* 5:123–9.

Brown, L.S. 1991. The Impact of AIDS on Drug Abuse Treatment. In *Improving Drug Abuse Treatment*, ed. R.W. Pickens, C.G. Leukefeld, and C.R. Schuster (385–93). Rockville, Md.: National Institute on Drug Abuse.

Catalano, R.F., J.D. Hawkins, E.A. Wells, J. Miller, and D. Brewer. 1991. Evaluation of the Effectiveness of Adolescent Drug Abuse Treatment, Assessment of Risks for Relapse, and Promising Approaches to Relapse Prevention. *International Journal of the Addictions* 20:1085–140.

Christensen, A., and N.S. Jacobson. 1994. Who (or What) Can Do Psychotherapy: The Status and Challenge of Nonprofessional Therapies. *Psychological Science* 5:8–14.

Colten, M.E. 1982. Attitudes, Experiences and Self-Perceptions of Heroin-Addicted Mothers. *Journal of Social Issues* 38:77–92.

D'Aunno, T., and R.A. Mohr. 1993. The Role of Drug Abuse Treatment Units in HIV Prevention (unpublished paper).

De Leon, G. 1985. The Therapeutic Community: Status and Evolution. *International Journal of the Addictions* 20:823–44.

De Leon, G., N. Jainchill, and M. Rosenthal. 1985. Addiction and Psychiatric Disorder: The Problem of Differential Diagnosis. Paper presented at the World Conference of Therapeutic Communities, San Francisco, June.

Dendy, R.F. 1979. Developments in Training. In *Handbook on Drug Abuse*, ed. R.L. DuPont, A. Goldstein, and J. O'Donnell (415–22). Washington: U.S. Government Printing Office.

Deren, S., and J. Randall. 1990. The Vocational Rehabilitation of Substance Abusers. *Journal of Applied Rehabilitation Counseling* 21:3–6.

Dickinson, K. and R. Maynard. 1981. The Impact of Supported Work on Ex-Addicts. New York: Manpower Demonstration Research Corp.

Dole, V.P. 1991. Interim Methadone Clinics: An Undervalued Approach. *American Journal of Public Health* 81:1111–12.

Dole, V.P., M.E. Nyswander, and A. Warner. 1968. Successful Treatment of 750 Criminal Addicts. In Proceedings of the First National Conference on Methadone Treatment, 11–22. New York: Rockefeller University.

Durlak, J.A. 1979. Comparative Effectiveness of Paraprofessional Helpers. *Psychological Bulletin* 86:80–92.

Eldred, C.A., and M.N. Washington. 1975. Female Heroin Addicts in a City Treatment Program: The Forgotten Minority. *Psychiatry* 38:75–85.

Fisher, D.G., and M.D. Anglin. 1987. Survival Analysis in Drug Program Evaluation: I. Overall Program Effectiveness. *International Journal of the Addictions* 22:115–34.

Friedman, L.N. 1978. The Wildcat Experiment: An Early Test of Supported Work in Drug Abuse Rehabilitation. Washington: National Institute on Drug Abuse.

Gearing, F.R. 1968. Progress Report of Evaluation of Methadone Maintenance Treatment Program – as of March 31, 1968. In Proceedings of the First National Conference on Methadone Treatment (1–10). New York: Rockefeller University.

Gerstein, D.R., and H.J. Harwood. 1990. *Treating Drug Problems*. Washington: National Academy Press.

Greenberg, R.M. and B.S. Brown. 1984. Agency Directors/Staff Views of the Changing Nature of Drug Abuse and Drug Abuse Treatment. In Clinical Research Notes, ed. National Institute on Drug Abuse (February): 10–12. Rockville, Md.

Gustafson, John S. 1991. Do More . . . and Do It Better: Staff-Related Issues in the Drug Treatment Field that Affect the Quality and Effectiveness of Services. In *Improving Drug Abuse Treatment*, ed. R.W. Pickens, C.G. Leukfeld, and C.R. Schuster (53–62). Rockville, Md.: National Institute on Drug Abuse.

Hall, S.M. 1983. Methadone Treatment: A Review of the Research Findings. In *Research on the Treatment of Narcotic Addiction*, ed. J.R. Cooper, F. Altman, B.S. Brown, and D. Czechowicz (575–632). Rockville, Md.: National Institute on Drug Abuse.

Hall, S.M., P. Loeb, K. Coyne, and J. Cooper. 1981a. Increasing Employment in Ex-Heroin Addicts: I. Criminal Justice Sample. *Behavior Therapy* 12:443–52.

———. 1981b. Increasing Employment in Ex-Heroin Addicts: II. Methadone Maintenance Sample. *Behavior Therapy* 12:453–60.

Hall, S.M., J.L. Sorensen, and P.C. Loeb. 1988. Development and Diffusion of a Skills-Training Intervention. In *Assessment and Treatment of Addictive Disorders*, eds. T.B. Baker and D.S. Cannon (180–204). New York: Praeger.

Hargreaves, W.A. 1980. Interest in Ancillary Services in Methadone Maintenance. *Journal of Psychedelic Drugs* 17:47–50.

Hawkins, J.D., R.F. Catalano, and E.A. Wells. 1986. Measuring Effects of a Skills Training Intervention for Drug Abusers. *Journal of Consulting and Clinical Psychology* 54:661–4.

Hubbard, R. 1993. Drug Abuse Treatment Outcome Study (DATOS) Research. Paper presented at NIDA Second National Conference on Drug Abuse Research and Practice, Washington, July 16.

Hubbard, R.L. 1994. Personal communication.

Hubbard, R.L. and H.J. Harwood. 1981. Employment Related Services in Drug Treatment Programs. Washington: U.S. Government Printing Office.

Hubbard, R.L., M.E. Marsden, J.V. Rachal, H.J. Harwood, E.R. Cavanaugh, and H.M. Ginzburg. 1989. *Drug Abuse Treatment: A National Study of Effectiveness*. Chapel Hill, N.C.: University of North Carolina Press.

Jaffe, J.H. 1979. The Swinging Pendulum: The Treatment of Drug Users in America. In *Handbook on Drug Abuse*, ed. R.L. DuPont, A. Goldstein, and J. O'Donnell, (3–20). Washington: U.S. Government Printing Office.

———. 1993. The Concept of Dependence: Historical Reflections. *Alcohol Health and Research World* 17:188–9.

Joe, G.W., B.S. Brown, and D.D. Simpson. 1995. Psychological Problems and Client Engagement in Methadone Treatment (submitted paper).

Kleber, H.D., and F. Slobetz. 1979. Outpatient Drug Treatment. In *Handbook on Drug Abuse*, ed. R.L. Dupont, A. Goldstein, and J. O'Donnell (31–38). Washington: U.S. Government Printing Office.

Kozel, N.J., and B.S. Brown. 1973. The Counselor Role as Seen by Ex-Addict Counselors, Nonaddict Counselors, and Significant Others. *Journal of Consulting and Clinical Psychology* 41:315.

Liebman, J., L. Knezek, K. Coughey, and S. Hua. 1993. Injection Uses, Drug Treatment and HIV Risk Behavior. In *Handbook on Risk of AIDS: Injection Drug Users and Sexual Partners*, ed. B.S. Brown and G.M. Beschner (355–73). Westport, Conn.: Greenwood Press.

Livingston, P., J. Randall, and E. Wolkstein. 1990. A Work-Study Model for Rehabilitation Counselor Education in Substance Abuse. *Journal of Applied Rehabilitation Counseling* 21:16–20.

Loeb, P., M. LeVois, and S.M. Hall. 1982. *Leader's Manual: Job Seekers' Workshop*. Rockville, Md.: National Institute on Drug Abuse.

Longwell, B., J. Miller, and A.W. Nichols. 1978. Counselor Effectiveness in a Methadone Maintenance Program. *International Journal of the Addictions* 13:301–15.

LoSciuto, L.A., L.S. Aiken, M.A. Ausetts, and B.S. Brown. 1984.

Paraprofessional versus Professional Drug Abuse Counselors: Attitudes and Expectations of the Counselors and Their Clients. *International Journal of the Addictions* 19:233–52.

Lowinsohn, J.H., and R.B. Millman. 1979. Clinical Aspects of Methadone Maintenance Treatment. In *Handbook on Drug Abuse*, ed. R.L. Dupont, A. Goldstein, and J. O'Donnell (49–56). Washington: U.S. Government Printing Office.

Lurie, P., and A.L. Rheingold. 1993. *The Public Health Impact of Needle Exchange Programs in the United States and Abroad*. San Francisco: University of California.

Mackay, P.W., and G.A. Marlatt. 1991. Maintaining Sobriety: Stopping Is Starting. *International Journal of the Addictions* 25:1257–76.

Manpower Demonstration Research Corp. 1980. Summary and Findings of the National Supported Work Demonstration. Cambridge, Mass.: Ballinger.

McAuliffe, W.E., and J.M.N. Chien. 1986. Recovery Training and Self Help: A Relapse-Prevention Program for Treated Heroin Addicts. *Journal of Substance Abuse Treatment* 3:9–20.

McCaughrin, W.C., and R.H. Price. 1992. Effective Outpatient Drug Misuse Treatment Organizations: Program Features and Selection Effect. *International Journal of the Addictions* 27:1335–58.

McLellan, A.T., L. Luborsky, G.E. Woody, C.P. O'Brien, and K.A. Druley. 1983. Predicting Response to Drug Abuse Treatment, Role of Psychiatric Severity. *Archives of General Psychiatry* 40:620–5.

Mulligan, D.H., D. McCarty, D. Potter, and M. Krakow. 1989. Counselors in Public and Private Alcoholism and Drug Abuse Treatment Programs. *Alcoholism Treatment Quarterly* 6:75–89.

National Institute on Drug Abuse. 1976. Summary Report. March 1976. National Drug Abuse Treatment Utilization Survey. Rockville, Md.

———. 1981. Trend Report. January 1977–September 1980. Data from the Client Oriented Data Acquisition Process. Rockville, Md.

———. 1982. *An Evaluation of the Impact of Employment Specialists in Drug Treatment*. Washington: Department of Health and Human Services.

Nurco, D. 1985. Unpublished data.

Nurco, D.N., P.E. Stephenson, and T.E. Hanlon. 1991. Aftercare/Relapse Prevention and the Self-Help Movement. *International Journal of the Addictions* 25:1179–200.

Pescor, M.J. 1938. A Statistical Analysis of the Clinical Record of Hospitalized Drug Addicts. (Public Health Reports (supp.) 143.) Washington: U.S. Public Health Service.

Platt, J.J., S.D. Husband, J. Hermalin, J. Cater, and D.S. Metzger. 1993. Cognitive Problem-Solving Employment Readiness Intervention for Methadone Clients. *Journal of Cognitive Psychotherapy* 7:21–3.

Platt, J.J., and C. Labate. 1976. Recidivism in Youthful Heroin Offenders and Characteristics of Parole Behavior and Environment. *International Journal of the Addictions* 11:651–7.

Platt, J.J., and D.S. Metzger. 1987. Cognitive Interpersonal Problem-Solving Skills and the Maintenance of Treatment Success in Heroin Addicts. *Psychology of Addictive Behaviors* 1:5–13.

Platt, J.J., D.O. Taube, M.A. Duome, and D.S. Metzger. 1988. Training in Interpersonal Problem-Solving (TIPS). *Journal of Cognitive Psychotherapy* 2:1–30.

Price, R.H., A.C. Burke, T.A. D'Aunno, et al. 1991. Outpatient Drug Abuse Treatment Services, 1988: Results of a National Survey. In *Improving Drug Abuse Treatment*, ed. R.W. Pickens, C.G. Leukefeld, and C.R. Schuster (63–92). Rockville, Md.: National Institute on Drug Abuse.

Price, R.H., and T.A. D'Aunno. 1992a. Drug Abuse Treatment System Survey. A National Study of the Outpatient Drug-Free and Methadone Treatment System. In *Drug Abuse Treatment System Survey: A National Survey of Outpatient Drug Abuse Treatment Services, 1988–1990. Final Report*, ed. R.H. Price and T.A. D'Aunno (3–10). Ann Arbor, Mich.: Survey Research Center.

——. 1992b. Drug Abuse Treatment System Survey. A National Study of the Outpatient Drug-Free and Methadone Treatment System, 1988–90. In *Drug Abuse Treatment System Survey: A National Survey of Outpatient Drug Abuse Treatment Services, 1988–1990. Final Report*, ed. R.H. Price and T.A. D'Aunno (27–34). Ann Arbor, Mich.: Survey Research Center.

——. 1992c. The Organization and Impact of Outpatient Drug Abuse Treatment Services. *Drug and Alcohol Abuse Reviews* 3:35–58.

Reissman, F., and H.J. Popper. 1968. *Up from Poverty: New Career Ladders for Nonprofessionals*. New York: Harper and Row.

Robins, L.N. 1979. Addict Careers. In *Handbook on Drug Abuse*, ed. R.L. DuPont, A. Goldstein, and J. O'Donnell (325–36). Washington: U.S. Government Printing Office.

Rounsaville, B.J., and H.D. Kleber. 1985. Psychotherapy Counseling for Opiate Addicts: Strategies for Use in Different Treatment Settings. *International Journal of the Addictions* 20:869–96.

Rounsaville, B.J., M.M. Weissman, K. Crits-Christoph, C.H. Wilber, and H.D. Kleber. 1982b. Diagnosis and Symptoms of Depression in Opiate Addicts: Course and Relationship to Treatment Outcome. *Archives of General Psychiatry* 33:151–6.

——. 1982a. Heterogenity of Psychiatric Diagnosis in Treated Opiate Addicts. *Archives of General Psychiatry* 39:161–6.

Substance Abuse and Mental Health Services Administration. 1993. National Drug and Alcoholism Treatment Unit Survey. 1991 Main Findings Report. Rockville, Md.

Selwyn, P.A., A. Feingold, A. Iezza, et al. 1989. Primary Care for Patients with Human Immunodeficiency Virus (HIV) Infection in a Methadone Maintenance Treatment Program. *Annals of Internal Medicine* 111:761–3.

Simpson, D.D., G.W. Joe, G. Rowan-Szal, and J. Greener. Forthcoming. Client Engagement and Change during Drug Abuse Treatment. *Journal of Substance Abuse* (in press).

Simpson, D.D., J.L. Savage, N.R. Lloyd, and S.B. Sells. 1978. *Evaluation of Drug Abuse Treatment Based on the First Year of DARP*. Rockville, Md.: National Institute on Drug Abuse.

Sobey, F.S. 1970. *The Nonprofessional Revolution in Mental Health*. New York: Columbia University Press.

Sorensen, J.L., S.M. Hall, P. Loeb, T. Allen, E.M. Glaser, and P.D. Greenberg. 1988. Dissemination of a Job Seekers Workshop to Drug Treatment Programs. *Behavior Therapy* 19:143–55.

Special Action Office for Drug Abuse Prevention. 1972. *Legislative History of the Drug Abuse Office and Treatment Act of 1972*. Washington: Executive Office of President.

Tucker, M.B. 1979. A Descriptive and Comparative Analysis of the Social Support Structure of the Heroin Addicted Woman. In *Addicted Women: Family Dynamics, Self Perceptions and Support Systems*, ed. National Institute on Drug Abuse (37–76). Washington: U.S. Government Printing Office.

Vaillant, G.E., and E.S. Milofsky. 1982. Natural History of Male Alcoholism. IV. Paths to Recovery. *Archives of General Psychiatry* 39:127–33.

Weinman, B.A. 1990. Treatment Alternatives to Street Crime (TASC). In *Handbook of Drug Control in the United States*, ed. J.A. Inciardi, 139–50. Westport, Conn.: Greenwood Press.

Winick, C. 1991. The Counselor in Drug User Treatment. *International Journal of the Addictions* 25:1479–502.

Woody, G.E., L. Luborsky, A.T. McLellan, et al. 1983. Psychotherapy for Opiate Addicts. Does it Help? *Archives of General Psychiatry* 40:639–45.

Woody, G.E., A.T. McLellan, L. Luborsky, and C.P. O'Brien. 1985. Sociopathy and Psychotherapy Outcomes. *Archives of General Psychiatry* 42:1081–6.

Woody, G.E., A.T. McLellan, L. Luborsky, et al. 1984. Severity of Psychiatric Symptoms as a Predictor of Benefits from Psychotherapy. The Veterans Administration – Penn Study. *American Journal of Psychiatry* 141:1172–7.

Woody, G.E., A.T. McLellan, C.P. O'Brien, and L. Luborsky. 1991. Addressing Psychiatric Comorbidity. *In Improving Drug Abuse Treatment*, ed. R.W. Pickens, C.G. Leukefeld, and C.R. Schuster, 152–66. Rockville, Md.: National Institute on Drug Abuse.

5

What We Know and What We Actually Do: Best Practices and their Prevalence in Substance Abuse Treatment

Richard H. Price

Introduction

Gaps between what we know and treatment practice. The basic premise of this chapter is that there is a substantial gap between what we know and what is actually practiced in the field of substance-abuse treatment. Furthermore, doing an inventory of what we know about best practices and the prevalence in practice can inform both research policy and treatment policy more generally (Frances 1988; Tims 1984). To address such questions a representative sample of treatment practice is essential (Price and D'Aunno 1992). When the prevalence of existing treatment practices can be compared with what is known about the effective ingredients of treatment, then gaps between knowledge and practice can be identified and systematically addressed.

Client career and treatment process. A second organizing premise of this chapter is that substance abuse is a chronic, relapsing disorder that unfolds over an entire lifetime. Indeed, the sociological concept of "career" is useful in providing a framework for understanding both the unfolding of substance-abuse problems over the life course and the corresponding treatment career of the individual client (D'Aunno and Price 1985; McCaughrin and Price 1992). Just as a substance-abuse career may unfold over time, so may treatment in its various stages be conceptualized as part of a client's lifetime treatment career. A treatment career may involve various episodes of engagement in treatment and withdrawal, and, in a particular episode, may also progress from early stages of assessment and treatment planning through actual treatment and, eventually, long-term maintenance of behavior change. Thus, a life course and career perspective can be useful not only for conceptualizing problems of substance abuse, but also in identifying the correspondence between stages both in the course of the disorder and its treatment.

Ideological debate. Much of the literature on the treatment of substance abuse has been marked by strong ideological commitments (D'Aunno, Sutton, and Price 1991) and considerably weaker data on effectiveness. At a broad policy level our national response to the problem of substance abuse has been driven by simple but powerful ideas that are typically about the nature of substance abuse and the remedies that seem to flow logically from our assumptions about the problem (Gerstein and Harwood 1990). The ideas have ranged from the libertarian view that substance abuse was private behavior, not to be governed by the state, to a medical conception emerging in the early 1800s that substance abuse was a disease. Similarly, criminal conceptions argue that control through the justice system is the preferred response. Today, a major policy debate is emerging in which the medical view predominates, but where the major question before us is whether or not substance abuse treatment should be regarded as a public good available to all (Weisner and Room 1984).

Within the various medical and helping professions a similar debate has ensued about the "best treatment approach" for substance abuse. The debate has divided rather sharply along ideological and professional lines, with advocates of psychodynamic, medical and pharmacological, behavioral, and self-help traditions each making strong claims for the effectiveness of their particular treatment approach (D'Aunno, Sutton, and Price 1991). To complicate matters somewhat, portions of the self-help movement regard substance-abuse problems as a disease, but advocate membership and adherence to the principles of mutual help groups such as Alcoholics Anonymous as the treatment of choice (Morgenstern and McCrady 1992).

This debate has not done much to clarify the question of which, if any, core treatment processes are essential for effective treatment. It has, however, frequently deflected attention away from broader questions concerning: (1) the importance of individual differences in patient characteristics; (2) whether certain staffing patterns are optimal for treatment effectiveness; (3) which organizational variables support or undermine the treatment process; and (4) whether certain basic procedural steps in the patient's treatment career are critical to treatment success.

Focus of the present review. In the current review we will argue that research knowledge is accumulating about each of these questions that allows the possibility of identifying the broad outlines of some best practices in the organization and delivery of substance abuse treatment. At the same time, data are now accumulating on the prevalence of these practices in the treatment field itself (Price et al. 1989). This places us in a position to compare what we know about best practices with what is actually being practiced.

The review that follows will confine itself to research on outpatient treatment. Recent National Drug Abuse Treatment Utilization Surveys indicate that the number of outpatient units in the United States has nearly doubled in the 1980s. At the same time, inpatient treatment has undergone a substantial decrease. Weisner and Schmidt (1992) suggest that cost containment pressures are responsible for much of this shift to outpatient treatment since it can be provided less expensively. Furthermore, Hayashida et al. (1989) as well as a recent Institute of Medicine report (1989) suggest that the weight of research evidence supports the proposition that outpatient treatment can be effective.

Within the outpatient treatment domain methadone treatment is offered for opiate abusers and counseling-oriented non-pharmalogical outpatient treatment is offered for a range of other substance-abuse problems. We will consider what is known about best practices in both methadone and non-methadone counseling-oriented forms of outpatient treatment. We will also examine the prevalence of those practices in the current national outpatient treatment system, relying in particular on the National Drug Abuse Treatment System Surveys conducted by the Institute for Social Research at the University of Michigan (Price et al. 1991; Price and D'Aunno 1992).

From a broad policy perspective the question of who has access to treatment for substance-abuse problems is fundamental to the overall effectiveness of the national treatment system. Although the question of access is obviously crucial to the larger question of the treatment effectiveness, the current review will confine itself to narrower questions of best treatment practices among those currently exposed to treatment. The chapter by Horgan in this volume will address the critical question of population need and access to substance-abuse treatment, while the chapter by Simpson will discuss the related and critical questions of identification, recruitment and engagement of substance abusers into the treatment process.

An Organizing Framework for Best Treatment Practices

Figure 5.1 provides an organizing framework for conceptualizing best practices in substance-abuse treatment and a corresponding organizing framework for the present review. Figure 5.1 portrays the treatment process as flowing from initial stages of *patient assessment* where addiction status, physical symptoms, mental health status, and AIDS risk among other things can be assessed, to a second stage where *treatment planning* and patient-treatment matching occurs. In this second stage information from patient assessment can be combined with knowledge about treatment technologies either delivered in the treatment setting itself or available through a referral mechanism. The third stage of the treatment-process model characterizes the delivery of treatment itself. It distinguishes between the *core treatment features*, whether they are pharmacological, behavioral or psychotherapeutic, and crucial *supplementary services* frequently needed by substance-abuse clients, such as employment counseling, legal counseling, family supportive services, and so on. Finally, an *aftercare* stage is demarcated in which continued client monitoring and relapse prevention measures can be undertaken. The term "aftercare" is used here to suggest the importance of continuing chronic or periodic care over the lifetime of a client in substance-abuse treatment. More recently, the view of treatment is shifting in the direction of seeing treatment as a life-long activity focusing on relapse prevention rather than one involving a period of acute treatment followed by aftercare. Consistent with the assumption that substance abuse is a chronic

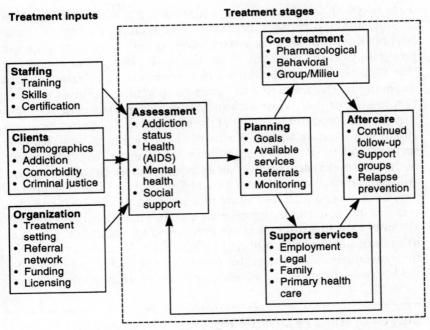

Figure 5.1   The substance-abuse treatment process: critical stages and inputs

relapsing disorder, a feedback loop is indicated, suggesting that periodic client reassessment and support may be optimal in the treatment process.

In addition to each of these four broad stages in the treatment process, figure 5.1 calls attention to three critical sets of input variables that substantially influence the impact of substance-abuse treatment. *Client variables*, including sociodemographic characteristics, addiction severity, family circumstances, availability of social supports, and a variety of other characteristics of clients, are widely agreed to have substantial impact on treatment outcome. A second major input to the treatment process itself is *treatment staffing*, including the nature, amount, and training background of the treatment staff. Background characteristics, education, and specialized training of treatment staff are critical issues for treatment effectiveness and are also characteristics of the treatment system that can be influenced by policy through training, certification, licensing, and a variety of other mechanisms. Finally, a third set of input variables broadly characterized as *organizational* factors are included in figure 5.1. These include not only characteristics of the treatment setting such as whether treatment is delivered in a medical or nonmedical setting, but also broader economic and policy variables that are beyond the scope of this review even though they may impinge powerfully on the actual delivery of services. In another chapter in this volume D'Aunno reviews questions of organizational and financing mechanisms that can be used to achieve services integration linking primary care with substance-abuse treatment.

Figure 5.1 is intended to reflect the organizing idea that substance-abuse clients may follow a *treatment career* and that particular services and/or treatment operations delivered at particular stages of the treatment career reflect an emerging consensus about known and desired standards of care. In addition, figure 5.1 is intended to portray *key inputs to the treatment process* that must also be taken into account in the design of broader substance-abuse treatment policy. We now turn to a discussion of what is known about best practices in each of the domains outlined in figure 5.1, focusing at the same time on information about the prevalence of such practices in the field of outpatient substance-abuse treatment in the United States.

Stages in the Treatment Process

Below we review relevant research on (1) *patient assessment,* (2) *treatment planning,* (3) *core treatment mechanisms* in both methadone and non-methadone outpatient treatment, (4) the role of *supportive services,* and finally, (5) *aftercare* in substance-abuse treatment. In each instance we review relevant research from the treatment literature and data on the prevalence of best practices in actual treatment practice from the National Drug Abuse Treatment System Survey (Price et al. 1991; Price and D'Aunno 1992).

Patient assessment in substance-abuse treatment
Recent advances in conceptualization and measurement of substance-abuse problems call into question any simplistic assumptions about patient uniformity. These advances also provide the basis for systematic patient assessment before treatment planning and the actual implementation of drug-abuse treatment. There are at least three important conceptual and measurement advances to consider. First, new diagnostic criteria and assessment instruments have been developed to measure both the presence and severity of alcohol and drug dependence. Most notably, measurement instruments based on the DSM III-R, including the Diagnostic Interview

Schedule (DIS), Robins et al. (1981), and the Psychiatric Diagnostic Interview (Othmer, Powell, and Penick 1980). Similarly this substance abuse module of the Composite International Diagnostic Interview (CIDI-SAM; Robins et al. 1988) and the Addiction Severity Index (McLellan et al. 1980b), as well as the individual assessment profile developed by Dr. Robert Hubbard and his colleagues at Research Triangle Institute (Hubbard et al. 1989), all can provide useful data on substance dependence syndromes and can be incorporated into systematic assessment of dependence and addiction patterns.

A second major critical development in the field of assessment has been the sharpening of the conceptual distinction between substance dependence and substance-related disabilities. In the case of alcohol dependence, for example, the dependence syndrome is seen as a relatively coherent pattern of symptoms that occur together and mutually reinforce each other. On the other hand, alcohol-related disabilities are seen as an often heterogeneous set of social, psychological, and physical impairments that may occur independently of the dependence syndrome itself. Treatment practice should be sensitive to this distinction.

A third development has been research on the value of patient-treatment matching (Institute of Medicine Report 1989). In the past, the dominant approach both in treatment research and in clinical practice has been to seek the "one best treatment" or to ask whether a particular treatment is better than no treatment at all. The matching hypothesis argues that various treatments may be differentially effective for different patterns of dependence or different subgroups of patients within the substance-abuse population. The working assumption is that adequate assessment combined with research and knowledge about differential outcomes for different subgroups should lead to "tailor made" treatment planning that matches patients with particular needs to particular types of treatments.

While the conceptual advances described above are of considerable importance to patient assessment, there remains the question of what particular types of information are most predictive of outcome and potentially most useful in treatment planning. At least four types of information appear to be of value. First, general diagnostic information is needed about the overall physical health of patients. Physical health information should include data about health effects of chronic substance abuse, as well as acute and other chronic disorders that may impair recovery or interact with various treatment regimens. Second, assessment of the social stability of patients and social supports available appears to be a major generic predictor of treatment response (McLellan et al. 1980b; McLellan 1983). A third key domain is psychiatric diagnosis, including information about severity and intensity of symptoms. Typically, greater severity is associated with poorer treatment response, and psychiatric diagnosis has also been a powerful generic predictor of response across a variety of patient populations (McLellan et al. 1980a; Rounsaville et al. 1987). Some investigators have indicated that the presence of antisocial personality disorder (Powell et al. 1985) is a key indicator of poor treatment response. Finally, and perhaps most important, is the measurement of the severity of drug dependence. In general, greater severity is associated with poorer treatment response and, in alcohol patients, more rapid return to drinking and drinking problems. This particular variable has been a reliable predictor of return to substance use but is a somewhat less good predictor of adjustment in other life areas such as family relations, employment and medical health (Babor et al. 1988).

In short, both conceptualization and measurement of patient status have developed considerably over the past decade. There is reason to believe that adequate assessment and conceptualization of patient patterns of dependence and disability could lead to a careful individualized and adaptive treatment planning that would be both more efficient and more effective. Indeed, McCaughrin and Price (1992) report that, in a national survey of outpatient drug-abuse treatment programs, clinics that utilize medical tests as part of their assessment have lower rates of continued use among outpatient populations. Similarly clinics that report higher rates of testing for AIDS also have higher proportions of clients that have met their treatment goals. It should be noted here, however, that higher levels of testing in these domains may also reflect a more general pattern of clinic adherence to high standards for assessment and treatment, resulting in more favorable client outcomes.

To what degree are these advances in conceptualization and assessment of substance-abuse problems actually reflected in improved practice in the field? One set of answers comes from the National Drug Abuse Treatment Systems data from a nationally representative sample of outpatient treatment programs collected in 1988 and 1990. In both 1988 and 1990 a very high percentage (between 80 and 90 percent) of outpatient treatment programs reported some assessment of mental health status. A smaller proportion (between 60 and 70 percent) reported that DSM III diagnostic procedures were employed for patients. On the other hand, the use of physical exams varied dramatically between methadone and drug-free outpatient treatment settings. Nearly 90 percent of methadone programs reported the routine use of physical exams for clients, while less than 30 percent of outpatient drug-free programs reported routine use of physical examinations. Some important portion of this difference between methadone and non-methadone programs is probably due to the fact that methadone programs are much more likely to have medical personnel and be located in medical settings. While assessment of HIV is relatively low across the outpatient treatment sector, increases were observed between 1988 and 1990 in methadone programs from approximately 20 to 40 percent of programs. On the other hand, drug-free programs continued to have extremely low levels of HIV assessment in both 1988 and 1990 with less than 10 percent of programs reporting any HIV testing.

It seems clear that patient-assessment technology has dramatically improved in the field of substance-abuse treatment. These improvements may actually stimulate differential treatment planning. This is clearly an area where routine practice in the field can be improved and can lead to more effective treatment planning and outcomes.

Treatment planning and patient–treatment matching
The idea that the substance-abuse population is far from homogeneous and that different treatments may well be differentially effective for different subgroups of patients has now become firmly established in the substance-abuse treatment research field. This new conceptual approach is reflected in treatment research in a number of ways. For example research that emphasizes multidimensional outcomes rather than a single outcome is now commonplace (Institute of Medicine Report 1989; Woody 1983). In addition to outcomes such as abstinence, mental health and family and occupational outcomes are also frequently measured. Similarly, multivariate analyses allow a variety of different combinations of patient–treatment matching strategies to be evaluated, and advances have been made in the area of assessment of client characteristics. Finally, it is evident that an emphasis on identifying and measuring core treatment processes is emerging rather than just outcomes in treatment research.

While this new, more differentiated conceptual approach to understanding the relationship between differences in addiction patterns and the assignment of patients to treatment appears promising, research results are still sparse. Furthermore, it is unclear to what degree new knowledge about patient–treatment matching is actually entering the field of treatment practice. However, some data are available on the types of treatment goals which appear to be most important in treatment planning in the field of treatment practice.

The National Drug Abuse Treatment System Survey conducted by the Institute for Social Research, University of Michigan (NDATSS) of 575 outpatient treatment programs (Price et al. 1991) included questions about the degree to which various treatment goals are important in outpatient substance-abuse treatment units. Results of the survey were quite uniform across both methadone and drug-free programs. Three goals dominated as major treatment objectives in the outpatient treatment sector. They included (1) complete abstinence, (2) the development of a stable personal relationship, and (3) the attainment and maintenance of good physical health. It is notable that the goal of "responsible use" was not perceived as a legitimate goal of treatment. A high proportion of outpatient programs gave "responsible use" low ratings of endorsement as a treatment goal.

Core treatment processes in outpatient drug-abuse treatment

The vast majority of previous research on drug abuse treatment has been focused on outcome evaluation (D'Amanda 1983). Considerably less attention focused on the actual processes and mechanisms of treatment. Moos, Cronkite, and Finney (1982) and Finney and Moos (1989) have criticized this traditional "summative approach to evaluation." Not only has measurement of actual treatment processes been undertaken infrequently, but seldom have studies attempted to link treatment processes to outcomes with the goal of identifying the most effective ingredients of treatment. A focus on effective treatment mechanisms is important for treatment research since knowledge about effective treatment mechanisms would be crucial in treatment planning (Allison et al. 1985).

Basic treatment processes in outpatient treatment. There appear to be major conceptual and ideological disagreements about which basic mechanisms are the most effective ingredients of substance abuse treatment (O'Brien et al. 1984). As Morgenstern and McCrady (1992) observe, there are strong disagreements between proponents of two major schools of thought. One approach, the "disease model," actually refers to the Alcoholics Anonymous approach (as distinguished from a narrow focus on biological and genetic vulnerabilities). Representative reviews have been published by Laundergan (1982), Cook (1988 a,b), Anderson (1981), and Wallace et al. (1988). A second major school of thought includes a variety of behavioral models exemplified by the work of Marlatt and

Gordon (1985), Annis (1986), Litman (1986), Azrin et al. (1982), Elkins (1980), and McCrady (1985). Of course, behavioral therapy can be utilized in the treatment of diseases as well. Some behavioral treatments use the strict application of learning principles, while others are "behavioral" only in the sense that they do not involve a biological intervention.

Randomized trials comparing these two treatment approaches directly against each other with appropriate control groups and long-term follow-up are not yet available. Nevertheless, substantial expert opinion from both camps on the nature of treatment mechanisms that are crucial to effective treatment are available. Morgenstern and McCrady (1992) conducted a study designed to illuminate expert understanding of which mechanisms were judged to be most critical in the treatment of alcohol and drug problems. After a detailed analysis of the literature in the general disease (AA) and behavioral approaches, they identified 35 processes in the research literature identified as crucial for improvement. By itself, this list of 35 processes represents an important taxonomy of potential treatment mechanisms and also offers hypotheses for further tests in treatment trials that emphasize both process and outcome.

Morgenstern and McCrady then surveyed experts in the alcohol/drug treatment field to obtain judgments about how beneficial or harmful each of these 35 processes would be in resolving an alcohol or drug problem. Overall, experts rated (1) client acceptance of responsibility for change as a critical component, (2) client preparation for dealing with relapse, and (3) reducing denial, as the three most important treatment processes. Predictably, behavioral experts tended to rate behavioral processes as important. However, surprisingly, disease-model/AA experts tended to rate both behavioral and disease-model processes highly. Morgenstern and McCrady (1992) conclude that the climate of opinion in the field is beginning to change, reflecting the impact of the behavioral approach on the treatment of alcohol and drug problems, even among those disease/AA experts who have been the opponents of the behavioral approach.

Data on the prevalence of various disease-oriented and more behavioral approaches to treatment in the outpatient treatment system in the United States do provide some information about the nature of the core drug-abuse treatment technology currently being provided. Results from the National Drug Abuse Treatment System Survey in the 1988 and 1990 surveys indicate that virtually 100 percent of outpatient drug-abuse treatment programs offer individual therapy as a core treatment technology, followed closely by approximately 95 percent of programs offering group therapy. A third and broadly prevalent core treatment modality is education about the nature of addiction. Approximately 90 percent of outpatient programs reportedly offer such educational services. These data do not, however, provide information about the degree to which outpatient programs are currently offering disease/AA-oriented treatment programs, behavioral programs, or a combination of the two.

Core treatment process in methadone outpatient treatment. While methadone treatment for narcotic addiction continues to provoke considerable scientific discussion and debate (Dole et al. 1982; Liappas, Jenner, and Cicente 1988; Hargreaves 1983), there is also substantial emerging agreement about appropriate program practices and core treatment mechanisms that lead to increased effectiveness. First, a variety of researchers have reported that relatively high-dose treatments that include client participation in decisions about dosage produce higher rates of retention in treatment (Dole 1988; Watters 1986; Cooper et al. 1983). Furthermore, research indicates that the longer methadone clients remain in treatment the less likely they are to return to illicit drug use and injections (Hubbard et al. 1989; Des Jarlais, Joseph, and Dole 1981). There is also an emerging consensus that methadone treatment for intravenous drug users is important for preventing transmission of HIV (Abdul-Quader et al. 1987; Schuster 1988; Des Jarlais et al. 1990; Ball et al. 1988; Cooper 1989). Thus, considerable research consensus is emerging about the value of relatively high methadone doses for retaining clients in treatment. High doses are, in turn, a major predictor of lower levels of relapse and also provide risk reduction for HIV infection. It also appears that active client participation in dosage planning and active participation in their overall treatment program is an important aspect of effective methadone treatment.

D'Aunno and Vaughn (1992) examined the extent to which outpatient methadone maintenance treatment units in the United States are actually engaging in treatment practices that previous research indicates are effective. They drew on a national random sample of 172 methadone treatment units and focused on a number of key treatment practices to assess the degree to which they conformed with what we know about effective outpatient methadone treatment. D'Aunno and Vaughn were concerned in particular on restrictive treatment practices that involved lower than optimal dose levels, reduced client influence on dose levels, and time limits set on detoxification. In addition, they examined the degree to which these restrictive treatment practices were related to important treatment outcomes, such as client time in treatment, one of the most important factors in treatment effectiveness.

D'Aunno and Vaughn (1992) found that there is substantial variation in methadone treatment practices across the nation. There was, for example, considerable variation in clients' awareness of their dosage and in their capacity to influence dose levels. Furthermore, methadone units varied considerably in the dose levels that they dispensed, with as many as 25 percent of units typically setting an upper limit on dose levels of 20–60 milligrams/d. Average dose levels for the majority of units is approximately 50 milligrams/d. Furthermore, 50 percent of units encouraged their clients to detoxify in less than six months and overall, methadone treatment tends to be less than 20 months for more than half the units. As D'Aunno and Vaughn observe, "to the extent that high dose levels and client participation in dose decisions contribute to client retention in treatment and abstinence from illicit drug use, the data suggest that the practices of many units are counterproductive" (p. 256). In an area of drug-abuse treatment where a fair amount is known about the optimal treatment technology, it appears that a substantial proportion of the nation's methadone units are delivering treatment in a suboptimal way.

D'Aunno and Vaughn also examined their data to identify client characteristics, organizational and environmental factors, and characteristics of treatment units themselves that were associated with less than optimal treatment practices. They found that units that had higher percentages of black clients had lower dosage levels, lower imposed limits on dosage levels, and were less likely to permit take-home dosages (characteristic of high levels of patient participation). Methadone units that were embedded in a mental health clinic, a hospital, or some other facility were more likely than free-standing units to have adequate dose levels and permit client influence on dosage levels.

Perhaps most significant from a policy point of view, D'Aunno and Vaughn reported that units indicating that their practices are influenced by government regulation were more likely to have higher dose limits and higher average dose levels than those that reported that government regulation was not as influential. Clearly, outpatient methadone treatment is an arena where there is a growing understanding of effective treatment technology, but where the field of practice clearly has not yet caught up with what we know. This is also an arena in which government licensing, regulation, and policy influence could improve treatment practices.

Supportive treatment services

As suggested in figure 5.1, treatment focusing narrowly on the goal of abstinence may not, by itself, result in successful substance-abuse treatment. The growing prevalence of multiple drug dependence, comorbidity with physical disorders, family conflict that may exacerbate dependence, vocational difficulties or legal problems may all substantially complicate the substance-abuse treatment picture in ways that compromise treatment. In a recent study of outpatient drug-abuse treatment in a national sample McCaughrin and Price (1992) reported that outpatient treatment units that offer a higher percentage of clients services in addition to core treatment services also have higher proportions of clients who meet treatment goals. These findings were obtained controlling for a wide range of client demographics, treatment practices, and organizational and treatment conditions. This suggests that additional services are not merely "ancillary", but important to successful rehabilitation. The chapter in this volume by Horgan suggests that multiple drug use, poverty, unemployment, and other major social and health problems can complicate the needs of drug-abuse treatment clients in critical ways.

Clearly, drug-abuse treatment units must either be able to deliver these additional services within the context of their own treatment program or have available highly reliable referral sources that can provide additional components of treatment (Price et al. 1991). To what degree are additional services actually provided in outpatient drug-abuse treatment? Again, the National Drug Abuse Treatment System Survey provides some crucial answers. In surveying 575 outpatient drug-abuse treatment units in 1988 and 1990, treatment administrators and clinical supervisors were asked about additional services provided to clients, including medical care, mental health treatment, multiple drug treatment, employment counseling, financial counseling, legal counseling, and counseling for persons convicted of driving while intoxicated. A striking and repeated finding in both 1988 and 1990 is that, with the exception of treatment for multiple drug problems (which was reported to be offered in about 60 percent of treatment units), all of these other services were offered in less than half of outpatient treatment units. While these additional services have been, in the past, viewed as critical components of "best practice" in the provision of substance-abuse treatment, recent reductions in the support of treatment have led to a "bare bones" approach which reduces or eliminates these services.

In addition, the recent AIDS epidemic raises the question of whether supplementary services relevant to AIDS risk are being provided in outpatient drug-abuse treatment programs. In the National Drug Abuse Treatment System Survey sample, both in 1988 and 1990, outpatient units were asked about the degree to which they engaged in various prevention practices for AIDS and whether they have specific staff or adequate funding. Outpatient units indicated that they engaged in counseling on sexual and needle risks to "some" or "a great" extent, but that considerably fewer had specific staff designated for AIDS prevention or adequate funds to carry out this crucial additional treatment service. Generally speaking, methadone outpatient clinics tended to have somewhat higher levels in each of these categories than did non-methadone drug-free outpatient settings.

Aftercare and continuity of care

There is increasing evidence that aftercare is an essential aspect of effective substance-abuse treatment and that relapse prevention is a critical aspect of the treatment process. Furthermore, relapse prevention and related treatment technologies (Marlatt and Gordon 1985) are now available, and research results are encouraging. In a national study of effective aspects of outpatient drug-abuse treatment programs, McCaughrin and Price (1992) obtained evidence that post-treatment processes and active efforts at client follow-up are important to positive treatment outcome. They found, for example, that outpatient treatment units that collect follow-up information on clients had higher rates of clients who met treatment goals over and above a variety of other predictors of treatment effectiveness. Similarly, units that collected follow-up information also produced lower rates of clients continuing to use alcohol or drugs. Again, these results were obtained controlling for client characteristics, organizational characteristics, quality assurance efforts and a variety of other aspects of the treatment program.

To what extent, then, are outpatient treatment units actually engaged in client follow-up and aftercare? Again the National Drug Abuse Treatment System Survey provides us with some important information. In the outpatient treatment sector, only 75 percent of drug-free treatment of clients ended treatment with written plans for continued care. For methadone clients only 45 percent of clients terminating treatment had written plans for continued care. Furthermore, the NDATSS survey (see Price et al. 1991) asked outpatient units about the degree to which they collected *any* follow-up information and found that only 63 percent of outpatient units collected any follow-up information whatsoever on clients. Among those who did, the most commonly sought information was about continued drug or alcohol abuse, with employment status, health status, and the client's evaluation of the treatment experience as less commonly collected types of information.

It seems clear that active aftercare and outreach is an important component of effective outpatient drug-abuse treatment and a clear best practice (Gilbert 1988). On the other hand, such efforts are not being undertaken in the outpatient treatment sector to the degree that research evidence indicates they should be.

Major Inputs to Effective Treatment Practice

As implied in figure 5.1, in addition to each of the treatment stages reviewed above, at least three additional inputs to effective substance-abuse treatment need to be considered. They are (1) *therapist characteristics and staffing patterns*, (2) *patient characteristics*, and (3) the *organizational context of treatment*.

Therapist characteristics and staffing patterns

The question of what skills, knowledge and personal characteristics of treatment personnel are most important for treatment effectiveness has received some attention in the research literature (Institute of Medicine Report 1989). This topic is reviewed by Brown in chapter 4 in this volume. Both professional opinion and the outcome research that is available suggest that staffing characteristics are important input variables influencing both the process and outcome of substance-abuse treatment. Staffing characteristics may influence a variety of outcomes, including treatment motivation, dropout rates, and more explicit measures of treatment success such as continued abstinence or success in meeting treatment goals.

One aspect of therapist interpersonal functioning that has received considerable attention is therapist empathy. Research by Miller, Taylor and West (1980), Valle (1981), and Kristenson et al. (1983) all indicate that empathetic understanding is a common element in effective brief interventions, particularly for alcohol problems. In related research, Oei and Jackson (1984) found greater improvement among individuals whose therapists engaged in self-disclosure while reinforcing clients' positive self-statements.

A second key issue in therapist skills and background has to do with the status of therapists as recovering substance abusers. Several research findings deserve comment. First, studies by Kirk, Best, and Irwin (1986) and Lawson (1982) reported that client perceptions of counselor empathy were unaffected by whether the counselor was a recovering substance abuser or not. Aiken et al. (1984) report no significant differences in treatment outcomes between counselors who are themselves recovering substance abusers and those who are not. The National Drug Abuse Treatment Systems Survey interviewed treatment unit directors and clinical supervisors from a representative national sample of 575 outpatient drug-abuse treatment programs to obtain their opinions about characteristics of staff who should be hired to ensure effective treatment. These respondents indicated that both specialized training in substance-abuse treatment and previous work experience were extremely important hiring criteria in selecting staff to ensure effective treatment. A personal history of substance abuse was perceived as a qualification of substantially less value.

What do staffing patterns actually look like in outpatient treatment? The same surveys of outpatient drug-abuse treatment programs provide no data on the distribution of empathic skills among treatment personnel, but do provide information on the distribution of educational qualifications, specialized training, and specialized certification for substance-abuse treatment. In addition, the surveys provide data on the prevalence of recovering addicts who serve as treatment staff. Data from both the 1988 and 1990 surveys indicate that outpatient units are staffed predominantly by bachelor's level and master's level staff. Ph.D. level staff and M.D.s occupy only a small minority (10 percent) of all staff positions. Recovering addicts represent nearly one-third of all treatment staff in non-methadone outpatient treatment, while the prevalence of recovering abusers is substantially lower in methadone settings. Our data also indicate that slightly more than half of all treatment staff have specialized training in substance-abuse treatment. Considerably less than 50 percent of all staff have special certification in substance-abuse treatment. Furthermore, specialized training and certification is considerably less prevalent in methadone clinics.

While therapist qualifications are an important aspect of staffing, client–staff ratios reflect another key aspect of staffing inputs into the treatment process. McCaughrin and Price (1992) reported that the ratio of treatment staff to clients is a significant predictor of treatment success when continued use of alcohol or drugs is the outcome measure. This finding remains significant after controlling for client characteristics, quality assurance efforts, and a variety of treatment variables.

What are we to conclude about staffing characteristics? It seems clear that some therapist skills are important in affecting substance-abuse treatment outcomes, particularly those having to do with the capacity to empathetically engage the patient. On the other hand, the value of being a recovering substance abuser appears moot. At the very least, professional opinion in the field and outcome studies suggest that unquestioning acceptance of the value of recovering addicts as treatment personnel is probably unwise. At the same time, while specialized training and work experience are viewed as key qualifications for treatment staff effectiveness, the prevalence of such training in a national sample of outpatient clinics appears considerably below what is possible. Finally, high ratios of clients to treatment personnel are associated with lower levels of treatment effectiveness. This finding is not unique to the field of substance-abuse treatment, but obviously has direct policy and economic implications in building an effective national substance-abuse treatment system.

Patient characteristics

Special issues for women in substance-abuse treatment. The special problems and vulnerabilities of women in need of substance-abuse treatment and the barriers they encounter in seeking treatment have only recently begun to be recognized in the research literature (Bell Unger 1988). For example Robertson (1991) argues that for some women with children, alcohol and drug use may be an important risk factor for homelessness. Policy decisions on homelessness need to be sensitive to the problems associated with a criminalization of drug use and the scarcity of appropriate treatment programs. Similarly, King (1991) has noted that drug policy for pregnant women has frequently taken on a coercive and punitive character, raising a variety of value issues in formulating drug and alcohol-abuse treatment policies for pregnant women. Furthermore, female drug users are at high risk of contracting and transmiting AIDS through heterosexual transmission. Schilling et al. (1991) have found that female methadone patients can benefit from skills training to develop a variety of prevention strategies, including condom use, that may alter risk-related sexual behavior.

Sexual victimization and sexual abuse represent another key issue for women that may both play a role in the etiology of substance abuse and have implications for effective treatment. Root (1989) has reviewed a variety of women's substance-abuse cases usually labeled as "treatment failures" and has identified sexual victimization as an issue that precipitates the use of substances to mitigate post-traumatic stress symptoms. Paone et al. (1992) report high rates of sexual abuse in chemically dependent women and argue that it is important to integrate therapy for sexual abuse into treatment for such women.

Age and cohort differences among women in their attitudes toward substance use appear to be an important factor to be taken into consideration in the design of treatment programs and in strategies for recruitment. Gomberg (1988) notes that older alcoholic women tend to have less liberal attitudes toward substance use than younger women, even though younger women report more rejection and stigmatization. In addition, Harrison and Belille (1987) report that, in a study of 1,776 adult women in treatment for chemical dependency, generational as well as age differences were critical in distinguishing chemical-dependency histories and attitudes. Younger women who grew up in the 70s had different experiences with substance use than did older women, which may have affected their attitude towards substance use.

Finally, a critical issue in treating women with substance-abuse problems has to do with their service utilization patterns. Weisner and Schmidt (1992) report that female problem drinkers were more likely than male problem drinkers to use non-alcohol health care settings, particularly mental health treatment services. Copeland and Hall (1992) report that women attending a treatment service designed to be gender sensitive were women who might not have otherwise sought treatment for their substance-dependence problems.

It is only in the recent past that the special issues confronted by women with substance-abuse problems have gained serious attention in the treatment research community. It is less clear how this new attention will affect the actual design and delivery of programs that are responsive to women's issues. The 1990 National Drug Abuse Treatment System reports that 22.5 percent of outpatient services had special services for pregnant women. Fifty-one percent of programs stated that they had some other services for women. Future national survey research should investigate the prevalence of such gender-sensitive services in the national treatment system.

Substance-abuse treatment for minority populations. Data from the 1988 and 1990 Drug Abuse Treatment Systems Survey (Price et al., 1991) clearly indicate that minority clients, particularly African-American and Hispanic clients, are substantially over-represented in the outpatient drug-abuse treatment population in the United States. Nevertheless, it is not clear that responsive services designed to recruit and to maintain minority clients in the treatment system are yet a broadly established feature of the national treatment system.

Rowe and Grills (1993) observe that in epidemiological and service studies, the variables of race, culture, and class are often confounded in collecting and interpreting data regarding the use of drug-abuse services. Rowe calls for a more sensitive and systematic capacity to recognize variation within minority communities. The authors argue that there is a need to be attuned to cultural differences between white and minority communities that may lead to higher rates of treatment dropout or failures in recruitment.

Further, a predominant drug-abuse treatment approach such as the twelve-step process may be resisted by African-American clients. Smith et al. (1993) observed that twelve-step fellowships may produce confusion over issues of the role of religion, the need to surrender and declare personal powerlessness, the role of family structure, and a variety of other issues that are major concerns to the African-American community. They note that some programs, such as African-American extended-family programs, represent positive alternative examples of culturally adaptive treatment programs. Rowe and Grills (1993) take an even stronger position, arguing that African-centered programs that emphasize cultural issues, community healing, and an orientation to positive potential may be a critical ingredient of success for some segments of the African-American community. Miller and Miller (1988) note that alcoholism is a major problem in Black urban areas, and they call for more responsive treatment and in particular increased representation of Black counselors in urban alcoholism programs.

Economic changes and changes in the financing of the treatment system may have important impacts on minority substance-abuse treatment utilization. Treatment services continue to experience privatization. As more services are supported by employee assistance programs, persons who are jobless, particularly in minority communities, may have to rely on publicly financed treatment that may not provide the services needed. In a similar vein, Thornton and Carter (1988) examined data on treating economically deprived Black female alcoholics over a decade in Durham, North Carolina. They conclude that a comprehensive care approach that uses the input of Black female therapists as case managers will have distinct advantages.

Finally, Schilling and his colleagues (1989) offer an extended discussion of strategies for AIDS prevention research in Black and Hispanic communities. While their discussion is focused primarily on issues of prevention strategies, a number of their observations about cultural issues in the Hispanic and Black communities are clearly relevant for treatment as well. For example, they note that cultural orientations such as machismo may be a key barrier to the use of condoms and the prevention of HIV transmission in the Hispanic community, while emphasis on family responsiveness may actually improve recruitment of Hispanic males. They also emphasize the importance of family support systems in the Black community, and observe that cultural differences may be masked once addiction begins to dominate the lives of minority clients and the biological patterns common to addiction predominate. Thus Shilling et al. (1989) observe that both experience drawn from drug and alcohol programs in general as well as culturally sensitive aspects of treatment need to be taken into account in designing culturally sensitive programs for minority clients. In 1990, the National Drug Abuse Treatment Systems Survey indicated that 1.2 percent of programs had started new services especially designed for Blacks, and 6.9 percent of programs started new programs for minority clients.

Organizational factors

The organizational context in which substance-abuse treatment is delivered can and does affect the quality and effectiveness of that treatment. In the National Drug Abuse Treatment System Survey (Price et al. 1989), hospital-based, community mental health-based and free-standing outpatient drug-abuse treatment programs were compared on a wide range of different aspects of service delivery. In general, and as might be expected, medically based and professionally based mental health systems both had a higher prevalence of professional and medical staff serving as substance-abuse treatment personnel. In addition, medically based settings such as hospitals and methadone programs had stronger emphases on physical examinations and other aspects of medical assessment of client problems. In addition, hospital-based and methadone programs were more likely to employ quality assurance programs and to be licensed by state or federal agencies. On the other hand, outpatient drug-abuse treatment programs that were not affiliated with medical or methadone treatment settings, but free-standing programs were more likely to use counselor certification as a mechanism for ensuring treatment staff quality.

Patterns of staffing and client–staff ratios were described earlier as staffing inputs but are of course, also, aspects of the organization of drug-abuse treatment. It should be clear that staffing patterns represent a major organizational factor potentially responsive to policy initiatives that can affect the kind and quality of substance-abuse treatment services delivered in the United States. In addition, adequate client–staff ratios represent another key organizational input that almost certainly will have implications for not only the quality of service delivery, but also, of course, its cost.

How does profit status and ownership affect treatment efficiency and access? Economic and organizational pressures to change treatment practices, and in some cases to compromise best practices, are critical to consider in a review of "best practices." Burke and Rafferty (1990) have shown that the most pervasive and persistent differences among drug-treatment units distinguish for-profit units from non-profit and public units. Private for-profit units are more likely to rely on private sources of funding, including client fees, and services supported by private insurance are less likely to depend on referrals from the courts, police, and social service agencies and serve a distinctly different clientele. For-profit clients are less likely to be young, unemployed, and unable to pay for treatment, and are less likely to have multiple drug problems. In general, for-profit units serve a less disabled, less vulnerable pool of clients who have a much wider range of financial resources available to them.

Wheeler et al. (1992) and Edlund et al. (1990) show that private for-profit units generate higher profits and charge higher prices, but may also operate at higher efficiency levels than public and private not-for-profit units. However, it is important to note that public treatment units provide better access to care for persons who are unable to pay for care. Furthermore, public and not-for-profit units appear to do more to facilitate access to care for people whose means of payment are limited and who must rely on public programs.

Wheeler et al. (1992) and Fadel and Wheeler (1991) also found that private for-profit treatment units increase their efficiency by providing a lower percentage of individual therapy sessions. This raises questions about whether this treatment strategy has an effect on the overall quality of care delivered. In another study, Wheeler, et al. (1992) found that for-profit units charge substantially higher prices for their services than do public units and that the treatment differences reported above remain, even after controlling for the effects of production, cost differences, differences in degree of competition for resources, differences in regulatory climate, and differences in patient characteristics.

In short, the incentive systems in the drug-abuse treatment sector, just as in the health care sector at large, are likely to have key effects on the quality of drug-abuse care, its effectiveness, and the degree to which "best practices" are actually carried out. A systematic analysis of what we know about treatment effectiveness from clinical studies must be combined with a richer understanding of the technical and economic constraints imposed on treatment practices in actual service systems. Only in this organizational framework can meaningful statements be made about policy recommendations and their likely impact.

Conclusion

Table 5.1 summarizes in brief form key findings from the literature review presented above following the various stages in the treatment process and focusing on key treatment inputs. Major gaps between what we know from treatment research and what is actually practiced in the outpatient drug-abuse treatment system are emphasized. It is clear that gaps exist in needed knowledge from treatment research and between what is already known and what is currently being practiced in the field of substance-abuse treatment.

The problem of implementing new knowledge from research in clinical practice is not unique to addiction medicine or addiction treatment. This problem exists throughout all of clinical medicine, and indeed, in all fields where basic science must inform a field of practitioners. A substantial amount of research has been devoted to knowledge utilization and application in a variety of fields. Research on "best practices" and their implementation in the practice context deserves full and detailed treatment in its own right.

A critical research need for the future is a better understanding of the factors that lead treatment systems to adopt or fail to adopt best practices and how these factors can be supported by national policy initiatives, particularly in light of attempts at health care reform. With the advent of managed care in drug-abuse treatment, there may be an increasing number of opportunities to implement changes that will narrow the gap between what we know and what we actually do in practice. To the degree that managed-care systems can actually provide incentives for effective care, managed-care health organizations should begin to focus on the gap between what is known about best practices and what is currently being carried out, and improve the effectiveness of service delivery.

Note
Chapter prepared for Milbank Memorial Fund/National Institute on Drug Abuse Workshop on Policy Implications of Current Knowledge about Treatment for Drug Abuse. Final Draft: 4 August 1995.

Table 5.1 Review Summary.

Treatment Processes and Inputs	What We Know and Current Practice
TREATMENT PROCESS	*REVIEW FINDINGS*
Assessment	Advances in assessment methods recently achieved
	Physical health not routinely assessed in drug-free outpatient treatment
	Mental health assessed, formal diagnosis less frequently
	Prevalence of addiction severity assessment unknown
	HIV assessment infrequent but growing
Treatment Planning	Research on patient–treatment matching increasing
	Prevalence of individualized treatment planning unknown
	Current treatment goals are abstinence, physical health, relationship improvement, not "responsible use"
Core Treatment Mechanisms	Expert opinion identifies acceptance of responsibility, relapse preparation, denial reduction as core mechanisms of effective treatment
	Current practice involves individual and group therapy and addiction education
	High-dose methadone treatment is effective but many programs restrict dosage levels and client participation in treatment planning
Supportive Treatment Services	Supportive legal, family, job, and medical services are important for effective treatment
	Less than half of treatment settings provide supportive services
	AIDS prevention and counseling infrequent

Aftercare

New relapse prevention treatment and education available
Follow-up and aftercare is critical to effective treatment
Less than three-quarters of outpatient and half of methadone units have formal written follow-up plans
Less than two-thirds of outpatient services collect any follow-up information at all

TREATMENT INPUTS

Staffing

Majority of staff are BA and MA level
Only half have special training or certification in substance-abuse treatment
Work experience and special training seen as important hiring qualifications
Recovering addict status not seen as special qualification. Effectiveness unclear
Understaffing and poor client–staff ratios produce poorer outcomes

Client Characteristics

Women substance-abuse clients have special service needs associated with pregnancy, sexual abuse, child care, and homelessness
Less than half of outpatient services have special services for women, one-fifth have services for pregnant women
Minority clients need culturally sensitive, supportive services to improve recruitment and reduce dropout
New services for minority clients are not being developed rapidly

Organization

Staffing, client assessment, client characteristics vary in methadone vs. outpatient drug-free programs
Hospital and mental health settings utilize more professionals in treatment
Public programs provide better access than private-for-profit programs
Private-for-profit programs may achieve lower cost by reducing individual treatment intensity

References

Abdul-Quader, A.S., S.R. Friedman, D.C. Des Jarlais, M.M. Marmor, R. Maslansky, and S. Bartelme. 1987. Methadone Maintenance and Behavior by Intravenous Drug Users that Can Transmit HIV. *Contemporary Drug Problems* 14:425–34.

Aiken, L.S., L.A. LoSciuto, M.A. Ausetts, et al. 1984. Paraprofessional versus Professional Drug Counselors: The Progress of Clients in Treatment. *International Journal of Addictions* 19:383–401.

Allison, M., R.L. Hubbard, S.G. Craddock, and J.V. Rachal. 1985. Drug Abuse Treatment Process: Preliminary Examination of the TOPS data (RTI/1901/01-06S). Research Triangle Park, N.C.: Research Triangle Institute.

Anderson, D.J. 1981. *Perspectives in Treatment.* Center City, Minn.: Hazelden.

Annis, H.M. 1986. A Relapse Prevention Model of Alcoholics. In *Treating Addictive Behavior,* ed. W.R. Miller, and N. Heather (407–21). New York: Plenum Press.

Azrin, N.H., R.W. Sisson, R. Meyers, and M. Godley. 1982. Alcoholism Treatment by Disulfiram and Community Reinforcement Therapy. *Journal of Behavior Therapy and Experimental Psychiatry* 13:105–12.

Babor, T.F., Z.S. Dolinsky, B.J. Rounsaville, et al. 1988. Unitary versus Multidimensional Models of Alcoholism Treatment Outcome: An Empirical Study. *Journal of Studies on Alcohol* 49:167–77.

Ball, J.C., W.R. Lange, C.P. Myers, and S.R. Friedman. 1988. Reducing the Risk of AIDS through Methadone Maintenance Treatment. *Journal of Health and Social Behavior* 29:214–26.

Bell Unger, K. 1988. Chemical Dependency in Women: Meeting Challenges of Accurate Diagnosis and Effective Treatment. *Western Journal of Medicine* 149(6):746–50.

Burke, A.C., and J. Rafferty. 1990. *Ownership Differences in the Organization and Provision of Outpatient Substance Abuse Services.* Ann Arbor, Mich.: University of Michigan, Survey Research Center, Institute for Social Research.

Cook, C.H. 1988a. The Minnesota Model in the Management of Drug and Alcohol Dependency: Part I. *British Journal of Addictions* 83:735–48.

———. 1988b. The Minnesota Model in the Management of Drug and Alcohol Dependency: Part II. *British Journal of Addictions* 83:735–48.

Cooper, J.R. 1989. Methadone Treatment and Acquired Immunodeficiency Syndrome. *Journal of the American Medical Association* 262:1664–8.

Cooper, J.R., F. Altman, B.S. Brown, and D. Czechowicz (eds). 1983. Research on the Treatment of Narcotic Addiction. DHHS pub. no. (ADM) 83-1281. Rockville, Md.: U.S. Department of Health and Human Services.

Copeland, J., and W. Hall. 1992. A Comparison of Women Seeking Drug and Alcohol Treatment in a Specialist Women's and Two Traditional Mixed-Sex Treatment Services. *British Journal of Addiction* 87:1293–302.

D'Amanda, D. 1983. Program Policies and Procedures Associated with Treatment Outcome. In *Research on the Treatment of Narcotic Addiction.*

DHHS pub. no. (ADM) 83-1281, ed. J.R. Cooper, F. Altman, B.S. Brown, and D. Czechowicz (637–79). Rockville, Md.: U.S. Department of Health and Human Services.

D'Aunno, T.A., and R.H. Price. 1985. Organizational Adaptation to Changing Environments: Community Mental Health and Drug Abuse Services. *American Behavioral Scientist* 28(5):669–83.

D'Aunno, T.A., R.I. Sutton, and R.H. Price. 1991. Isomorphism and External Support in Conflicting Institutional Environments: A Study of Drug Abuse Treatment Units. *Academy of Management Journal* 34(3):636–61.

D'Aunno, T., and T.E. Vaughn. 1992. Variations in Methadone Treatment Practices: Results from a National Study. *Journal of American Medical Association* 267(2):253–8.

Des Jarlais, D.C., S.R. Friedman, and C. Casriel. 1990. Target Groups for Preventing AIDS among Intravenous Drug Users: 2. The "Hard" Data Studies. *Journal of Consulting and Clinical Psychology* 58:50–6.

Des Jarlais, D.C., H. Joseph, and V.P. Dole. 1981. Long-Term Outcomes after Termination from Methadone Maintenance Treatment. *Annals of the New York Academy of Sciences* 362:231–8.

Dole, V.P. 1988. Implications of Methadone Maintenance for Theories of Narcotic Addiction. *Journal of the American Medical Association* 260:3025–9.

Dole, V.P., M.E. Nyswander, D. Des Jarlais, and H. Joseph. 1982. Performance-based Rating of Methadone Maintenance Programs. *New England Journal of Medicine* 306:169–72.

Edlund, M., J.R.C. Wheeler, and T.A. D'Aunno. 1990. Payment Systems and Payment Incentives in Outpatient Substance Abuse Treatment. *Public Budgeting and Financial Management* 4(1):107–23.

Elkins, R.L. 1980. Covert Sensitization Treatment of Alcoholism. Contributions of Successful Conditioning to Subsequent Abstinence Maintenance. *Addictive Behaviors* 5:67–89.

Fadel, H., and J.R.C. Wheeler. 1991. Pricing Behavior of Outpatient Substance Abuse Treatment Organizations. Drug Abuse Treatment System Survey Working Paper. Ann Arbor, Mich.: University of Michigan, Survey Research Center, Institute for Social Research.

Finney, J.F., and R.H. Moos. 1989. Theory and Method in Treatment Evaluation. *Evaluation and Program Planning* 12:307–16.

Frances, R.J. 1988. Update on Alcohol and Drug Disorder Treatment. *Journal of Clinical Psychiatry* 49(9, suppl.):13–17.

Gerstein, D.R., and H.J. Harwood (eds) 1990. *Treating Drug Problems: Vol. 1. A Study of the Evolution, Effectiveness and Financing of Public and Private Drug Treatment Systems.* Washington: National Academy Press.

Gilbert, F.S. 1988. The Effect of Type of Aftercare Follow-up on Treatment Outcome among Alcoholics. *Journal of Studies on Alcohol* 49:149–59.

Gomberg, E.S. 1988. Alcoholic Women in Treatment: The Question of Stigma and Age. *Alcohol & Alcoholism* 23(6):507–14.

Hargreaves, W.A. 1983. Methadone Dose and Duration for Maintenance

Treatment. In *Research on the Treatment of Narcotic Addiction*. DHHS Pub. No. (ADM) 83-1281, ed. J.R. Cooper, F. Altman, B.S. Brown, and D. Czechowicz (19–79). Rockville, Md.: U.S. Department of Health and Human Services.

Harrison, P.A., and C.A. Belille. 1987. Women in Treatment: Beyond the Stereotype. *Journal of Studies on Alcohol* 48(6):574–8.

Hayashida, M., A.I. Alterman, A. McLellan, and C.P. O'Brien. 1989. Comparative Effectiveness and Costs of Inpatient and Outpatient Detoxification of Patients with Mild-to-Moderate Alcohol Withdrawal Syndrome. *New England Journal of Medicine* 320(6):358–65.

Hubbard, R.L., M.E. Marsden, J.V. Rachal, H.J. Harwood, E.R. Cavanaugh, and H.M. Ginzburg. 1989. *Drug Abuse Treatment: A National Study of Effectiveness*. Chapel Hill, N.C.: The University of North Carolina Press.

Institute of Medicine Report. 1989. *Prevention and Treatment of Alcohol Problems: Research Opportunities*. (Publication IOM-89-13). Washington: National Academy Press.

King, P.A. 1991. Helping Women Helping Children: Drug Policy and Future Generations. *Milbank Quarterly* 69(4):595–621.

Kirk, W.G., J.B. Best, and P. Irwin. 1986. The Perception of Empathy in Alcoholism Counselors. *Journal of Studies in Alcohol* 47:834–8.

Kristenson, H., H. Ohlin, M.B. Hulten-Nosslin, et al. 1983. Identification and Intervention of Heavy Drinking in Middle-Aged Men: Results and Follow-Up of 24-60 Months of Long-Term Study with Randomized Controls. *Alcoholism and Clinical Experimental Research* 7:203–9.

Laundergan, J.C. 1982. *Easy Does It! Alcohol Treatment Outcomes, Hazelden and the Minnesota Model*. Center City, Minn.: Hazelden.

Lawson, G. 1982. Relation of Counselor Traits to Evaluation of the Counseling Relationship by Alcoholics. *Journal of Studies on Alcohol* 43(7):834–9.

Liappas, J.A., F.A. Jenner, and B. Cicente. 1988. Literature on Methadone Clinics. *International Journal of the Addictions* 23(9):927–40.

Litman, G. 1986. Alcoholism Survival: The Prevention of Relapse. In *Treating Addictive Behaviors*, ed. W.R. Miller and N. Heather (391–405). New York: Plenum Press.

Marlatt, G.A., and J.R. Gordon. 1985. *Relapse Prevention: Maintenance Strategies in the Treatment of Addictive Behaviors*. New York: Guilford Press.

McCaughrin, W.C. and R.H. Price. 1992. Effective Outpatient Drug Abuse Treatment Organizations: Program Features and Selection Effects. *International Journal of the Addictions* 27(11):1335–58.

McCrady, B.S. 1985. Alcoholism. In *Clinical Handbook of Psychological Disorders: A Step-by-Step Manual*, ed. D.H. Barlow (245–98). New York: Guilford Press.

McLellan, T.A. 1983. Patient Characteristics Associated with Outcome. In *Research on the Treatment of Narcotic Addiction*. DHHS pub. no. (ADM) 83-1281, ed. J.R. Cooper, F. Altman, B.S. Brown, and D. Czechowicz (541–64). Rockville, Md.: U.S. Department of Health and Human Services,

McLellan, A.T., L. Luborsky, F. Erdlen et al. 1980a. The Addiction Severity Index. In *Substance Abuse and Psychiatric Illness*, ed. E. Gottheil, A.T. McLellan, and K.D. Druley. New York: Pergamon Press.

———. 1980b. An Improved Diagnostic Evaluation Instrument for Substance Abuse Patients: The Addiction Severity Index. *Journal of Nervous and Mental Disorders* 168:26–33.

Miller, J.M., and J.M. Miller. 1988. Alcoholism in a Black Urban Area. *Journal of the National Medical Association* 80(6):621–3.

Miller, W.R., C.A. Taylor, and J.C. West. 1980. Focused versus Broad-Spectrum Therapy for Problem Drinkers. *Journal of Consulting and Clinical Psychology* 48:590–601.

Moos, R.H., R. Cronkite, and J.W. Finney. 1982. A Conceptual Framework for Alcoholism Treatment Evaluation. In *The Encyclopedia Handbook of Alcoholism*, ed. E.M. Pattison and E. Kaufman (1120–39). New York: Gardener Press.

Morgenstern, J. and B.S. McCrady. 1992. Curative Factors in Alcohol and Drug Treatment: Behavioral and Disease Model Perspectives. *British Journal of Addiction* 87:901–12.

O'Brien, C.P., G.E. Woody, and A.T. McLellan. 1984. *Psychotherapeutic Approaches in the Treatment of Drug Abuse*. DHHS Publication No. (ADM), Research Monograph 51. Rockville, Md.: National Institute on Drug Abuse

Oei, T.P.S., and P.R. Jackson. 1984. Some Effective Therapeutic Factors in Group Cognitive-Behavioral Therapy with Problem Drinkers. *Journal of Studies on Alcohol* 45:119–23.

Othmer, E., B.J. Powell, and E.C. Penick. 1980. *Psychiatric Diagnostic Interview* (PDI), 9th rev. Kansas City, Kans.: University of Kansas Medical Center.

Paone, D., W. Chavkin, I. Willets, P. Friedmann, and D. Des Jarlais. 1992. The Impact of Sexual Abuse: Implications for Drug Treatment. *Journal of Women's Health* 1(2):149–53.

Powell, B.J., E.C. Penick, M.R. Read, et al. 1985. Comparison of Three Outpatient Treatment Interventions: A Twelve-Month Follow-up of Men Alcoholics. *Journal of Studies on Alcohol* 46:309–12.

Price, R.H., A.C. Burke, T. D'Aunno, et al. 1991. Outpatient Drug Abuse Treatment Services, 1988: Results of a National Survey. In *Improving Drug Abuse Treatment*. NIDA Research Monograph 106, ed. R.W. Pickens, C.G. Leukefeld, and C.R. Schuster (63–92). Rockville, Md.: National Institute on Drug Abuse.

Price, R.H., and T. D'Aunno. 1992. The Organization and Impact of Outpatient Drug Abuse Treatment Services. In *Drug and Alcohol Abuse Reviews, vol. 3: Treatment of Drug and Alcohol Abuse*, ed. R.R. Watson (37–60). Clifton, N.J.: The Humana Press, Inc.

Price, R., T. D'Aunno, C. Burke, and J. Wheeler. 1989. National Drug Abuse Treatment System Survey 1988: Preliminary Results. Presented to the Director, National Institute on Drug Abuse (October 19). Rockville, Md.

Robertson, M.J. 1991. Homeless Women with Children: The Role of Alcohol and Other Drug Abuse. *American Psychologist* 46(11): 1198–204.

Robins, L.N., J.E. Helzer, J. Croughan et al. 1981. National Institute of Mental Health Diagnostic Interview Schedule: Its History, Characteristics, and Validity. *Archives of General Psychiatry* 38:381–9.

Robins, L.N., J. Wing, H.U. Wittchen et al. 1988. The Composite International Diagnostic Interview. *Archives of General Psychiatry* 45:1069–77.

Root, M.P.P. 1989. Treatment Failures: The Role of Sexual Victimization in Women's Addictive Behavior. *American Orthopsychiatry Association* 59(4):542–9.

Rounsaville, B.J., Z.S. Dolinsky, T.F. Babor, et al. 1987. Psychopathology as a Predictor of Treatment Outcome in Alcoholics. *Archives of General Psychiatry* 44:505–13.

Rowe, D., and C. Grills. 1993. African-centered Drug Treatment: An Alternative Conceptual Paradigm for Drug Counseling with African-American Clients. *Journal of Psychoactive Drugs* 25(1):21–33.

Schilling, R.F., N. Ei-Bassel, S.P. Schinke, K. Gordon, and S. Nichols. 1991. Building Skills of Recovering Women Drug Users to Reduce Heterosexual AIDS Transmission. *Public Health Reports* 106(3):297–304.

Schilling, R.F., S.P. Schinke, S.E. Nichols, et al. 1989. Developing Strategies for AIDS Prevention Research with Black and Hispanic Drug Users. *Public Health Reports* 104(1):2–11.

Schuster, C.R. 1988. Intravenous Drug Use and AIDS Prevention. *Public Health Reports* 103:261–6.

Smith, D.E., M.E. Buxton, R. Bilal, and R.B. Seymour. 1993. Cultural Points of Resistance to the 12-Step Recovery Process. *Journal of Psychoactive Drugs* 25(1):97–108.

Thornton, C.I., and J.H. Carter. 1988. Treating the Black Female Alcoholic: Clinical Observations of Black Therapists. *Journal of the National Medical Association* 80(6):644–7.

Tims, F.M. 1984. Introduction. In *Drug Abuse Treatment Evaluation: Strategies, Progress and Prospects*. National Institute on Drug Abuse Research Monograph no. 51, DHHS pub. no. (ADM) 84-1329, ed. F.M. Tims and J.P. Ludford (9–11). Rockville, Md.

Valle, S.K. 1981. Interpersonal Functioning of Alcoholism Counselors and Treatment Outcome. *Journal of Studies on Alcohol* 42:783–90.

Wallace, J., D. McNeil, D. Gilfillan, K. Maclean, and F. Fanella. 1988. Six-Month Treatment Outcomes in Socially Stable Alcoholics. *Journal of Substance Abuse Treatment* 5:247–52.

Watters, J.K. 1986. Treatment Environment and Client Outcome in Methadone Maintenance Clinics. Unpublished doctoral dissertation. Ann Arbor, Mich.: University of Michigan.

Weisner, C., and R. Room. 1984. Financing and Ideology in Alcohol Treatment. *Social Problems* 32(2):167–84.

Weisner, C., and L. Schmidt. 1992. Gender Disparities in Treatment for

Alcohol Problems. *Journal of the American Medical Association* 268(14):1872–6.

Wheeler, J.R.C., H. Fadel, and T.A. D'Aunno. 1992. Ownership and Performance in Outpatient Substance Abuse Centers. *American Journal of Public Health* 82f(5):711–18.

Woody, G.E. 1983. Treatment Characteristics Associated with Outcome. In *Research on the Treatment of Narcotic Addiction.* DHHS pub. no. (ADM) 83-1281, ed. J.R. Cooper, F. Altman, B.S. Brown, and D. Czechowicz (541–64). Rockville, Md.: U.S. Department of Health and Human Services.

Part II

Financing of Drug-Abuse Treatment

6

Drug-Abuse Treatment Costs: An Interpretive Essay

*Allen C. Goodman, Janet R. Hankin,
and Eleanor Nishiura*

Introduction

The cost and utilization effects of ADM (alcoholism, drug abuse, mental health) treatments are important areas of health services research. Indeed, the apparent decrease in utilization and/or spending that accompanies increased ADM treatment, labeled the *offset effect* (Holder 1987; Jones and Vischi 1979; Luckey 1987), has been used as a major justification for increasing resources for ADM treatment. The premise for this argument is that additional treatment for ADM conditions results not only in improved health for beneficiaries, but also in decreased utilization and/or spending for other types of health-care services.[1] Some researchers, however, (e.g., Mechanic 1983) have argued that ADM coverage must be evaluated on its own merits and not solely, or even primarily, on its ability to offset other costs.

Research on the relationship between drug-abuse treatment utilization or costs, and other ADM and non-ADM treatments and costs, requires attention to several important analytical issues. First, it is important to control for selection bias, i.e., who receives ADM specialized treatment. If only certain people receive such care, generalizing about the impact of ADM treatment is problematic unless one can determine why they, and not others, were treated.

Second, the impacts of comorbidities on both the treatment choice and the treatment costs must be considered. Comorbidities may increase costs. They may also be important determinants of location of treatment (inpatient, outpatient, or alternative settings).

Third, costs should be examined separately by location. Outpatient vs. inpatient care may represent different levels of resource allocation. Alternatively, outpatient vs. inpatient may be a proxy for severity of condition.

Fourth, because different treatment locations and combinations may suggest wholly different types of treatment (for example, inpatient treatment only, outpatient only, or a combination of the two), the location and combination of treatment and (subsequently) treatment costs should be examined as separate, albeit related, processes. Costs may vary depending on whether entry into the system is by inpatient or outpatient status. Sequencing of care (e.g., outpatient follow-up of inpatient care) may also be important.

Fifth, substitution among various treatments (e.g., drug abuse, alcoholism, mental health, and non-ADM), and among locations (outpatient, inpatient, provider's office) must also be considered. Analysts must examine whether general health-care services can take the place of specialty care for drug-abuse treatment. They must also address the substitution between inpatient and outpatient care, and between drug-abuse and nondrug-related care.

Finally, all of these effects must be evaluated within the context of the availability and the structure of third-party payments for ADM coverage. Benefits may be paid by both private and social insurance (federal and state plans). Appropriate analysis of drug-abuse treatment costs and offsets could provide important information to aid in the formulation of a national health-care policy designed to stem the recent increases in health-care costs. With substantive substitution among treatments, mandated drug-abuse coverage could dampen the expenditure increases that would otherwise occur with increased levels of health-care coverage for increased numbers of people. In contrast, limited substitution among treatments would yield more modest dampening effects on total health-care costs, because the ADM treatments would be used with, rather than instead of, other treatments.

This chapter attempts to address the issues raised above in a manner that reflects both recent research efforts and current policy imperatives. It recognizes both the development of health-care cost research, and the linkage of this research to health policy concerns. It tries, as well, to link research questions developed in the health services arena with analytical methods that economists have found to be useful.

Analytical Issues

Selection of subjects

As noted above, the analysis of treatment costs, utilization, and cost offsets is replete with selection problems. In just about all research there is an absence of controlled experiments, and researchers are frustrated by several selection problems. Who receives ADM specialized treatment, and who does not? For those who receive ADM treatment, when do they receive it, and what type do they receive? Is the ADM treatment followed up in subsequent periods, and if not, why not?

In the alcoholism literature, Hayami and Freeborn (1981) found no cost offset associated with more generous alcoholism treatment insurance coverage in an HMO. The motivation to use treatment must be considered. Those induced to use more treatment because it is covered by insurance are likely to have different cost offsets compared with those who used more treatment for some other reason (e.g., a decision to stop taking drugs), a serious selection bias. There has essentially been no analysis of the selection problem in the drug-abuse literature.

Importance of comorbidities

As illustrated in figure 6.1 (not to scale), drug disorders frequently occur with other conditions (shaded areas represent comorbidities in which two or more conditions are presented). According to the Epidemiologic Catchment Area Study, 6.1 percent of a combined community and institutional population had drug-abuse disorders in their lifetimes. Of these, 53.1 percent also had a mental disorder, 47.3 percent had an alcohol-abuse problem, and 71.6 percent had either mental or alcohol disorders in their lifetimes. Among persons treated for drug disorders, the 6-month prevalence rates were 34.1 percent for alcohol disorders, 64.4 percent for mental illness, and 79.2 percent for either alcohol or mental disorders (Regier et al. 1990). Other studies have shown similar rates (Ross et al. 1988).

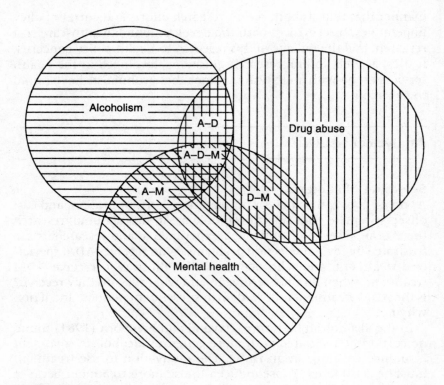

Figure 6.1   ADM comorbidities.

Just as alcohol and psychiatric disorders are common among persons treated for drug-abuse problems, drug problems are frequently noted among those being treated for alcoholism or mental illness. Regier et al. (1990) reported that 16 percent of persons treated for alcohol disorders and 8 percent of persons treated for mental disorders also had drug disorders. In a review of several studies, Galanter et al. (1988) found that as many as 40 percent of patients with mental illness were identified with drug problems (in psychiatric specialty settings).

ADM comorbidities often mean higher costs for drug-abuse treatment. Costs may be higher with comorbidities because the more serious, and hence more costly, drug-abuse problems are most likely to have comorbidities (McLellan 1983; Hesselbrock et al. 1985; Rounsaville 1987; Schuckit 1985; Walsh et al. 1991). Thus any "target outcome" (specified by health status at time of release) becomes more costly to attain.

Second, costs may be higher because the treatment of comorbidities requires more complex regimens. Psychiatric treatment may not be possible until a patient has been detoxified, or disruptive psychiatric symptoms may need to be treated before drug treatment can occur.

Finally, higher costs may occur because drug-abuse treatment is less effective when a comorbidity is present. For example, persons with psychiatric problems often respond poorly to typical drug-abuse treatments (U.S. Department of Health and Human Services 1993, p. 48). A result of the poorer outcomes is higher utilization.

In another example, mental health patients with drug problems are more likely to be rehospitalized after initial treatment (Drake and Wallach 1985; Lyons and McGovern 1985) and they have shorter lengths of stay, but more total hospital days, than mental health patients without a drug disorder (Richardson 1985; Lyons and McGovern 1985). These studies suggest more episodic patterns of care, resulting in greater utilization, for persons with dual diagnoses.

As the importance of comorbidities is increasingly recognized, treatment for these conditions is frequently merged and attempts to develop protocols appropriate for multiple problems are increasing (Weisner 1992; Institute of Medicine 1989; Ridgely et al. 1990). With the interrelationship of symptoms of comorbidities, and the difficulty of determining the primary ADM diagnosis (Lehman et al. 1989; Galanter et al. 1988), treatments which emphasize the duality of the disorder, rather than a specific primary diagnosis, are needed. Perhaps because the present health-care and financing systems often present barriers to this kind of treatment (Ridgely et al. 1990), there is little known about the effect these protocols could have on treatment outcomes and health-care costs.

Location of care

In recent decades there has been a consistent increase in the use of outpatient substance-abuse services (Knowles 1983; Institute of Medicine 1990a). According to the National Drug and Alcoholism Treatment Unit Survey (U.S. Department of Health and Human Services 1993), 87.9 percent of clients receiving drug-abuse treatment were in outpatient settings. Much of this trend is undoubtedly due to lower costs for outpatient drug-abuse treatment when compared with inpatient treatment. For example, costs ranging from $2,300 for outpatient drug-free (i.e., nonmethadone) treatment to $18,000 for inpatient drug-free treatment have been reported (Butynski 1991).

The emphasis on the lower costs of outpatient care has

encouraged Utilization Reviews to identify unnecessary substance-abuse admissions. Strumwasser et al. (1991), for example, reported that 75 percent of the inpatient substance-abuse admissions they reviewed were unnecessary. The Institute of Medicine (1990b) reported that one-third of inpatient admissions for alcoholism treatment could be treated in the outpatient setting. However, issues regarding the cost advantages of the outpatient setting remain.

Much of the substance-abuse research on the location of care deals with alcoholism treatment. After reviewing several studies, Miller and Hester (1986) concluded that outpatient care is usually as effective as inpatient care and much less expensive. Although it is often assumed that research results from studies of alcoholism costs and utilization will also apply to drug disorders (Jones and Vischi 1979), we do not know that this is true. For example, the possibility that clients with drug disorders have poorer outcomes than clients with alcoholism (Hoffman and Harrison 1987) suggests that more research is needed which deals specifically with issues related to drug abuse, including treatment location.

Cost savings of particular locations must be evaluated in terms of the intensity of treatment and treatment outcomes. The Treatment Outcome Prospectus study shows, however, that outpatient drug-abuse treatment outcomes are dependent on length of time in treatment, and that retention is often less in outpatient nonmethadone programs than in methadone programs and therapeutic communities (National Institute on Drug Abuse 1992, pp. 102, 132). Further research on the effect of location on retention rates for drug treatment programs would be useful.

Intensity of service may be less for outpatient treatment (McLellan et al. 1993a), affecting both cost and outcome. Research showing less drug use following more intense psychosocial services (McLellan et al. 1993b) suggests that the kinds of services which are offered at different treatment settings can have important influences on outcomes, and on the total treatment costs.

Although comparisons by treatment location are often limited to actual health-care costs, it may sometimes be important to consider the indirect costs of the different locations. For example, the room and board costs that are associated with inpatient care may be absorbed by the family and community when outpatient care is used. On the other hand, outpatient treatment may allow patients to continue work, education, and household responsibilities during the treatment period and thus, to increase the productivity of the individual. Alterman et al. (1994) included a consideration of indirect costs in their comparison of Day Hospital and Inpatient treatment costs. They found, even with Day Hospital treatment including the costs of transportation and meals, that total costs for traditional inpatient care were much higher than for Day Hospital treatment.

Finally, conclusions about outpatient-care cost advantages must consider the changes in total costs that result from an increase in outpatient utilization and not just a comparison of the separate costs of outpatient and inpatient episodes. An increase in the use of outpatient substance-abuse care will result in total health-care cost savings, however, only if outpatient care is substituted for inpatient care, and *not* added to the total amount of health care that is used (Jensen and Morrisey 1991). Goodman et al. (1994), for example, suggest that different locations for alcoholism treatment are *complements*, being used together, rather than substitutes for each other. Similar research for drug abuse or dependence does not exist.

Offset and substitution effects

The literature on health-care offset effects has suggested that use of some ADM treatment can lead to decreased usage and/or spending on other ADM treatments, as well as on non-ADM utilization and costs. An offset effect is claimed when the use of one treatment appears to be related to a reduction in total health-care costs. Applied to drug-treatment services, an offset effect refers to the apparent reduction in utilization and costs of non-drug services following the receipt of drug treatment.

In economic terms, offset effects imply substitution among treatments; appropriate studies must examine both the extent to which one treatment substitutes for another in the provision of health care, and the effect of this substitution on total costs. The greater the substitution of drug treatment for other general health care, the more likely that liberalized drug-treatment benefits in insurance policies may pay for themselves by reducing other health-care costs. Drug-treatment costs (services) are defined as costs (services) related to treatment provided under a diagnosis of drug disorder. General health-care costs (services) refer to all other health care and treatment.

The various forms of drug treatment can have substitution effects for the individual with drug disorders in many ways. First, treatment that results in recovery from drug-related disorders, in and of itself, leads to improved health, thus reducing use of other treatments. Second, other disorders that are exacerbated by drug disorders may also be alleviated, and their treatment avoided. Third, drug treatment may be substituted for more expensive treatments. In addition, other family members may also see numbers of visits and costs reduced through reduction of the stress brought on by a family member who abuses drugs.

Few studies have examined the effect of drug abuse or dependence on the use and costs of other medical services, although, as noted by Jones and Vischi, it is usually assumed that the effect for drug abuse will be similar to that of treatment for alcoholism. However, at least one study has shown that patients with drug disorders and their families use more health-care services than non-users (Needle et al. 1988). Bartels et al. (1993) reported greater inpatient and emergency room utilization and costs for schizophrenic outpatients with substance-abuse problems, than for persons with no current substance-abuse problems. Baldwin et al. (1993) suggest that costs associated with ICU admissions for substance-abuse related disorders are high. Illicit drug-related disorders accounted for 5 percent of admissions, but 10 percent of costs.

More research has been completed on offset effects in alcoholism treatment than on drugs. These studies of the offset effect of alcoholism treatment have usually not provided an explicit model of the process under which nonalcoholism costs and utilization change with the initiation of alcoholism treatment, and the methodologies of studies have differed. Offsets have been determined by comparing total health-care costs of treated and untreated alcoholics before and after their referrals to alcoholism treatment (Reiff et al. 1981; Sherman et al. 1979); costs before and after alcoholism treatment for the same individuals (Holder and Blose 1986; Holder and Hallan 1986; Reutzel et al. 1987; Hayami and Freeborn 1981); and pre-treatment and post-treatment costs of treated alcoholics and nonalcoholics (Holder and Hallan 1986; Forsythe et al. 1982). Offsets are implied when total health-care costs are less after alcoholism treatment than before; when alcoholics have lower costs than nonalcoholics or untreated alcoholics in a period after they are treated; or when treatment costs decline more after treatment for alcoholics than for a comparison group, regardless of the final costs.

Although all of these studies have methodological problems (Holder 1987; Jones and Vischi 1979), their combined results have led many to conclude that total health-care costs are less with alcoholism treatment than they would be without this treatment (Holder 1987; Jones and Vischi 1979; Luckey 1987). Some studies have failed to find treatment offset, however, rendering equivocal the conclusion that increased alcoholism treatment inevitably leads to lower costs (Institute of Medicine 1990b). Given the dearth of literature on drug-abuse treatment, it is unclear whether a treatment offset effect might be found.

Availability of benefits

Many observers have felt that the mandating and/or coverage of ADM conditions through health insurance could have important effects on overall health-care expenditures, as well as on peoples' health. Analysis of these policies have yielded mixed findings. Although the financing of drug treatments by private health insurance benefits has increased considerably in the past two decades (Institute of Medicine 1990a; Jensen and Morrisey 1991), the benefits both vary widely and are frequently less than for other types of health care (Rogowski 1992). There has been little analysis of the costs and utilization associated with this type of coverage (Institute of Medicine 1990a, p. 274).

There is some evidence that limiting inpatient days for mental health and substance abuse results in lower costs. This may result, however, from changes in diagnoses or cost shifting, rather than from lower utilization (Frank et al. 1991; Frank and Lave 1985).

The RAND Health Insurance Experiment made major progress in addressing a wide range of questions relating to health insurance in an experimental setting, but it was less helpful in assessing the impact of insurance benefits with respect to drug-abuse treatment. Researchers (Newhouse et al. 1994) found a wide variety of substantive own-price impacts with respect to coinsurance rates. Manning et al. (1986) find that insurance plans with higher coinsurance rates cause significantly lower use of outpatient psychotherapy services; they find no evidence of any offsetting utilization or expenditures on other services. The RAND studies do not examine drug-abuse treatment separately from other types of ADM care.

Other studies often provide limited information about drug-abuse costs because alcoholism, drug, and mental health treatments are combined in the analysis (Institute of Medicine 1990a, p. 274). If accompanied by information on benefits, analysis of health insurance claims can provide an important resource for a separate analysis of drug-treatment costs.

Economic Analyses

Selection problems

With the considerable literature on the selection biases as related to the utilization and expenditure on health services, it is more important to concentrate on those related to ADM treatments, most particularly drug abuse. It is well known (Heckman 1979) that inferences drawn from samples that have been non-randomly selected are likely to be statistically biased. Following Heckman, a substantial technical literature (and set of sophisticated statistical packages) have developed to handle such biases. There are two important types of selection biases in the ADM literature. The first regards coverage for treatment; the second involves the site (inpatient, outpatient, self-help clinic) and time (one time period as opposed to another) of treatment.

Selection issues regarding treatment coverage involve the joint choice of insurance plan (irrespective of whether the insurance is provided privately or by government programs) and the treatment that is received. Studies of HMOs, fee-for-service, or VA (Veteran's Association) clinics that fail to consider this joint decision are suspect, since the treatment decision (when, where, and how much) is most certainly jointly related to the type of coverage available. Studies such as the RAND Health Insurance Experiment would be excellent for addressing this issue, but this one-time experiment is unlikely to be repeated.

The second issue for sample selection involves site and time of treatment. Ignoring the issue of why treatment was initiated, consider the measurement of subsequent treatment. Whether subsequent treatment occurs is almost certainly related to coverage availability, seriousness of the complaint, and comorbidities. So are the costs of treatment, *if* treatment occurs (with costs presumably higher the more serious the complaint and/or comorbidities). Analysis that ignores the selection criteria almost certainly biases the inferences about when, whether, and how much treatment is used.

Importance of comorbidities
Economists have only recently recognized the importance of comorbidities in the analysis of treatment costs. There are several aspects to this interest. First, patients with drug abuse may also be treated for related conditions such as alcoholism and mental health problems. Simply adding up the costs for one condition may underestimate the larger set of costs that accrue to individual patients.

Second, patients with comorbidities may be sicker, thus requiring inpatient care, more visits, or treatment of longer duration. In studies of alcoholism treatment costs Goodman et al. (1992a; 1993) find that increased comorbidities, all else equal, are related to higher cost treatment.

Third, the fact that conditions and treatments among comorbidities are related suggests that there are substitution possibilities among treatments for comorbidities which might not be apparent among more heterogeneous groups of treatments. Recognizing in particular that people suffering from alcoholism, drug abuse, or mental health disorders may all receive their treatments at the same location (e.g., VA hospitals or state mental hospitals), and/or from the same providers, suggests significant substitution possibilities within a given setting.

In research currently in progress, examination of an insurance claims database suggests the pervasive nature of comorbidities. The database is a nationally based selection of insurance claims for 36 companies for January 1989 through December 1991. All covered employees or dependants who had an ADM diagnosis at any time during that period are included in the database.

The vast majority (93.1 percent) of the persons with at least one ADM diagnosis were treated for mental illness. Approximately 5.34 percent of those with ADM diagnoses presented a drug diagnosis, and 7.45 percent presented an alcoholism diagnosis. Overall, 5.15 percent of the ADM patients had comorbidities.

Table 6.1 considers the four categories in the Drug Abuse section of figure 6.1, based on primary diagnoses during the three-year period.[2] During the three-year period 16,811 subjects had drug abuse diagnoses. Of these, 15.5 percent (2,609 persons) also had an alcoholism diagnosis, 29.0 percent (4,876) also had a psychiatric diagnosis, and 13.8 percent (2,329) had all three. Thus, although drug abuse was a fairly small percentage of total ADM diagnoses, over 58 percent of all drug-abuse diagnoses came with comorbidities.[3]

The availability of 36 different employers allows us to examine

Table 6.1 Comorbidities among patients treated for drug-abuse disorder from 1989 through 1991.

Comorbidity	No.	%
Drug Only	6,997	41.63
Drug and Psych	4,876	29.00
Drug and Alc	2,609	15.52
Drug, Alc and Psych	2,329	13.85
Total	16,811	100.00

the incidence of comorbidities across different industrial and insurance settings. Among persons with at least one drug-abuse diagnosis, the incidence of having only a diagnosis of drug abuse varies from 29.18 percent for Employer 3, to 60.85 percent for Employer 19. These differences in the likelihood of comorbidities may stem from different work conditions, locations, benefits packages and/or employee attitudes toward drug-abuse treatment. Future research will examine these differences in more detail.

Cost Modeling

Health economics provides a considerable literature on the estimation of health-care costs, much of it related to hospitals. Health economists attempt to explain health-care outputs (such as number of visits or days spent) by levels of both labor and capital inputs. Alternatively, they may seek to use the health-care outputs to explain either the total, or the variable, production costs. Both types of analyses lead to estimates of production or cost functions, and to inferences regarding substitution among inputs.[4]

Much of the early research on treatment costs used groups as units of analysis. To model treatment costs for *individuals*, it is necessary to relate costs of different treatment modalities to treatment location, number of treatment events, sociodemographic risk factors, and comorbidities. A cost model developed by Goodman, Holder, and Nishiura (1991) provides a useful approach for analyzing both cost and utilization, at inpatient and outpatient settings, over time.

In this analysis it is essential to consider the definition of output. With measures of treatment results unavailable, the amount of treatment may serve as an alternative measure of output. Hence, outpatient output is defined by number of *visits*, and inpatient output is defined by number of *days*. Cost per unit output is then measured either as cost per outpatient visit, or cost per inpatient day.[5]

This approach responds to several important cost-measurement issues:

1   Cost *functions* relating individual treatment costs to number of treatment events (for outpatient care, visits; for inpatient care, days) should be estimated separately for inpatient and outpatient care, over time.
2   Different treatment locations and combinations may suggest

wholly different patterns of care. A patient may have inpatient treatment only (no outpatient), outpatient treatment only (no inpatient), or mixed treatment (both).[6] This suggests that treatment location and combination of locations, and (subsequently) treatment cost, should be modeled as separate, albeit related processes.

3 Comorbidities may have substantive, and differing, impacts on both choice of treatment and treatment costs. By choice of treatment we refer to the "yes/no" decisions of whether there is treatment, treatment modality (if treated), and location of treatment (inpatient vs. outpatient). Treatment costs, conditional on choice of treatment, may also be related to the prevalence and severity of comorbidities.

It is useful to characterize the cost function for drug-abuse treatment (DR) in two stages. The first stage involves treatment choice, and the second stage estimates cost functions, conditional on treatment choice. The cost of treatment in any given period (calendar or episode) is conditional on *whether* treatment was used. If treatment was used, the analysis proceeds to the second stage, where one estimates the cost based on treatment location, and the amount of treatment, *given* the location. For example, patients exhibiting certain comorbidities may be put into either some inpatient, or outpatient-only treatment. Once in that treatment type, the impact of the comorbidity may be marginal in the estimation of the second-stage cost functions. Yet, clearly the comorbidity was important in the first-stage choice.

Treatment is most easily characterized as occurring at inpatient or non-inpatient settings. The model presented here uses two branches of treatment for convenience although more branches are easily handled.[7] The upper branch includes outpatient treatment only. The lower branch combines inpatient only, and mixed treatment into "some inpatient."

Figure 6.2 shows the branching schematically for drug-abuse treatment DR. Within any given period, cost is a function of the probability of any treatment, the location of the treatment, and the cost if treated. It is plausible that all three decisions are related to the severity of the complaint, comorbidities, sociodemographic characteristics, prices of alternatives, insurance benefits, and/or payment mechanisms. How these interact can have substantive impacts on annual treatment costs measured either for individuals or by treatment locations.

What is essential to interpreting overall costs, and their relations

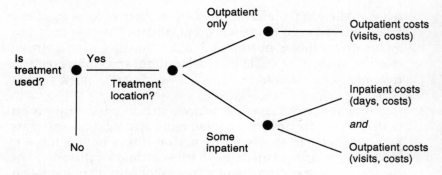

Figure 6.2 Treatment branches and costs.

to health-care policies, is the realization that many sorts of costs are conditional on a decision to treat, and the location of treatment. Concentrating on conditional costs ignores the probability of incurring those costs. Since total costs depend on both the costs and their probabilities, it is critical to model each, as well as their relationship.

Treatment – whether and/or where?
The first stage of the model determines whether treatment occurs in a given period. Whether a person initiates ADM treatment may be related to overall health, age, sex, and other sociodemographic characteristics, as well as non-ADM comorbidities. Availability and comprehensiveness of ADM coverage is also of prime concern. Subsequent treatment is related to similar factors as well as to the level and effectiveness of ADM and non-ADM treatments in earlier periods.

Given treatment initiation or continuation, location of treatment is modeled next. As noted above, the model uses the branches of (1) some in-patient, with or without accompanying outpatient care, and (2) outpatient only, again considering individual-specific morbidity factors. It also might include chronological time, in recognition that cost considerations or pressure from insurers may lead to a drift toward less inpatient care over time.

With insurance claims data, drug-abuse disorders can be summarized in three broad categories. The first category distinguishes drug abuse and drug dependence. If dependence is a substantively different condition than abuse, type of drug-abuse disorder may be significantly related to choice of treatment location. Selection into certain types of treatment (for example, inpatient treatment) may be more likely with dependence than with abuse diagnoses.

The second category refers to the type of drug being abused (for example, heroin vs. codeine). Knowing the type of drug will affect both the model of treatment and the setting necessary for treatment (Saxe and Shusterman 1991). Detoxification from particular drugs may require inpatient care.

The third category refers to the set of comorbidities such as psychiatric problems or alcoholism disorders which occur with drug abuse. The inter-relationship of these comorbidities among themselves, as well as coupled with the diagnoses of drug abuse or dependence, may have substantial impacts on the treatment location. For example, a patient with alcohol and heroin dependence *plus* a major depression may need inpatient rather than outpatient care.

Costs of the component parts

From this framework, it follows that the total treatment cost is the sum of treatments at various locations over a longer-term period. This suggests that treatment costs should be carefully interpreted within any given limited time period. The policy implications related to this caution may turn out to be critical.

Consider a simple example. Suppose that an individual is in treatment for two years. In the first year there are inpatient treatment costs of $1,500, and outpatient treatment costs of $600. In the second year there are inpatient treatment costs of $1,000, and outpatient treatment costs of $500. Clearly, the total treatment costs are $3,600; 69 percent go to inpatient care and 31 percent go to outpatient care.[8]

Suppose that an analyst seeks to examine the impacts of a change in governmental health-care policy and/or private insurance coverage. All else equal, this change increases outpatient use (and hence expenditures) in the second year from $500 to $700. The report may state that outpatient costs increased by 40 percent. Yet, total Year Two costs increase from $1500 to $1700, or about 13.3 percent. Costs for the entire two-year episode increase from $3,600 to $3,800 or by 5.5 percent. Thus, the smaller the individual share in the total cost (total vs. outpatient only; two years vs. one year), the smaller its impact, or elasticity (5.5 percent vs. 40 percent).

This example demonstrates the importance of considering changes in costs within the framework of the *totality* of care. Data on costs of care have most often been collected by location, conditional on those receiving treatment. Those who do not receive further treatment become "non-observations" rather than observations with values of zero costs. As a result the expenditures of treated samples may represent considerable overestimates of population costs. Correspondingly, changes in expenditures at any given location might be interpreted as large percentages when they may in fact represent only small portions of the whole.

Cost measurement is problematic. Outpatient events that are measured in visits should be aggregated separately from inpatient events that are measured jointly by stays and days per stay. Moreover the costs must be estimated jointly with the probability of having any treatment, and the probability of treatment at a specific location.

This joint determination of treatment costs has two important impacts. First, if treatment location is omitted, items that determine treatment location may mistakenly be attributed to the resulting costs. Goodman et al. (1992a; 1992b; 1993) have found that many impacts of comorbidities occur at the point of determining whether to be treated and which treatment to have, as opposed to the number of treatment events or the costs of treatment.

Second, date and location of one type of treatment feed back on the use of other types of treatment. Increased numbers of ADM treatment events at the time of treatment initiation, for example, may substitute for non-ADM events in that same time period, or for ADM and/or non-ADM treatments in subsequent time periods. Goodman, Holder, and Nishiura (1991) use a recursive model in which treatment decisions are made sequentially (figure 6.3) to identify *usage effects*. The usage effects measure the impact of alcoholism treatment initiation (point A) on future alcoholism treatment (point B), and on current (point D) and future (point E) nonalcoholism treatment. In subsequent analyses, the direct and the indirect effects were estimated separately and compared. As with the cost functions, both duration of the treatment period, and individual-specific demographics were included in the estimation.

The + (increased stimuli lead to increased responses) and − (increased stimuli lead to decreased responses) signs in figure 6.3 show the alcoholism-treatment effects that were estimated by Goodman, Holder, and Nishiura (1991). Although the direct effect (path *AE*) of short-term alcoholism treatment on subsequent non-alcoholism treatment is negative, the indirect effect is positive and large. An indirect effect occurs through the interactions of various types of care. For example, *increased* short-term alcoholism treatment is related to *decreased* short-term nonalcoholism treatment (path *AD*), but the *decreased* short-term nonalcoholism treatment, in turn, implies *increased* subsequent nonalcoholism treatment (path *DE*). Hence the resulting indirect increment of short-term alcoholism treatment to subsequent nonalcoholism treatment is

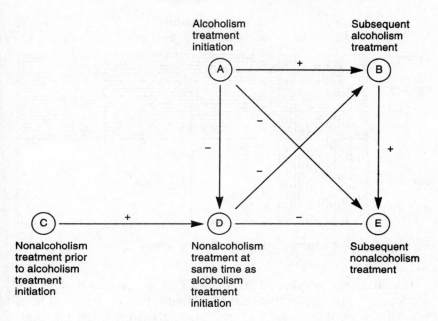

Figure 6.3 Impacts of alcoholism treatment initiation.

positive. In other words, increased short-term alcoholism treatment is indirectly related to increased subsequent nonalcoholism treatment. Thus, short-term impacts of ADM care must be distinguished from those occurring in the longer term.

A Demand Model

The cost models described above allow us to *predict* the use of health inputs without the often difficult computation of price or coinsurance terms. They do *not*, however, consider how patients and their providers, as health-care *demanders*, substitute among drug, mental health, or alcoholism treatments, surgery, or nonsurgical treatments, or among inpatient, outpatient and office care. Nor do they consider how providers, as health-care *suppliers*, may substitute among physicians, therapists, self-help groups, inpatient and/or non-inpatient care. The economics literature provides a useful set of analyses to measure demand substitution explicitly, through reactions to prices and expenditures.

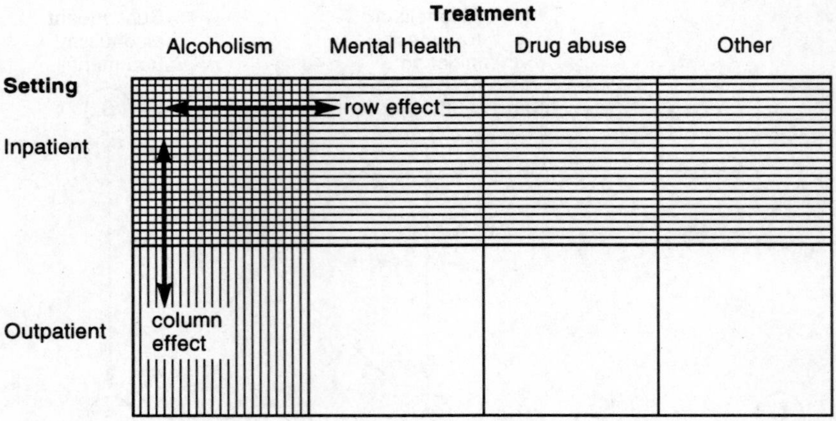

Treatment

	Alcoholism	Mental health	Drug abuse	Other

Figure 6.4 Column (setting) and row (treatment) effects.

The analysis presented here looks at a consumer-demand approach, following Deaton and Muellbauer (1980). Referred to as the Almost Ideal Demand System, this analysis considers expenditure shares as determined by total expenditures and the prices of the various treatments. The system offers an alternative to number of visits for measuring treatment levels. When comparing treatments for different illnesses, units of treatment may differ, and more visits do not necessarily imply better care or greater offset effects. Use of budget shares helps to surmount the units of treatment problem, if treatment levels can be properly defined through the shares.

The matrix in figure 6.4 provides four treatment categories and two treatment settings. The four columns represent alcoholism, mental health, and drug-abuse treatment, with the fourth column representing non-ADM treatments (which could be subdivided into surgery, non-surgical injuries, etc.). The two rows represent inpatient and outpatient care. In this example, then, there are eight types of care (4 columns x 2 rows).

The matrix format provides a natural ordering for settings down columns (*column* effects), or for treatments across rows (*row* effects). Much of the literature suggests that column effects would provide the best possibilities of substitution; e.g., outpatient drug care is a good substitute for inpatient drug care. Goodman et al. (1994), however, find that for short-term alcoholism treatment, column effects (between inpatient and outpatient care) are modest. Inpatient and outpatient alcoholism treatments substitute less well for each other than do inpatient and outpatient psychiatric treatments. The best substitute for inpatient alcoholism treatment is inpatient psychiatric treatment, a *row effect*.

These short-term findings, based on the comprehensive coverage of a single company, suggest only limited opportunities (in the early to mid-1980s) for alcoholism-treatment cost saving by shifting from inpatient to outpatient settings. Generalizing to the case of drug abuse, substitution between drug abuse and psychiatric inpatient treatment may be more promising from a cost-saving perspective. It would be valuable to test for substitution across ADM treatments and settings, and between ADM and non-ADM treatments.

Two instances arise in which one might question the applicability of standard economic demand analysis. The first concerns "supplier-induced demand," or SID, in which the provider may be an imperfect agent for the patient, ordering additional treatment that may increase the provider's income (Roemer 1961; Reinhardt 1989). In a detailed discussion, Folland, Goodman, and Stano (1993, ch. 8) acknowledge the possibility of SID, but note that many attempts to measure SID suffer from substantive statistical problems. They conclude that the magnitude of SID is very small.

A second critique of the standard demand analysis might arise from recent work on "rational addiction," following Becker and Murphy (1988). In this analysis, addictive drugs are assumed to provide some pleasure, or else people would not use them. An individual who optimizes in a rational-addiction framework may choose to undergo substance-abuse treatment, to reduce his or her habit, and its cost, *rather* than to eliminate it altogether. Rational-addiction literature has been applied to prevention initiatives (e.g., raising the price of cigarettes, Chaloupka 1991), rather than to treatment demand, but future treatment-related analysis may find it to be a productive approach.

Design and Data Problems

Research on the impacts of health-care policies on the costs and utilization associated with substance abuse has been limited by several data and design problems. First, existing data sets are often inadequate to answer specific research questions. Clinic data are often limited to utilization at only one site and may lack outcome information. Insurance claims are not linked to outcomes data and the insurance coverage information that is needed to interpret these data are sometimes not available. Survey data can be costly to obtain and may suffer from issues of recall and lost records. Individuals may not have at their fingertips the kind of information needed for these kinds of studies.

A second set of problems relates to the design of research projects and hypothesis testing. By traditional experimental standards, the impacts and costs of substance-abuse treatment must be tested against a group of substance abusers who did not receive treatment. Laboratory animals provide an ideal group of subjects for such research, since treatment can be withheld from them. *People* emphatically do not provide such a test, as it is considered unethical to withhold treatment from those who need it.

Moreover, even if one can find an untreated population, there are sample selectivity problems related to insurance coverage, severity of the problem, or denial of the need for treatment. In some experimental designs, comparison groups are drawn, which are matched by sociodemographics and other factors, but such matches are always tenuous.

It is incumbent on researchers to present innovative ways of comparing treatments, costs, and outcomes, under these conditions. Where data permit, analyzing the impact of more generous vs. less generous ADM benefits for those who are treated, may also enable one to examine how quantity and quality of care might impact on utilization, costs, and patient outcomes. Again, however, the problem of an untreated population is not addressed. Alternatively, appropriate matching groups may be formed, with the proper modeling of sample selection attempted. The difficulties inherent in modeling these behaviors suggest that those who evaluate research design, as well as those who refer to the research for policy guidance, must acknowledge that "people research" will inevitably differ from "animal research" in protocols, in experimental design, and ultimately in the strengths of the resulting inferences. It is exceedingly difficult to randomize patients to treatment/nontreatment conditions.

Applications to Health Policy

The earlier discussion referred to health-care costs and health-care substitution in the abstract, ignoring policies that related either to the design of health insurance policies, or to the potential impacts of so-called "managed care" alternatives. The following two sections address these two items in order, with particular reference to the legacy and to the future of ADM research as related to health-services policy.

ADM health insurance impacts

The legacy of the offset literature has been to claim significant impacts for ADM therapy on the use of both ADM and non-ADM care. Early ADM research asserted that ADM therapy not only addressed ADM conditions, but also led to reduced (or offset) treatment levels and/or costs for other conditions. Expectations for non-ADM treatment have usually been different. Although these treatments might reduce prevalence of psychiatric, drug-abuse, or alcoholism conditions, as when surgery relieves pain that has led to addictions to painkillers, evaluations do not require this in order for the treatment to be deemed effective.

In contrast, ADM treatment must not only address ADM conditions, but must also reduce other utilization and/or costs. Freund (1994) provides an example of this imperative, in reviewing Newhouse et al. (1994) on the RAND Health Insurance Experiment (HIE). In particular, she notes a failure of the HIE and its analyses "to acknowledge the potential of good mental health care to offset other medical spending."

A belief in health-care cost and utilization offsets almost certainly leads to a policy prescription suggesting that comprehensive ADM coverage be included in private insurance contracts or, alternatively, that social insurance, including Medicare and Medicaid, cover ADM conditions. It would seem that if cost offsets do occur, then insurers might be expected to include coverage voluntarily. With regard to national health-care policies, both the Clinton Administration health-care proposals and those that followed have also proposed comprehensive ADM coverage.[9]

The impacts of such coverage have not been extensively examined. The early aggregate studies are not adequate for examining the policy impacts on individuals. If one is investigating the possibilities of offset effects regarding individual behavior, demand cross-elasticities must be modeled explicitly. This has not been done. The RAND study concentrated on "own-price" elasticities, referring to the impact of changes of price or coinsurance for a given ADM treatment on its *own* usage, but ignoring the impact of ADM prices or insurance on the usage of non-ADM treatments. Most other studies have concentrated on changes in own usage that would accompany changes in coinsurance, deductibles, maximum coverage, and the like.

Moreover, policy changes for individuals must be aggregated in a "market" context. Increased coverage for ADM would lead to increased individual demand. When such increased individual demands are aggregated, the resources to supply such treatment must necessarily be attracted from other types of care, either through some type of market bidding, or alternatively from the taxation to build facilities such as Veterans Administration hospitals and clinics. These market impacts almost certainly increase the incremental cost of providing treatment services, thus raising societal costs.

Managed care
Managed care represents the various attempts to affect and to control price, volume, quality, and accountability of medical services (Boland 1991). The term refers to a set of practices by insurers and providers, including HMOs and PPOs, that include prospective pricing, bundling of services, peer review, mandatory-use review, benefit redesign, capitation payments, channeling, and shared clinical decisions (Curtiss 1990). To develop and to maintain effective systems of managed care, managers need information on the costs and utilization typically associated with the programs they are using.

There has been no rigorous analysis of managed care as it applies to drug-abuse treatment. An appropriate general model of drug-abuse managed care would provide information on how resources substitute for each other in all settings. Measured utilization and costs of various treatments must then be compared with what *might* occur with various controls such as maximum utilization requirements, controls on treatment location, limitations on provider choice, and increased employee cost sharing.

It is essential, in providing guidance to care managers, to examine practices over a wide range of organizational structures and payment mechanisms. We contrast this "wide range" approach with narrower analyses that focus on managed care through HMOs, because HMO analysis shows *only* how HMO managers manage. The wider approach provides a menu of possibilities that are available to *all* managers, within a setting that is not constrained like HMOs.

Conclusions

The analysis and understanding of drug-abuse treatment costs have lagged behind comparable work in mental health and alcoholism treatment, even though the three are closely related through comorbidities, treatment locations, and treatment modalities. Recent initiatives sponsored by the National Institute on Drug Abuse seek to close this gap.

It is essential to link such cost analysis with treatment outcomes. Such linkages are tenuous due to the nature of the morbidities. If, for example, the patient halts his or her pattern of substance abuse for a year, and then starts again, has the treatment been successful or not? Insights might be gained from examining other chronic diseases such as asthma, or diabetes.[10]

It is also essential to examine the totality of care. Costs aggregated for individuals by treatment location almost certainly underestimate the total health-system related component, because they do not follow individuals through other ADM or non-ADM treatments. Aggregation by treatment location almost certainly imposes a selection effect that has been recognized. Examining costs by payer, rather than by recipient, may help to address this problem.

Finally, substance-abuse costs and treatments must be evaluated *on their own*, instead of by whether they serve to offset other costs, care, or behaviors. Careful measurement suggests that treatment-related impacts are likely to be very small. Including criminal behavior as an external benefit requires a measurement of crimes *not committed*, as a result of drug treatment.[11] Counting subsequent crime as a failure of drug-abuse treatment ignores the fact that there are a multiplicity of nondrug-related factors that cause crime.

Moreover, evaluating ADM treatment by the presence of an offset imposes standards that are considerably more stringent than are required of most other treatments. Literature on the evaluation of non-ADM treatment does not create standards for offsets, either implicitly or explicitly. Cardiology care, for example, is not evaluated by its impact on other sorts of utilization, such as gynecological or ENT care. The evaluation of ADM treatment, the impacts of insurance coverage, and the inclusion of ADM in a national health policy should not depend on the presence, or the size, of offset or external effects, but rather on the improved health of people suffering from ADM disorders.

Notes

The research reported in this chapter was supported in part by NIAAA grant AA-07694 and NIDA grant DA-08711. The opinions stated do not represent the National Institute of Alcoholism and Alcohol Abuse, the National Institute on Drug Abuse, or Wayne State University. We thank Carol Cowell, Gabrielle Denmead,

Cherry Lowman, and an anonymous referee for comments and suggestions regarding our work. All errors are our own.

1 Decreased criminal activity by those who have undergone drug treatment is sometimes enumerated as a reduced cost, or as an external benefit. We do not address this aspect explicitly in this chapter, although we will discuss it when considering criteria for evaluating drug-abuse treatment policies.
2 Identities of subjects and employers are confidential. More detail is available on the nature of the database from the authors.
3 It is possible that due to social stigmas relating to drug abuse, some number of drug and alcoholism problems were classified as mental illness diagnoses. Without independent clinical verification, it is impossible to know the extent of this problem.
4 See Folland, Goodman, and Stano (1993) for a presentation and a critique of such analyses. Jensen and Morrisey (1986), for example, use treated cases as a measure of output.
5 Such measures are also independent of the length of the calendar period of the episode.
6 Even this is a simplification since it does not address the sequencing of treatments.
7 It is an empirical question as to how finely to differentiate the different types and combinations of treatment. Self-help groups, for example, might form another setting, although claims data would be unlikely to contain useful information regarding this alternative.
8 We concentrate on the costs that would occur at clinics or hospitals, ignoring costs such as foregone wages or impacts on families. Including these other costs would strengthen our conclusions regarding the need to consider the totality of care.
9 See Section 1115 of the 1993 version of the Health Security Act as an example.
10 Dr Thomas McLellan made this point at the parent conference to this volume.
11 One might examine whether populations with better coverage for ADM commit fewer crimes, all else equal, than populations with lesser coverage. Controlling for other influences on criminal behavior, this method might provide some analytical insights.

References
Alterman, A.I., et al. 1994. Effectiveness and Costs of Inpatient vs. Day Hospital Cocaine Rehabilitation. *Journal of Nervous and Mental Diseases* 182:157–63.
Baldwin, W.A., et al. 1993. Substance Abuse Related Admissions to Adult Intensive Care. *Chest* 103:21–5.
Bartels, S.J., et al. 1993. Substance Abuse in Schizophrenia Service Utilization and Costs. *Journal of Nervous and Mental Disease* 181:227–32.

Becker, G.S., and K.J. Murphy. 1988. A Theory of Rational Addiction. *Journal of Political Economy* 96:675–700.

Boland, P. 1991. *Making Managed Health Care Work: A Practical Guide to Strategies and Solutions.* New York: McGraw-Hill.

Butynski, W. 1991. Drug Treatment Services: Funding and Admissions. In *Improving Drug Abuse Treatment.* NIDA Research Monograph 106, ed. R.W. Pickens, C.G. Leukefeld, C.R. Schusters (20–52). Rockville, MD: National Institute on Drug Abuse.

Chaloupka, F.J. 1991. Rational Addictive Behavior and Cigarette Smoking. *Journal of Political Economy* 99:722–42.

Curtiss, F.R. 1990. Managed Care: The Second Generation. *American Journal of Hospital Pharmacy* 47:2047–52.

Deaton, A., and J. Muellbauer. 1980. An Almost Ideal Demand System. *American Economic Review* 70:312–26.

Drake, R.E., and M.A. Wallach. 1985. Substance Abuse among the Chronic Mentally Ill. *Hospital and Community Psychiatry* 40:1041–6.

Folland, S., A.C. Goodman, and M. Stano. 1993. *The Economics of Health and Health Care.* New York: Macmillan.

Forsythe, A.B., B. Griffiths, and S. Keiff. 1982. Comparison of Utilization of Medical Services by Alcoholics and Non-Alcoholics. *American Journal of Public Health* 72:600–2.

Frank, R.G., D.S. Salkever, and S.S. Sharfstein. 1991. A New Look at Rising Mental Health Insurance Costs. *Health Affairs* 10:116–23.

Frank, R.G. and J.R. Lave. 1985. The Impact of Medicaid Benefit Design on Length of Stay and Patient Transfers. *Hospital and Community Psychiatry* 36:749–53.

Freund, D.A. 1994. Looking Back to Move Forward. *Health Affairs* 13:293–5.

Galanter, M., R. Castaneda, and J. Ferman. 1988. Substance Abuse among General Psychiatric Patients: Place of Presentation, Diagnosis, and Treatment. *American Journal of Drug and Alcohol Abuse* 14:211–35.

Goodman, A.C., H.D. Holder, and E. Nishiura. 1991. Alcoholism Treatment Offset Effects: A Cost Model. *Inquiry* 28:117–28.

Goodman, A.C., H.D. Holder, E. Nishiura, and J.R. Hankin. 1992a. An Analysis of Short Term Alcoholism Treatment Cost Functions. *Medical Care* 30:795–810.

——. 1992b. A Discrete Choice Model of Alcoholism Treatment Location. *Medical Care* 30:1097–110.

——. 1993. Long-Term Alcoholism Treatment Cost Functions. Detroit: Wayne State University (unpublished).

Goodman, A.C., H.D. Holder, E. Nishiura, J.R. Hankin, and J. M. Tilford. 1994. Short Term Alcoholism Treatment: Prices, Demand, and Substitution Effects. Detroit: Wayne State University (unpublished).

Hayami, D.E., and D.K. Freeborn. 1981. Effect of Coverage on Use of an HMO Alcoholism Treatment Program, Outcome, and Medical Care Utilization. *American Journal of Public Health* 71:1133–43.

Heckman, J.J. 1979. Sample Selection Bias as a Specification Error. *Econometrica* 47:153–61.

Hesselbrock, M.N., R.E. Meyer, and J.J. Keener. 1985. Psychopathology in Hospitalized Alcoholics. *Archives of General Psychiatry* 42:1050–5.

Hoffman, N.G., and P.A. Harrison. 1987. Patient Variations in Alcoholism Treatment Utilization. *Business and Health* 5:16–18.

Holder, H.D. 1987. Alcohol Treatment and Potential Health Care Cost Saving. *Medical Care* 25:52–71.

Holder, H.D., and J.O. Blose. 1986. Alcoholism Treatment and Total Health Care Utilization and Costs: A 4-Year Longitudinal Analysis of Federal Employees. *Journal of American Medical Association* 256:1456–60.

Holder, H.D. and J.B. Hallan, 1986. Impact of Alcoholism Treatment on Total Health Care Costs: A Six-Year Study. *Advances in Alcohol and Substance Abuse* 6:1–15.

Institute of Medicine. 1989. *Prevention and Treatment of Alcohol Problems: Research Opportunities.* Washington: National Academy Press.

——. 1990a. *Treating Drug Problems.* Washington: National Academy Press.

——. 1990b. *Broadening the Base of Treatment for Alcohol Problems: Report of a Study by a Committee of the Institute of Medicine.* Washington: National Academy Press.

Jensen, G.A., and M.A. Morrisey. 1986. The Role of Physicians in Hospital Production. *Review of Economics and Statistics* 68:432–42

——. 1991. Employer-Sponsored Insurance Coverage for Alcohol and Drug Abuse Treatment. *Inquiry* 28:393–402.

Jones, J.R., and T.R. Vischi. 1979. Impact of Alcohol, Drug Abuse and Mental Health Treatment on Medical Care Utilization. *Medical Care* 17:1–26.

Knowles, P.L. 1983. Inpatient vs. Outpatient Treatment of Substance Misuse in Hospitals, 1975–1980. *Journal of Studies on Alcohol* 44:384–7.

Lehman, A.F., C.P. Myers, and E. Corty. 1989. Assessment and Classification of Patients with Psychiatric and Substance Abuse Syndromes. *Hospital and Community Psychiatry* 40:1019–25.

Luckey, J.W. 1987. Justifying Alcoholism Treatment on the Basis of Cost Savings, The 'Offset' Literature. *Alcohol Health and Research World* 12:8–15.

Lyons, J.S., and M.P. McGovern. 1985. Use of Mental Health Services by Dually Diagnosed Patients. *Hospital and Community Psychiatry* 40:1067–9.

Manning, W.G., et al. 1986. How Cost Sharing Affects the Use of Ambulatory Mental Health Services. *Journal of the American Medical Association* 256:1930–4.

McLellan, A.T., et al. 1983. Predicting Response to Alcohol and Drug Abuse Treatments *Archives of General Psychiatry* 40:620–5.

——. 1993a. Private Substance Abuse Treatment: Are Some Programs More Effective Than Others? *Journal of Substance Abuse Treatment* 10:243–54.

——. 1993b. The Effects of Psychosocial Services in Substance Abuse Treatment. *Journal of American Medical Association* 26:1953–9.

Mechanic, D. 1983. Does Psychiatric Care Reduce the Demand for Medical Care Services? *Medical Care* 21:1126–7.

Miller, W.R., and R.K. Hester. 1986. Inpatient Alcoholism Treatment. Who Benefits? *American Psychologist* 41:794–805.

National Institute on Drug Abuse. 1992. *Extent and Adequacy of Insurance Coverage for Substance Abuse Services: A Study of the Evolution, Effectiveness, and Financing of Public and Private Drug Treatment Systems.* DHHS Publication No. (ADM) 92-1778. Rockville, Md.

Needle, R., et al. 1988. Costs and Consequences of Drug Use: A Comparison of Health Care Utilization and Social-Psychological Consequences for Clinical and Nonclinical Adolescents and Their Families. *International Journal of Addictions* 23:1125–43.

Newhouse, J.P., et al. 1994. *Free for All: Lessons from the RAND Health Insurance Experiment.* Cambridge, Mass.: Harvard University Press.

Regier, D.A. et al. 1990. Comorbidity of Mental Disorders with Alcohol and Other Drug Abuse: Results from the Epidemiologic Catchment Area (ECA) Study. *Journal of American Medical Association* 264:2511–18.

Reiff, S., B. Griffiths, and A.B. Forsythe. 1981. Utilization of Medical Services by Alcoholics Participating in a Health Maintenance Organization Outpatient Treatment Program: Three-Year Follow-Up. *Alcoholism: Clinical and Experimental Research* 5:159–62.

Reinhardt, U.E. 1989. Economists in Health Care: Saviors, or Elephants in a Porcelain Shop. *American Economic Review* 79:337–42.

Reutzel, T.J., F.W. Becker, and B.K. Sanders. 1987. Expenditure Effects of Change in Medicaid Benefit Coverage: An Alcoholism and Substance Abuse Example. *American Journal of Public Health* 77:503–4.

Richardson, M.A., T.J. Craig, and G. Haugland. 1985. Treatment Patterns of Young Chronic Schizophrenic Patients in the Era of Deinstitutionalization. *Psychiatric Quarterly* 57:104–10.

Ridgely, M.S., H.H. Goldman, and M. Willenbring. 1990. Barriers to the Care of Persons with Dual Diagnoses: Organizational and Financing Issues. *Schizophrenia Bulletin* 16:123–32.

Roemer, M.I. 1961. Bed Supply and Hospital Utilization: A National Experiment. *Hospitals* 35:36–42.

Rogowski, J.A. 1992. Insurance Coverage for Drug Abuse. *Health Affairs* 11:137–48.

Ross, H.E., F.B. Glaser, and T. Germanson. 1988. The Prevalence of Psychiatric Disorders in Patients with Alcohol and Other Drug Problems. *Archives of General Psychiatry* 45:1023–31.

Rounsaville, B.J. et al. 1987. Psychopathology as a Predictor of Treatment Outcomes in Alcoholics. *Archives of General Psychiatry* 44:505–13.

Saxe, L., and G. Shusterman. 1991. *Drug Treatment Modalities: A Taxonomy to Aid Development of Services Research.* Drug Abuse Background Papers on Drug Abuse Financing and Services Research, Research Series no. 1. Rockville, Md.: National Institute on Drug Abuse

Schuckit, M.A. 1985. The Clinical Implications of Primary Diagnostic

Groups among Alcoholics. *Archives of General Psychiatry* 42:1043–9.

Sherman, R.M., S. Reiff, and A.B. Forsythe. 1979. Utilization of Medical Services by Alcoholics Participating in an Out-Patient Treatment Program. Alcoholism: *Clinical and Experimental Research* 3:115–20.

Strumwasser, I., et al. 1991. Appropriateness of Psychiatric and Substance Abuse Hospitalization: Implications for Payment and Utilization Management. *Medical Care* 29 (suppl.):AS77–AS90.

U.S. Department of Health and Human Services. 1993. *Eighth Special Report to the U.S. Congress on Alcohol and Health.* NIH pub. no. 94-3699. Washington.

———. 1993. *National Drug and Alcoholism Treatment Unit Survey (NDATUS): 1991 Main Findings Report.* DHHS pub. no. (SMA) 93-2007. Washington DHHS.

Walsh, D.C., et al. 1991. Associations between Alcohol and Cocaine Use in a Sample of Problem-Drinking Employees. *Journal of Studies on Alcohol* 52:17–25.

Weisner, C. 1992. The Merging of Alcohol and Drug Treatment: A Policy Review. *Journal of Public Health Policy* 13:66–80.

7

Cost-benefit and Cost-effectiveness Analysis: Issues in the Evaluation of the Treatment of Illicit Drug Abuse

Jody L. Sindelar and
Willard G. Manning, Jr.

1 Introduction

Society is increasingly aware of the scarcity of resources and the need to limit how much money is spent on health care. Given this environment, there are greater efforts to direct resources toward medical treatments and programs that give the greatest value per dollar. The trend toward setting cost-conscious priorities is evident in several related trends in health care: the growth of managed care; the increasing reliance on capitation; the explicit rationing of the sort found in the Oregon Medicaid plan; and the increasing use of pharmaceutical formularies. Further, the recent debate on health-care reform has been motivated in part by concerns about the high and rapidly rising cost of health care, and the strains these costs place on the financial well-being of both the general public and government.

In the area of treatment for substance abuse, there is mounting pressure on treatment modalities to demonstrate their cost-effectiveness in order to maintain funding. The recent and swift movement in the alcohol treatment field away from 28-day inpatient treatment to "brief treatment" is one example of this. However, currently the evidence about the cost-effectiveness or cost-benefits of treatment of illicit drug abuse is insufficient to direct public policies on funding.

In a cost-conscious environment, the tools and techniques of cost-benefit and cost-effectiveness analysis (CBA and CEA) can be productively applied to the drug-treatment field. Society needs to know which types of treatment to fund (e.g., methadone maintenance (MM), therapeutic community (TC), or detoxification only), to what extent and for how long to fund them, and for whom to provide them. Society is also concerned with the trade-offs of funding drug treatment versus a variety of other ways of achieving some of its specific and broad goals. Other ways of reducing the consequences of drug abuse might include greater efforts at international drug interdiction, greater police presence, and new educational programs. CBA and CEA can be helpful to society in allocating its resources among the possible alternatives in order to reduce the costs associated with substance abuse.

Society at large is only one of the identifiable groups that will be concerned about decision-making and substance abuse. Public and private payers can ask questions similar to those of society; however, they may use different criteria in answering questions about which programs to fund, for how long, and for whom? They can ask, given a specific budget, how should they spend their money? Or, they may wish to determine the size of their optimal budget. Patients can ask similar questions but will evaluate the alternatives in terms of benefits and costs to themselves (and their family) rather than those that accrue to taxpayers, payers, or other members of society.

CEA and CBA can also be used to evaluate questions from the perspective of the drug-abuse treatment program itself. Drug-treatment programs may want to know whether or not to expand their facilities and if so, how? Should they add an extra counselor? Should the group size for counseling be increased? Should the dosage of methadone be increased? Should job training be emphasized? How long should the standard treatment regime last? After how many infractions should clients be asked to leave the program? The answers to these and other questions may vary depending on whether the programs have predetermined budgets or can increase revenues by providing and billing for different services. These questions could all be answered by a properly designed and implemented cost-benefit analysis, assuming that sufficiently good data were available.

Although there is a well-developed and specified set of technologies available to apply cost-benefit and cost-effectiveness analyses to health care of any sort, the actual application itself can be difficult. Such applications may be even more problematic in the case of substance abuse than they are in other health areas. The small but growing literature on the cost-effectiveness of different drug treatments is testimony to the difficulties (see Apsler and Harding 1991 and Peele 1990 for recent reviews). The small, extant "first generation" literature is plagued with problems such as inconsistencies in the perspectives taken, use of intermediate goals instead of ultimate goals, and too narrow a perspective of outcomes; see the Appendix to this chapter for a review of the specific studies.

Two inter-related issues make CBA and CEA difficult to conduct for the economic evaluation of programs for the treatment of drug abuse. One issue is that there are multiple outcomes of concern, for example, reduced drug use, reduced crime, greater social functioning by the patient, and greater self-esteem of the patient. Consequently, focusing on only one outcome may be misleading. Unfortunately, it is also difficult to aggregate the many disparate outcomes. A second issue is the different and sometimes conflicting perspectives of society, patient, payers, and programs. These two issues and their implications for CBA and CEA will be the focus of this chapter. Each is discussed in greater detail below.

Multiple goals and outcomes

Drug-treatment programs are aimed at reducing the use of illicit drugs, often focusing on one drug alone. The reduction of drug use can be the direct goal of the program but may be an intermediate goal from the perspective of society. There are many other important goals that can be considered the "ultimate" goal; some of these affect the patient per se and others affect society at large. Societal effects include, among others, reductions in drug-related crime and reduced spread of AIDs and other diseases. Effects falling directly on the patients and their families include improved self-esteem, better employment and more stable financial situations, better physical health, and better family functioning and less violence at home. The number and variety of goals make it difficult to conduct a simple comparison of alternative programs because different treatment approaches may yield very divergent patterns of outcomes. For example, therapeutic communities (TCs) may have different long-run effects on each of the many outcomes as compared with methadone maintenance.

Perspective
The priority placed on each of the goals to be achieved by drug treatment will vary depending on whether the perspective of the decision-maker is that of society as a whole, the individual under treatment, the payer, or the program. In fact, whether or not to consider some of these goals at all will depend on the perspective taken. For example, the reduction in crime is of great importance from the societal perspective, but not necessarily from that of a third-party health insurance payer.

Plan of chapter
The plan of the chapter is as follows. Although there are many interesting and important methodological, technical, and data-related issues concerning the economic evaluation of alternative drug treatments, we cannot treat them all in depth here. Instead, our aim is to emphasize the two key issues on perspective and multiplicity of outcomes which we think must be addressed prior to dealing with some of these other issues. We start with a brief overview of the principles of cost-benefit and cost-effectiveness analysis. We then turn to the role of perspective in evaluating of treatment alternatives and the complexities of dealing with multiple goals. The Appendix reviews details of several cost-effectiveness and cost-benefit analyses in the literature.

---

2   Tools of Cost-Benefit and Cost-Effectiveness Analysis

The goal of conducting a CBA or CEA is to provide information that will lead to achieving the greatest value per dollar spent on a treatment or program. The issue underlying a CBA or CEA inquiry could be framed as how to get the greatest gain for a given budget, could be aimed at determining the optimal amount to be spent on a treatment or project, and/or could be aimed at project selection. The literature on CBA, CEA, and related approaches provides a set of tools to conduct such an evaluation and hence achieve these goals (Drummond et al. 1992). It is important to note that the goal of both cost-benefit and cost-effectiveness analysis is not cost-minimization per se; they both are directed at getting the best value for given resources.

Here we briefly describe CBA and CEA to provide the framework for the more specific application of these methods to treatment for substance abuse. We start with CBA for several reasons. First, it is the broadest and most comprehensive of a set of related methods that include CBA, CEA, cost-utility analyses and other newer developments. CBA was the first method of this group to be developed. Many of the tools of CEA and the other related methods are derived directly from CBA and share a common theoretical framework.

Before turning to the tools of CBA and CEA it is useful to keep in mind that these tools are embedded in a broader decision-making setting. First, the goals of inquiry should be specified. If a particular program is under investigation, it should be established that the program has been effective; it does not make sense to conduct a cost-benefit analysis on an ineffective program. Further, establishing that the program caused the effect is a requisite to further inquiry. Then alternatives to achieving the stated goals should be considered. That is, one program may be cost-beneficial, but would not necessarily be the most cost-beneficial approach. Thus the broad set of alternative methods should be kept in mind. The perspective of the decision-maker is also important and is an issue that we deal with extensively in this chapter. The other area of our focus is the potential for far-ranging costs and benefits. By far-ranging, we mean to imply far-ranging in terms of both time frame and breadth of costs and benefits.

The theoretical basis for the approach used in both CBA and CEA is established in welfare economics, using the Kaldor–Hicks Criterion; see Gramlich (1990), Little (1958), and Starrett (1988). The principle is that if the winners gain enough to potentially compensate the losers for their losses, then the project is worth doing. The winners do not, in fact, have to compensate losers; the criterion is only that there is the potential to do so. An alternative principle, that of the Pareto Principle, requires that the compensation in fact be achieved. That is, under the Pareto Principle, society should implement all changes in which at least one person can be made better off, and no one is worse off after the compensation has taken place. However, due to the difficulties of implementing the compensation (e.g., measuring and enforcing redistribution), in practice this requirement would be very difficult to implement and few initiatives would be enacted.

Cost-benefit analysis (CBA)

In its simplest interpretation, CBA is an analytic method designed to help decision-makers. In CBA, the analyst considers, quantifies, and when possible and appropriate, values in monetary terms all of the costs and benefits associated with a specific program. In a CBA, all costs and benefits are considered and then a determination is made as to whether the benefits outweigh the costs (in present value terms). The analyst values all costs and benefits in monetary terms in order to aggregate the costs and benefits into a single indicator. Using the aggregate figures, one can then make comparisons based on the net benefits.

Sometimes, as in the case of treatment for drug abuse, determining which benefits to include and how to measure, value, and aggregate them is difficult. Outcomes of interest in the area of drug treatment tend to be resistant to quantification in any terms (e.g., increased self-esteem), and particularly to valuation in monetary terms. Many of the potential benefits are non-pecuniary (e.g., reduced transmission of HIV) and intangible (e.g., better family functioning, reduced fear of crime, and better parenting). Attempting to place a monetary value on these outcomes is highly problematic because of the absence of markets for these activities, and because of the ethical/equity issues raised. Because these non-pecuniary and intangible benefits are real and important, any analysis that includes only benefits that can be quantified in monetary terms would be incomplete and possibly badly biased. Furthermore, although intangible themselves, some of these intangible outcomes have real dollar costs associated with them; personal expenses to deter crimes and foster care for abused children are examples. These related costs can be helpful in finding pecuniary measures for the intangibles.

Willingness-to-pay surveys, or as they are sometimes referred to, contingent valuation surveys, could be used to place monetary values on outcomes (see Tolley et al. 1994). In willingness-to-pay surveys, individuals are asked to report how much they would be willing to pay to achieve a specific outcome. These responses can then be used to value outcomes. A strength of this method is that individuals themselves are valuing the outcomes and may be using a broad spectrum of benefits in their assessments (e.g., value to self, to friends, and to family). There are also weaknesses. Because the achievement of an outcome may be hypothetical, the individual may not have a realistic idea as to how he or she would value the outcome if actually faced with the decision. Further, each individual may be responding without actually considering their own actual income limitations. In the case of treatment for substance abuse, there will be multiple beneficiaries from effective treatment: society at large, the payer, the patient, and the friends and families of the patient. A thorough assessment from society's perspective would involve surveying all parties on their willingness to pay.

Turning to costs, cost components would include program costs, costs to the patient, and opportunity costs, more generally. Program costs are easily understood and are generally reflected in an operating budget of the program. Program costs may be paid for by public or private insurance, by the individual, or by charity from the provider. Costs to patients may include their share of the bill for treatment, their travel costs to treatment, other out-of-pocket costs (e.g., babysitting), and their time lost due to treatment. One way in which an economist's view of costs may differ from the common view is that costs could include foregone opportunities; these are called opportunity costs. Both patients and programs can incur opportunity costs. Opportunity costs of treatment to individuals could be the inability to simultaneously partake of another treatment. Other opportunity costs of treatment would be that patients' time in treatment would not be available for other activities such as working for pay, leisure pursuits, or time spent on household activities.

Cost-effectiveness analysis (CEA)

Because the goals of drug-treatment programs and other medical interventions are often difficult to value in monetary terms and hence to aggregate, CEAs are often conducted to make an economic evaluation of alternative treatments. This is a simpler and narrower approach, but may be more feasible to implement and may be quite appropriate for certain situations. A CEA examines only one outcome or one outcome at a time and measures that outcome in its natural units. A CEA determines which treatment produces a single desired outcome at the lowest per unit cost; it does not attempt to aggregate benefits into a summary, monetary measure. Costs, however, are still typically analyzed in monetary terms.

In the case of treatments for illicit drug use, cost-effectiveness ratios, for example, could indicate how much it costs to produce one drug-free day per patient, and which intensity of treatment is more cost-effective per drug-free day on average. CEAs could be employed to direct governmental funding toward the most cost-effective treatment with a specific outcome in mind.

A strength of a CEA relative to a CBA is the ease of measuring the outcome in natural units and that one does not have to aggregate unlike outcomes. However, that only one outcome at a time can be examined is a limitation. Cost-utility analysis or CUA is an extension of both CEA and CBA that allows for aggregation of multiple outcomes without placing monetary values on the outcomes. In CUAs, a utility measure, such as "quality of life" may be employed. See Kamlet (1992) for a comprehensive discussion of cost-utility analysis, its linkage of cost-effectiveness, and the sorts of valuations embedded in traditional economic approaches, based on the von Neumann-Morgenstern axioms. Although quality-adjusted life years may be used to aggregate some benefits, it may not aggregate all of the potential effects in many cases. For example, in the case of substance-abuse treatment, an assessment of utility by the patient would fail to capture the utility to the rest of society, which is also effected.

Below when we refer to CEA, we include both cost-utility analysis and the more narrowly defined CEA construct. This is a common use of the term CEA.

CBA or CEA

For both CBA and CEA, the primary issue is one of obtaining good value for resources used. The choice of using CBA versus CEA depends upon the question to be asked as well as availability of data and ease of valuing costs and outcomes. Sometimes the analysis may be conducted with a budget in mind, in which case the question becomes: how can a program or treatment achieve the greatest benefit given the budget? At other times, a particular goal may be desired and then the issue is how to achieve the goal by the cheapest method. In some cases the question could include an evaluation of the optimal level of treatment.

In the case of treatment for drug abuse that has multiple consequences, each CEA and CBA has advantages in trying to determine the best overall treatment program. In the case of CEA one would have to either select a single goal, rank order the goals, or use a summary measure, such as health-related quality of life measure (QALYs). Failure to capture all of the consequences in a CEA of a single outcome could lead to a biased assessment of the relative merits of alternative treatments. This would occur unless the other consequences of these treatments were identical or substantially positively correlated with the dimension studied. However, neither is likely. Further, it has been shown that the multi-dimensional goals such as crime reduction, increased employment, and greater self-esteem are not correlated within treatment regimes; for evidence on the independence of outcomes, see Simpson et al. (1978), Rounsaville et al. (1982), and Kosten et al. (1987). Thus, a CEA on a single outcome could be quite misleading and, consequently, could misdirect resources. CEAs of multiple outcomes, taking each outcome in turn as the one of interest (and ignoring the rest) could provide inconsistent results across outcomes. That is, one treatment might be most cost-effective for increasing employment while another might be most cost-effective for reducing crime. A feasible CBA could overcome the problems associated with the narrowness of a CEA. In CBA, one would aggregate the total dollar valuation of all outcomes. However, a CBA would be extremely difficult to conduct for treatment of substance abuse because of the difficulty of aggregation to a summary statistic. Willingness-to-pay methodology has been used in some circumstances, but could be difficult in the case of substance abuse. The difficulty would be in part due to the multiple perspectives involved, that is, one might have to survey the many parties, including "society" who would be affected.

To some extent, the literature on economic evaluations for general medical treatments has dealt with the issue of multiple outcomes of interest by using summary measures such as the years of health-related quality of life (QALYs); see Patrick and Erickson (1993). This approach also shifts the focus from a specific outcome or a set of outcomes to the utility of these outcomes, and away from intermediate outcomes to the ultimate measure of their value. We know of no comparable literature for drug-abuse treatment, however.

When CBA and CEA analyses are conducted carefully with meaningful decisions as to how to conduct the study, they can be extremely informative. Of course, neither are helpful if they are poorly conducted or if they are based on poor or inappropriate data. Also, neither of these two methodologies deals explicitly with issues of equity or the distribution of costs and benefits across subgroups. These issues must be dealt with separately.

Although it is very difficult, it is also quite useful, given the dearth of knowledge in this field, to conduct economic evaluations of treatment programs for drug abuse.

Effectiveness and causality
The undertaking of a CEA or CBA analysis is predicated on the effectiveness of the treatment program. If the treatment is not effective, there is no point in a CBA or CEA evaluation. Further, a basic underpinning of any cost-benefit analysis is that the treatment *caused* the observed changes; this is in contrast to a simple correlation between treatment and outcomes. The assumption in such analyses is that changes in the health outcome of interest are a direct result of the treatment, e.g., the changes in outcome were not due to patient selection effects, and would not have occurred without the intervention. If, for example, the patient entered a treatment program

because he or she had "bottomed out" and had decided to make changes, then entering into the program might have been correlated with the reduced drug abuse that would have occurred even in the absence of treatment. In such a case, the program and the reduction in illicit drugs are correlated. However, the program itself may not have facilitated the improvement.

Establishment of causation should be a prerequisite in any evaluation of effectiveness prior to the formulation of CBA or CEA. However, causation can be difficult to establish. Randomized clinical trials are used in order to ascertain causality. Even in these settings, causality may be questioned if there are selection biases in the patient's willingness to participate and to remain in the trial. Outside of an experimental setting, causation is even more difficult to show. Appropriate natural experiments could be useful but not typically available. For a further discussion, see Mullahy and Manning (1995).

3   Issues of Perspective

Several different groups can be affected by a treatment program. Society, for example, may be asked to bear part of the costs of a program and may benefit as well through reduced crime, reduced spread of AIDS and TB, among other benefits. The patient may be asked to pay monetarily and clearly devotes time and effort to the program; the patient would expect to benefit in multiple, but different dimensions. Which treatment provides the best value may depend upon the perspective from which the decision is to be made. What may be costly, or alternatively of value to one group, may not be so to another group. The analyst must know the perspective or viewpoint from which the study is to be conducted in order to determine whose benefits and costs are to be considered. The perspective of the analysis determines which costs and benefits, by whom, for whom are to be counted in the evaluation of the alternative treatments. Eisenberg (1989) and Warner and Luce (1982) discuss the relationships between perspective, study design/type, and cost types to be included. The perspective may also determine what constraints are in effect, if budget or political constraints are relevant.

Several different perspectives are frequently used for both CBA and CEA. These include the broader societal perspective, the payer's perspective, the patient's perspective, and the provider's perspective. The broadest of these perspectives is the social one. It considers the implications of the alternative treatments for all of the possible parties or individuals affected by the treatment alternatives, not just some special subset of actors.

Social perspective

Under the social perspective, a CBA of a treatment would enumerate all the changes in outcomes for all affected individuals, value these changes, assess the quantity of resources used in providing treatment, and place values on the resources used. In the case of costs, both direct and opportunity costs of the treatment should be considered. If the value of the benefits exceeds the costs of the resources used, then the treatment is worth doing from a CBA social perspective. This single evaluation, however, does not address the issue as to whether this is the best of all possible uses of resources. In order to make broader conclusions, one would have to compare across alternative programs and other uses of resources. CBAs and especially CEAs are often conducted comparing one program with another. This still does not give a global view of optimal resources, but may give practical direction to decision-makers.

A CEA is used to analyze an outcome of interest to society and to compare costs from a societal perspective. Two policies might be considered and ranked according to costliness per unit of that outcome; the least costly alternative would be preferable. The same process could occur for each of several different outcomes. However, it may be that no program or policy dominates in terms of achieving each single outcome in the least costly way.

Note that as mentioned above, even when the perspective is that of society, how the program or treatment affects the *distribution* of costs and benefits is not valued in the CBA or CEA analyses. That is, although society may especially value a redistribution toward the poor or those in poor health, this is not typically reflected in the calculation or evaluation of the costs and benefits. Instead, all of the costs and benefits are aggregated and who benefits and loses is not factored in, rather the emphasis is on the magnitude of the benefit.

Payers, patients, and programs

The other perspectives consider a smaller set of actors as relevant to the decision. Instead of considering the benefits and costs for all of the affected parties, each of the other perspectives considers only those benefits and costs that are relevant to their decision-makers. Sometimes the cost and benefit accruing to each perspective can be clearly delineated. Other times it may be more difficult. Take for example, the perspective of a private third-party insurance payer (such as Blue Cross/Blue Shield). The payer could consider only the benefits to itself of a well-served constituency (that is, the enrolled population is content enough not to switch plans), and the charges for treatment that must be paid by the insurer as the only relevant costs. Thus the private third-party payer would ignore the benefits or costs to others except to the extent that these indirectly affect the payer. As an example of an indirect effect, consider copayments borne by the enrollees; large copayments could make the enrollees sufficiently unhappy with the services of their payer that they might switch insurers, thus hurting the third-party payer. Alternatively, the third-party payer may directly consider costs and benefits borne by the enrollees. In the latter case, copayments by the enrollees and improved productivity on the job, for example, would be of direct concern to the third-party payer in a cost-benefit analysis. It is somewhat difficult to characterize the interest of the private third-party payer because of the complexities of direct and indirect effects.

Although there is some uncertainty surrounding the concerns of a third-party, private payer, it is unlikely that this perspective on treatment for heroin addiction would consider the financial and personal effects of the resulting reduction in criminal activity, or the effect on welfare payments. Further, it might not consider the time costs of treatment faced by its enrollees or their families. To the extent that the private insurer must pay for inpatient and outpatient medical costs, but not the costs of family care-giving or an outpatient pharmaceutical treatment (if it were not a benefit of the insurance plan), it would tend to favor policies which would shift the burden of treatment away from covered services onto uncovered ones. Thus, it is possible that what is optimal from a third-party payer's perspective may not be socially optimal, and vice versa.

The perspectives for Medicare and Medicaid may be even more complex. At one level, these are public institutions, which should have the public welfare at heart; thus, they should follow the social perspective. However, their formal responsibilities, the limitations of the budgeting process, and political realities will tend to give these programs a more limited view of the benefits and costs. For example, to the public payer with society's well-being in mind, welfare and disability payments and health plan costs are clearly relevant to the analysis, but these are often not considered in medical assessments by the federal government. Furthermore, the effects of crime reduction and time costs are rarely, if ever, considered by public payers of health programs.

Similarly, individual states may have a complex set of goals embedded in their perspective. State governments often provide some funding for drug treatment. They should have the well-being of the citizens of their state in mind. This could result in the state paying for drug treatment both to help the addicted as well as to reduce the crime and other related adverse effects of the state. On the other hand, the bureaucrats in charge of such decisions may invoke a more parochial view.

Treatment programs may also have some mixture of motives. They may have the societal goal of reducing the adverse affects of drug use, but would also have the narrower view of their program, its financial stability, and its staff as well as its patients. Patients would have their own benefits and costs in mind in their decisions regarding treatment, e.g., initiating and stopping treatment and where to seek what kind of treatment.

To illustrate concretely the importance of the perspective taken, we contrast and compare the differences in which costs and benefits would be of concern to which parties. In tables 7.1, 7.2, and 7.3 we have listed a number of potential gains (benefits) and losses (costs) from the treatment for substance abuse. Benefits and costs can be either positive or negative, depending on whether the treatment considered increases or decreases that outcome or cost. Table 7.1 lists potential benefits, ranging from the intermediate and direct outcomes of reduced drug use to reduced need for transfer payments. Table 7.2 deals with ultimate outcomes. We will discuss these distinctions in section 4 below. Table 7.3 indicates cost components. Our intent here is to list major issues, and not necessarily to provide an exhaustive list of all possible benefits and costs. Separate columns are provided for three of the more common perspectives that an analyst might employ – social, private payer, and patient. In each cell of the table we have indicated with an "a" or a "p" those benefits and costs that are relevant from the vantage of a particular perspective. The "a" indicates that all of the item should be included, while the "p" indicates that only part is relevant. A dash (–) or a blank indicates that the item is not relevant to that perspective. For example, all of the health-status and functioning effects are relevant to the social perspective, but a private payer (such as Blue Cross/Blue Shield) may only be interested in those which directly affect its clients.

The entries in the tables illustrate some interesting issues.

Transfer costs. The first issue has to do with government transfer payments – cases in which the government taxes one group of individuals and transfers money to another group, without

Table 7.1   Benefits of treatment for drug abuse.
(a = applies; p = partly applies; − = inapplicable)

		Perspectives		
	Benefits	Society	Patient	Private Payer
1	**Reduced Drug Use by Drug User**			
	Illicit drug being treated	a	a	a
	All other illicit drugs	a	a	a
	Alcohol	a	a	a
2	**Better Psychiatric Functioning and Mental Health of Drug User**			
	Antisocial personality	a	a	p
	Depression	a	a	p
	Anxiety	a	a	p
	Self-esteem	a	a	p
3	**Improved Physical Health of Drug User**			
	Own health status (e.g., hepatitis and overdoses)	a	a	p
	Reduced use of med. care paid by:			
	Self	a	a	−
	Private insurer	a	−	a
	Public insurer	a	−	−
	Charity	a	−	−
	HIV status and other communicable diseases	a	−	p
	Drug-related accidents			
	Self	a	a	a
	Others	a	p	p
	[Needle sharing (can be separate from AIDS or HIV as a behavior)]	a	p	p
4	**Better Employment and Other Use of Time by Drug User**			
	Establish initial employment and better job performance	a	a	−
	Attending school or vocational training	a	a	−
	Other constructive activities (e.g., family, friends hobbies)	a	a	−
	Reduced time in jail	a	a	−
5	**Better Fulfillment of Role in Family**			
	Reduced family violence	a	p	−
	Better family functioning	a	p	−
	Good upbringing for children (not pass on the drug habit)	a	p	−
	Better housing and food for family (better spending patterns)	a	p	−
	Financial stability and better planning	a	p	−

	Perspectives		
Benefits	Society	Patient	Private Payer
6 Better Functioning in Society and Market Place			
Better self-esteem	a	a	–
Better role model for peers and children	a	p	–
More educated consumer	a	p	–
Long-run planning	a	p	–
Pay-bills	a	p	–
Tax payer	a	p	–
7 Reduced Crime			
Harm against property	see text	p	–
Harm against persons (lives saved, hospital bills)	a	–	–
Reduced pressure on criminal justice system; jail, courts, and police	a	–	–
Reduced fear and less change in behavior by citizens due to fear of crime	a	–	–
Less need for protection (eg. private security)	a	–	–
8 Less Use of Transfer Programs			
Income transfers	–*	p	–
Health and support services	a	p	–
Administrative expenses	a	–**	–
Deadweight loss of tax and transfer	a	–**	–
Deadweight loss due to disincentive of welfare programs	a	–**	–
9 Program-Related Outcomes – Intermediate Outcomes*			
Retention			
Attendance and interaction at groups			
No. of infractions			
Counselor ratings			
Patient satisfaction with program			

*   Excludes part that is effectively a transfer payment. Includes administrative expenses and welfare losses due to taxation.

**   Only includes the small part that affects the patient directly.

*** Difficult to classify because these are proxies for outcomes which may be fully or partly of value depending on the perspective.

Table 7.2 Attributes of the quality of life of treatment of drug abuse.
(a = applies; p = partly applies; − = inapplicable or not directly)

	Perspectives		
Attributes	Society	Patient	Private Payer
Well-Being of:			
1 Drug Addict, Better:			
Enjoyment of time	a	a	−
Physical functioning	a	a	−
Psychiatric functioning	a	a	−
Productivity			
home	a	a	−
labor market	a	a	−
Self-esteem	a	a	−
Role fulfillment and enjoyment			
family	a	a	−
friends	a	a	−
Financial stability	a	a	−
Planning for long run	a	a	−
Housing situation	a	a	−
2 Family and Friends of Drug Addict			
Better enjoyment of family and friends, less			
violence, more involvement	a	p	−
Better role models for children, care of children,			
nutrition, housing	a	p	−
3 Rest of Society*			
Reduced worry about crime	a	−	−
Reduced need to change behavior out of fear			
over crime	a	−	−
Reduced personal harm and violence	a	−	−
Greater ability to devote financial resources to			
other priorities*			
private resources	a	−	−
public resources	a	−	−
Newly generated tax revenues from addicts			
working	p**	−	−

* Greater resources are available because there is a reduced need for public money to be spent on police, courts, jail, and charitable medical care necessary for victims of crime, violence, and accidents, and a reduced need for private money to be spent on private crime deterrence and medical care.

** Includes only the administrative costs and deadweight losses as negative benefits (or positive costs). The rest should be considered a transfer payment.

Table 7.3 Costs of treatment for drug abuse.
(a = applies; p = partly applies; – = inapplicable or not directly)

		Perspectives		
Costs		Society	Patient	Private Payer
I Program Costs				
(a)	Staff	a	p**	p**
	Clinical			
	Training and recruitment			
	Medical			
	Support (administrative, security, custodial)			
	Volunteers (counselors, teaching, Board of Directors)			
(b)	Medical	a	p**	p**
	(Methadone or other drugs			
	Physical exams			
	Urinalysis			
	Other)			
(c)	Building and Capital Equipment	a	p**	p**
	Rent or equivalent			
	Equipment (medical equipment, copy machines, computers, etc.)			
	Furniture, security system			
(d)	Variable Expenses	a	p**	p**
	Office supplies			
	Utilities			
	Insurance			
	Meals or stipends for patients			
2 Patient				
	Opportunity costs of time of treatment (time with family, friends, working)	a	a	–
	Direct costs (transportation, babysitting, etc.)	a	a	–

** Patient and payer care about program costs to the extent that they are charged for them.

compensating those who were taxed. The most common example is
that income taxes are transferred to the poor through welfare
payments. For example, disability payments are a transfer from the
non-disabled to the disabled. To a much more limited degree, theft
could be considered a transfer payment to the extent that goods are
being transferred from one individual to another. From a social
perspective, transfer payments are a redistribution of income, not a
net gain or a loss. Transfers per se do not change welfare because
what the gainers gain offsets what the losers lose, and, with an
exception discussed below, no resources are consumed in the
process.

There is, however, what is called the "deadweight loss" of the
taxes used to finance these transfer payments. Taxes contribute to
inefficient use of resources by distorting behavior, for example, the
labor-supply decisions of individuals. Transfer programs also incur
administrative expenses. Distortions in behavior and administrative
costs are the disadvantages of transfer payments. Alternatively,
some transfer programs can have side welfare gains. Those programs
that in essence offer some "insurance" value to individuals by
protecting them against adverse and unexpected outcomes (e.g.,
disability, unemployment, and poverty), reducing the ex-ante
financial risk to the individual of disability and unemployment.

Thus, with the exception of deadweight losses, administrative
expenses, and changes in risk-bearing, there are no net gains or
losses due to transfer programs from a social perspective. However,
from the perspectives of particular parties, the entire amount of the
transfer payments can constitute losses or gains. For instance, if a
treatment reduces the need for the Federal or State Government to
transfer payments, this is a budgetary benefit for them. For example,
individuals who are taxed would consider it a benefit if, due to an
effective treatment, they no longer had to pay so much in taxes to
support the needy. Recipients of a transfer payment consider the
payment to them a benefit.

Time costs of treatment. The time costs of treatment (the total value
of time consumed by treatment itself) are very real costs both from
a social perspective and from the patient's perspective. Time spent
in treatment diverts time from other possible uses, e.g., leisure, or
working for money to buy other goods and services. This is the
opportunity cost of time. Opportunity costs of time can be associated with money-making alternatives, such as working for wages,
and also can be associated with non-pecuniary uses, such as time
spent with one's family. Both pecuniary and non-pecuniary alternative uses of time should be considered. Thus collecting and

including only information on work-related income losses is inadequate for an analysis from the social and/or personal perspectives because it misses some non-market opportunities.

In the case of treatment for illegal drugs, the opportunity cost of patients' time spent in treatment has been considered by some to be a benefit rather than a cost; the reasoning is that time spent in a program is time off the streets for addicts. Thus there would be less of an opportunity for the individual to harm him or herself and less opportunity to commit crimes. However, if one takes the full social perspective, then time costs to the patient and the reduction in undesirable activities should each be enumerated separately and both should be included in the analysis. The time of the patient could be valued as zero or even negatively if the patient considered his or her activities outside of treatment to be self-destructive.

Note that while the opportunity cost of patients' time is a cost from the perspectives of the patients and society, it is not relevant from the perspective of the payer. An insurer does not have to pay for the time of patients and thus does not consider this to be a relevant cost. How the treatment program considers the time cost of individuals is more uncertain. It does not directly bear the time cost of the individual in treatment, but the program may have to be concerned about the amount of treatment time in order to attract and keep patients in the program, so they may care in indirect ways.

4   Issues of Multiple Outcomes

In order to correctly conduct a CBA or CEA, one needs to consider carefully the benefits and costs that should be included in such an evaluation. As discussed above, one critical step in this process is the identification of the correct perspective for the analysis. The perspective will help to dictate the set of benefits and costs that should be considered. Once the perspective has been determined, there are still decisions to be made as to what benefits to include.

The decision as to which benefits to consider is particularly pertinent for evaluations of treatments for drug abuse because there are multiple outcomes that are considered to be of importance. Some may consider reduction in or abstinence from illicit drug use as the primary focus, while others may consider the primary concern to be reduced crime. Some patients and programs may consider reduced drug use as the primary goal while much of the funding for methadone maintenance and other drug-treatment programs may have been promoted on the grounds of reduced crime.

We pose three stylized possibilities as to which of the multi-dimensional outcomes should be included in evaluations. The first view might be called the traditional, uni-dimensional approach of focusing only on drug use. This is seen in the first entry of table 7.1. The second, more recent approach emphasizes a multi-dimensional view of the outcomes, including reduction in illicit drug use and crime, as well as other outcomes related to better psychiatric functioning, reduced fear of crime in society, better self-esteem, better family functioning, and others as listed in table 7.1.

The third approach would be to use quality of life or utility measures to summarize or capture the value of all of the attributes of the program to both society and the drug users. Table 7.2 provides an example of the dimensions or attributes that this perspective might encompass for drug-treatment studies. Although this approach has not yet been used in drug-treatment studies, there are many analogies to this approach found in evaluations of other medical treatments. Instead of measuring effectiveness of medical treatment in clinical units, one would use functioning, the quality of life, or the individual's utility. Further, one would consider the utility gains of other beneficiaries from the reduced spread of disease and crime. A general medical example would be where, instead of considering the outcome of visual acuity after cataract surgery, the concern was with the quality of the individual's life as measured by their improved ability, due to surgery, to enjoy such activities as reading newspapers and books, and their ability to conduct their daily life because they can now drive, read, etc. In the case of drug treatment, the utility of the patients' and their family, and/or of society would be relevant, depending on the perspective taken.

The three frameworks are discussed below in a progression from the earliest to most recent developments. Also, in that order, they represent outcomes that are easiest to hardest to quantify.

Traditional, uni-dimensional view
The most obvious and direct benefit from drug-treatment programs is the reduced use of illicit drugs. Many effectiveness studies have used reduced drug use as the sole measure of outcome. Further, some studies on treatment effectiveness use retention in treatment as a proxy for future reduction in use of illicit drugs; the reasoning is that retention predicts later reduction in drug use.

Consistent with this uni-dimensional outcome would be the view that drug addiction is a progressive disease that should be stopped or many adverse outcomes for the addict and society will be felt; see Kosten et al. (1987) for more on this. The implication is that drug use is causally linked to the adverse outcomes of ultimate concern, thus stopping drug use will stop the cascade of ill effects. Drug use is seen as a sufficient statistic that captures all of the other consequences of drug abuse. Even in this uni-dimensional view, there are measurement issues and debates about this outcome. For example, should complete abstinence be the goal, should only the drug that is being treated (e.g., heroin) be considered, and should self-reported drug use be considered a valid measure or would objective measures such as urinalysis have to be employed? Other considerations are how to consider dropouts of the program, those who repeatedly seek treatment, and relapse.

If a single measure of outcome is to be used as a summary of all outcomes of interest, the outcome measure must not only capture the full benefit at a specific point of interest, but it must also be complete over time. Because different treatments may have different time courses of benefits and costs, a complete analysis should track or model such courses. Unfortunately, many studies of effectiveness and cost-effectiveness have not been comprehensive in modeling the time course of effects. Some studies use one-year quit rates, or the lack of criminal activity after a year, as measures of outcome. This approach of using an outcome from a limited time frame, such as a one-year quit rate, is a legitimate way of conducting the CEA as long as: (1) all other programs that are competing for consideration can be summarized or compared using the same metric; and (2) differences in the outcome at this point in time fully capture differences in all possible subsequent events (the mid-term outcome is a complete and sufficient statistic). Both must hold for the mid-term outcome to be an adequate summary measure. An example of what could be a problem is a comparison of two treatments with very different time paths of costs and benefits. If the survival curves for drug abstinence are different by more than a proportional factor – that is, if the shapes of the survival functions are quite different – then the one-year quit rates or any other intermediate outcome will provide a very incomplete and potentially misleading assessment of future outcomes of interest. Fisher and Anglin (1987) provide displays of survival curves that indicate very different shapes for the survival curves for different treatments.

Most of the studies that we reviewed only measure the benefits and/or costs of drug-abuse treatment over a relatively limited time frame. For example, Hubbard et al. (1989) reported their costs and benefit analysis for the period from one year prior to treatment to one year after treatment; they did report some outcomes (e.g., prevalence of criminal activity) for longer periods. Goldschmidt (1976) and McGlothlin and Anglin (1981) also reported results spanning just a few years of experience. Although these are relatively long time frames as compared with many medical studies, they might not capture the full range of the benefits that accrue to reduced drug use.

Reporting benefits and costs for a time period shorter than the full span of benefits is understandable given the costs and difficulty of conducting long-run follow-up studies. Some questions can be fully answered using a relatively short period of observation. For example, will a treatment pay for itself over a specified period or, which is the most cost-effective treatment over this period? The problem is that the overall best alternative may not be selected if the time period under observation is not representative of future periods. An alternative to actually following individuals for a long period is to use modeling to capture the longer-run impacts. For an example of the approach, see the article by Maidlow and Berman (1972).[1] Further, Hser and Anglin (1991) provide an interesting discussion of the course of disease and the role of survival analyses.

Multi-dimensional view
An alternative to the uni-dimensional view is that there are multiple outcomes of concern. This view is substantiated in the large domain of outcomes that are commonly surveyed in clinical trials for drug treatments and in treatment programs themselves (McLellan et al. 1980, 1982). These domains of outcomes are indicated in table 7.1 where categories one through five and seven compose the sub-parts of the commonly used Addiction Severity Index (McLellan et al. 1980, 1982). French, Rachel and Hubbard (1991) also provide a list of consequences of drug abuse and consider a variety of outcomes. Although considering a larger set of outcomes is more difficult and more costly to measure, the information on some of these categories is often gathered in drug-treatment settings through standardized assessments, e.g., the Addiction Severity Index (ASI). Categories six and eight, those of societal and welfare costs, are not part of the ASI, but have been discussed in evaluations of the social costs of drug users and the benefits of treatment. The ninth category of "program outcomes" (e.g., retention in the program) is the set of intermediate outcomes discussed previously. In fact it should not properly be considered in this list of multi-dimensional outcomes but is sometimes discussed in this framework, again as a proxy for more long-term success.

The multi-dimensional perspective is obviously the most comprehensive, and use of the different dimensions would best measure the total impact of the program. However, aggregating the disparate measures is difficult, if not impossible. Nonetheless, ignoring the multiple outcomes could severely bias choices of the best program. Weisbrod, Test, and Stein (1980) and Test and Stein (1980) provide an example of how to incorporate the many outcomes that may be useful in evaluating drug-treatment programs. They presented a quite comprehensive view of costs and benefits in their CBA analysis of the then experimental in-community treatment of severely mentally ill patients, as an alternative to the then more commonplace treatment in mental hospitals. Although the study did not deal with drug abuse or its treatment, it provides an interesting contrast to some of the drug-abuse literature because of the comprehensiveness of their assessment of costs and benefits.

They compared two different programs on the costs and the benefits of treating the chronically disabled psychiatric patient. The commonality of their topic with that of substance-abuse treatment is that in both cases there are several potentially important domains of outcomes. They calculated the costs of each program in monetary terms when they could. In addition to the direct costs of treatment, the justice system costs and the criminal activity tallied in some of the drug-abuse literature; they also included: (1) indirect treatment costs from social service agencies, community agencies, and sheltered workshops; (2) cash transfer payments, and in-kind food and lodging costs, as well as earned (employment-based) income; (3) family burden; (4) patient mortality; (5) patient mental health status and functioning. Health-care costs included direct treatment costs and emergency room use. They listed all of the relevant outcomes in their natural units. Some were easily placed in monetary terms; they included aspects such as improved decision-making and improvements in labor-market outcomes such as days worked and number of times job changes occurred.

They then compared each of the benefit categories across the two programs. The overall assessment of the program did not yield a single summary measure but rather compared the costs of each program and the relative benefits in each category. This method provided, as they said, "a structure for weighing advantages and disadvantages." In some cases such a structure with substantial quantitative information will be sufficient for making well-informed decisions.

Quality of life approach

The quality of life approach attempts to combine multiple outcomes into a single indicator. In this approach, the ultimate goal of drug-treatment programs would be to increase the well-being of the drug user and his/her family, as well as possibly the rest of society. These increases in well-being or utility gains occur through intermediate outcomes such as reduced drug use. In this approach, what matters is not drug use per se but the utility placed on the ability of the patient and others affected to function well in the various dimensions of his or her life, and to enjoy his or her life. Attempts are made to measure the utility or "quality of life" through surveys. Analyses combining the methods of CBA and CEA and utility indicators are referred to as "cost utility analyses."

This utility-based approach has not been used in the current drug-abuse effectiveness literature, but it is employed elsewhere; see Drummond et al. (1992) and Kamlet et al. (1992) for a discussion and examples. Table 7.2 lays out some outcomes that would be of concern in utility analyses of substance-abuse treatment programs. Note that as in table 7.1, there are several different parties that may be affected in utility terms: the drug users, family and friends, and society. Individuals' utility could be affected through their roles as a family member, a productive member of society, as a friend, and as an independently capable individual. These and others are among the attributes to be valued in utility terms. Society's well-being could be improved by an effective treatment through, among other things, reduced fear of crime, a reduced need for individuals to change their behavior due to crime, a release of resources that would have otherwise been spent on crime deterrence, and better health through reduced public health risks.

The idea of focusing on the ultimate goals is appealing. The difficulty in this approach is that of measurement, which may be more difficult as compared to the other two approaches discussed above. However, there is a large and growing literature on measuring utility and quality of life. There are now many standardized quality of life scales (Patrick and Erickson 1993). Of course, in this case of a large spillover of effects to those other than the drug abusers alone, a utility assessment should include the utility of other members of society as well as of the drug abuser. One would need to survey individuals who are affected by the crime caused by drug use to be able to capture the effects of drug abuse that are external to the drug abuser.

5   Directions for Future Research

There is great potential for carefully conducted cost-benefit and cost-effectiveness analyses of drug-treatment programs to guide policies and programs to achieve the greatest gain per dollar spent. The existing literature has provided useful initial information on the major elements in the evaluation of the effectiveness and cost-effectiveness of alternative treatments for the abuse of illicit drugs. But as with any first generation of studies, there are a number of methodological and data issues that need to be addressed before we can be confident about conclusions as to the cost-effectiveness or cost-benefits of drug treatment in general, or the relative merits of individual treatment approaches. Below we discuss several areas that need to be addressed in future work.

Perspective. Analysts need to decide on and consistently maintain an explicit perspective of the study so that they can properly determine which benefits and costs merit inclusion. This would help to avoid a number of conceptual errors that exist in the current literature, e.g., the inclusion of transfer payments and the exclusion of patients' opportunity costs of time in studies that purport to take a social perspective.

Multi-dimensional outcomes. Analysts need to provide a more complete enumeration, measurement, and valuation of the benefits related to treatment for illicit drug use. The literature tends to focus on retention in treatments, and reduction in drug use, or criminal activity. Retention in treatment is used as a proxy indicator for other outcomes and, itself, is not an ultimate goal. Reduced drug use and reductions in crimes should be important elements of any evaluation of drug-treatment programs, but the current literature often ignores a number of the other potentially important benefits, many of which are listed in tables 7.1 and 7.2. The work by Weisbrod et al. (1980) on the treatment of the seriously mentally ill provides a useful example of a more comprehensive approach.

Summary measures of outcomes. New methods should be devised to summarize and to value in common units the multiple outcomes of drug-abuse treatment. Without a summary measure of outcomes, determination of an overall preferred program is not ensured. Using only one (or only one at a time) can lead to biased evaluations unless the outcomes are perfectly correlated or the omitted outcomes are equivalent across treatments. In the drug-abuse treatment literature, the outcomes have been shown to be largely uncorrelated, so the use of outcomes one at a time is likely to be misleading in many cases.

Longer-term outcomes. The analysts need to be more complete in their enumeration and valuation of the longer-term consequences of drug treatment. Much of the current literature relies on outcomes at relatively short follow-up periods as proxies for longer-term results. These should only be used if they meet the specific conditions of being "complete and sufficient statistics" in the sense of being perfect predictors of future consequences of concern. If treatments have different time courses of costs and benefits, then a shorter-term horizon could unfairly penalize programs that tend to have the costs up front and the benefits downstream. It is understandable, however, that studies use intermediate outcomes, given the difficulties and costs of follow-up. This suggests that future studies should strive for innovations in collecting data from longer-term follow-ups in a more efficient manner.

Causality. Future studies should be sure to establish that the direction of causality flows from treatment to outcome. Outcomes and treatments can be correlated but not necessarily causally linked. The issue of causality, of course, presupposes that a treatment is effective. If a treatment is not shown to be effective, there may be little need for a cost-benefit evaluation.

Summary

In this chapter we have focused on the importance of perspective and multiple outcomes and have discussed a number of other issues, and, hopefully, have provided some guidance to future research on CBA and CEA in the evaluation of treatment programs for abuse of illicit drugs. Cost-benefit and cost-effectiveness analyses that are comprehensive and carefully conducted could make substantial contributions to the policy debate on drug-abuse treatment, providing guidance on priorities for program-related decisions and for public funding.

Appendix

Although "cost-benefit" and "cost-effectiveness" are issues of broad concern in the evaluation of drug-abuse treatment, we could find very little literature that attempts to specifically deal formally with both effectiveness and costs. There are numerous studies that examine treatment efficacy, fewer that analyze treatment costs, and very few that have attempted to do both. In their review of the literature, Apsler and Harding (1991) identified two studies, McGlothlin and Anglin (1981) and Hubbard et al. (1989). In addition, we found the Goldschmidt (1976) study, a series of RTI studies that are patterned on the Hubbard et al. (1989) study, and more recently, the Alterman et al. (1994) study. The review of the CBA and CEA literature (Elixhauser 1993) provided additional articles on screening and methodology, but none on the cost-benefit of treatment for the use of illicit drugs.

Goldschmidt. One of the earliest CEA on drug effectiveness that we could find was the 1976 analysis of methadone maintenance (MM) and therapeutic-community treatment (TC) conducted by Goldschmidt. This effectiveness analysis focused on abstaining from heroin, as measured by the norm-abider criteria and the heroin-free criterion; the former includes recent drug use (other than cannabis), abuse of alcohol, criminal activity, or lack of employment as evidence of treatment failure. None of the other benefits from tables 7.1 and 7.2 were reported. His analysis did correct for the "durability" or survival of successful treatment for a period of over two years for methadone maintenance (MM), but not for therapeutic community (TC). His cost analysis was limited to the program costs of treatment, excluding most of the other costs listed in table 7.3.

McGlothlin and Anglin. McGlothlin and Anglin (1981) conducted an analysis of the effect of the 1976 closing of a methadone maintenance program in Bakersfield, California, using patients in ongoing treatment in Tulare County as a control group. The strength of this study is the natural experiment that involuntarily ended access to treatment for a set of clients; this study thus avoids the "volunteer" bias present in some evaluations. The two samples were followed up with interviews and record checks after a period of approximately two years. The terminated sample exhibited higher re-addiction rates, criminal activity, and abuse of alcohol during the period between discharge and interview. At the time of the follow-up survey, there were only small differences between the two groups, other than a doubling of the fraction of the terminated group being under legal supervision.

McGlothlin and Anglin adopted a social perspective for their cost analysis which included treatment, justice system costs, property and other crime, and welfare costs. The crime costs are the income realized by the addict, not the costs to the victim or the aversive costs of non-addicts. The differences in costs between the terminated group from Bakersfield and the comparison group from Tulare shows slightly lower net costs for the terminated group. However, when readmissions to treatment were included, the comparison group exhibited lower cost and higher measures of effectiveness.

This analysis was more comprehensive in its assessment of both benefits and costs than the earlier Goldschmidt analysis. Its time frame of nearly two years was roughly comparable, but still somewhat incomplete in capturing the full longer-term implications of treatment. There was evidence that some of the patients were still relatively drug free after two years in both the comparison and involuntarily terminated group. Despite the stated social perspective of the analysis, the list of benefits and costs was incomplete compared with those in a full social perspective; see tables 7.1, 7.2, and 7.3. The effects of the treatment on family and others are only captured in criminal activity, and then under-counts the extent of these effects. The beneficial effects of treatment on the individual patient's health status and functioning and employment activity were not included. The effects on other medical costs that are related to either drug addiction or drug-related violence were not captured. The inclusion of welfare payments was inappropriate from a social perspective because this is a transfer payment. The welfare payments should be included as a benefit if the perspective is that of the patients', and as a cost if the perspective is that of the rest of society, but should be excluded if using a social perspective.

Hubbard et al. and succeeding RTI studies. Hubbard et al. (1989) examined the course of treatment and outcome for nearly 11,000 individuals enrolled in 41 different programs of treatment for drug abuse in 1978 through 1981 in the Treatment Outcome Prospective Study (TOPS). The programs were grouped into methadone maintenance, therapeutic community, and outpatient drug-free programs. Using multiple waves of interviews, they found evidence that treatment led to decreases in drug use and in criminal activity and suicide attempts. They also found substantial reductions in crime and other costs related to drug abuse, reductions large enough to cover the costs of treatment.

In Hubbard et al. (1989), they did not limit themselves to any particular perspective for the analysis. Instead, they presented components of economic impacts from a number of important perspectives. In framing their research, they listed three goals: (1) reduction or elimination of drug abuse; (2) reduced criminal activity associated with addiction; and (3) restoration of drug abusers to productive lives. These objectives recognize the fact that there are multiple parties affected by the alternative treatment regimens. Nevertheless, their social perspective analysis does not appear to be complete.

From the nature of the data available, they were only able to consider the relatively short-term effects of treatment (up to a year after treatment). Thus, if a particular episode of treatment has either positive or negative health, crime or other effects/costs that extend beyond the window of the study, their approach will omit those items. The risk is that the resulting statements about whether the treatment is cost effective, let alone effective could be incorrect because the omissions could lead to a systematic bias in the evaluation. If treatment costs are largely at the beginning of the period of time, but the benefits stretch out over a number of years, as Hser and Anglin (1991) conjecture, then the net value of a specific treatment will be understated.

Further, the conclusions could have been biased because not all of the affected parties, let alone all of the effects and costs, were included. Some of the costs enumerated here and in Harwood et al.'s documentation (1988) of crime "costs" include things which are essentially transfer costs from a social perspective, although they are very real costs from the perspective of the victims of crime. The costs of behavior to avoid crime and the pain and suffering of victims of crime were excluded. Losses in income, if that income is not from a job (legal or illegal), are really transfers and should be neglected, unless the perspective is that of the public payer of costs or the patient's perspective. Indirect costs of treatment (time lost due to treatment) were not fully accounted for, although they are required for both the social and patient's perspective. To the extent that current drug abuse has medical costs other than current drug-abuse treatment, the results were also incomplete. To the extent that patients may substitute alcohol or other substance abuse for the substance being treated, the estimates presented would be incomplete, and tend to overstate the social, patient, and public-payer net gains to be had from a particular substance-abuse treatment.

Alterman et al. Alterman et al. (1994) recently reported a comparison of results on the costs and effectiveness of a day treatment and inpatient rehabilitation program for the treatment of a cocaine-dependent group of men. Although the study is not a formal cost-effectiveness study, it does report results on both outcomes and costs. For example, one conclusion of the study was that although inpatient treatment was much more expensive as compared with day hospitalization, the two treatments had rather similar outcomes. Outcomes of concern were reduced alcohol and cocaine use and improved psycho-social and health functioning. In addition, they determined the program completion rates and the number of days of cocaine use in the past 30 days. The study examined two types of costs: (1) treatment costs based on various VA records; and (2) lost wages by patients. Subjects were randomly assigned to either of the two programs. The population was VA clients from the inner city of Philadelphia and was largely black and had low incomes.

The study had several advantages. First, the treatments compared were established programs offered by a major provider of such services (the VA), and thus dealt with effectiveness, rather than efficacy. Second, the use of randomization avoided selection biases and allowed the study to address causality in an unbiased way.

The study also had a number of disadvantages. First, because of the limited term of the study, the results may provide an incomplete enumeration of the full, longer-term outcomes and the costs of the alternative treatment regimens. Further, the comparisons could be biased if the outcomes and/or costs had different time paths for different treatments. Second, the list of benefits and costs did not form a complete list of the possible consequences to the provider, the patient, or to society at large. Further, research costs and costs that would typically fall on patients were not carefully and appropriately handled. Third, the sample sizes were small enough that some relatively large differences could not have been detected with suitable statistical precision. In addition, as the sample was all male and drawn from a poor VA population, the results may not generalize.

Summary

Many of the articles in the literature on drug-abuse treatment focus on a more limited set of benefits than is necessary for any of the major perspectives for either CBA or CEA – society, payer, or patient. Sometimes, instead of maintaining a stated perspective, the perspectives were mixed. Although the focus on treatment and crime costs does deal with major elements of public concern, the other costs and benefits need to be enumerated and included in the analyses.

Notes
We would like to thank Louise Russell and an anonymous reviewer for helpful comments.

1   This chapter illustrates the approach of modeling, but makes a number of serious errors that limit its usefulness. First, many of the benefits and costs discussed in this chapter are altogether absent. Instead, they rely on treatment costs and theft. Second, they use discounted cost and benefits assuming that each individual lives the average number of years. Instead, they should have calculated the discounted sum of *expected* costs and benefits, using a life table for the probabilities. Because discounting is nonlinear, the sum of the discounted amount over the average number of years is not equal to the sum of the discounted expected benefits and costs.

References

Alterman, A., et al. 1994. Effectiveness and Costs of Inpatient versus Day Hospital Cocaine Rehabilitation. *Journal of Nervous and Mental Diseases* 182:157–63.

Anglin, M.D., and D.G. Fisher. 1987. Survival Analysis in Drug Program Evaluation. Part II: Partitioning Treatment Effects. *International Journal of the Addictions* 22:377–87.

Anglin, M.D., and Y.I. Hser. 1990. Treatment of Drug Abuse. In *Drugs and Crime*, ed. M. Tonry and J.Q. Wilson (13, 393–460). Los Angeles: University of Southern California Press.

Anglin, M.D., G.R. Speckart, M.W. Booth, and T.M. Ryan. 1989. Consequences and Cost of Shutting off Methadone. *Addictive Behaviors* 14:307–26.

Apsler, R. 1991. Evaluating the Cost-Effectiveness of Drug Abuse Treatment Services. In *Economic Costs, Cost-Effectiveness, Financing, and Community-Based Drug Treatment* (NIDA Research Monograph Series 113). Rockville, Md.: National Institute on Drug Abuse.

Apsler, R., and Harding, W.M. 1991. Cost-Effectiveness Analysis of Drug Abuse Treatment: Current Status and Recommendations for Future Research. In *Drug Abuse Services Research Series, No. 1: Background Papers on Drug Abuse Financing and Services Approach.* DHHS pub. no. (ADM). Rockville, Md.: National Institute on Drug Abuse.

Ball, J.C., W.R. Lang, C.P. Myers, and S.R. Friedman. 1988. Reducing the Risk of AIDS through Methadone Maintenance Treatment. *Journal of Health and Social Behavior* 29:214–26.

Ball, J.C., L. Rosen, J.A. Flueck, and D. Nurco. 1981. The Criminality of Heroin Addicts when Addicted and when off Opiates. In *The Drugs-Crime Connection*, ed. J.A. Inciardi (39–65). Beverly Hills: Sage Publications.

Ball, J.C., and A. Ross. 1991. *The Effectiveness of Methadone Maintenance Treatment.* New York: Springer-Verlag.

Ball, J.C., J.W. Shaffer, and D.N. Nurco. 1983. The Day-to-Day Criminality of Heroin Addicts in Baltimore: A Study in the Continuity of Offense Rates. *Drug and Alcohol Dependence* 12:119–42.

Battjes, R.J., and R.W. Pickens. 1988. *Needle Sharing Among Intravenous Drug Abusers: National and International Perspectives.* NIDA Research Monograph No. 80. Rockville, Md.: National Institute on Drug Abuse.

Bradley, C.J., M.T. French, and J.V. Rachal. 1991. *Costs and Financing of Standard and Enhanced Methadone Treatment.* Research Triangle Park, N.C.: Research Triangle Institute.

Campen, J.T. 1986. *Benefit, Cost, and Beyond.* Cambridge: Ballinger.

Clifford, P.R. 1991. *Manual for the Administration of the Important People and Activities Instrument.* Providence, R.I.: Brown University.

Deschenes, E.P., M.D. Anglin, and G. Speckart. 1991. Narcotics Addiction: Related Criminal Careers, Social and Economic Costs. *Journal of Drug Issues* 21:383–411.

Des Jarlais, D.C., and S.R. Friedman. 1989. AIDS and the IV Drug User. *Science* 245:578.

Dole, V.P., and M. Nyswander. 1965. A Medical Treatment for Diacetylmorphine (Heroin) Addiction: A Clinical Trial with Methadone Hydrochloride. *Journal of the American Medical Association* 193:80–4.

Drummond, M.F. 1980. *Principles of Economic Appraisal in Health Care.* Oxford: Oxford University Press.

———. 1981a. *Studies in Economic Appraisal in Health Care.* Oxford: Oxford University Press.

———. 1981b. Welfare Economics and Cost-Benefit Analysis in Health Care. *Scottish Journal of Political Economy* 28:125–45.

Drummond, M.F., G.L. Stoddart, and G.W. Torrance. 1992. *Methods for the Economic Evaluation of Health Care Programs.* Oxford: Oxford University Press.

Eisenberg, J.M. 1989. Clinical Economics: A Guide to the Economic Analysis of Clinical Practices. *Journal of the American Medical Association* 262:2879–86.

Elixhauser, A. (ed.) Health Care Cost-Benefit and Cost-Effectiveness Analysis (CBA/CEA) from 1979 to 1990: a Bibliography. *Medical Care* 31:JS1–JS150.

Fisher, D.G., and M.D. Anglin. 1987. Survival Analysis in Drug Program Evaluation. Part I: Overall Program Effectiveness. *International Journal of the Addictions* 22:115–34.

French, M.T., and J.A. Fairbank. Forthcoming. Patterns of Drug Use, Criminal Activity, and Employment Status among Patients in Federally-Funded Drug Abuse Treatment Programs. Substance Abuse (in press).

French, M.T., and Zarkin, G.A. 1992. The Effects of Drug Abuse Treatment on Legal and Illegal Earnings. *Contemporary Policy Issues* 10:98–110.

French, M.T., J.V. Rachal, and R.L. Hubbard. 1991. Conceptual Framework for Estimating the Social Cost of Drug Abuse. *Journal of Health and Social Policy* 2:1–22.

French, M.T., G.A. Zarkin, R.L. Hubbard, and J.V. Rachal. Forthcoming. The Effects of Time in Drug Abuse Treatment and Employment on Post-Treatment Drug Use and Criminal Activity. *American Journal of Drug and Alcohol Abuse* (in press).

———. 1991. The Impact of Time in Treatment on the Employment and Earnings of Drug Abusers. *American Journal of Public Health* 81:904–7.

Fuchs, V.R. 1980. What is CBA/CEA, and Why are They Doing This to Us? *New England Journal of Medicine* 303:937–8.

Goldschmidt, P.G. 1976. A Cost-Effectiveness Model for Evaluating Health Care Programs: Application to Drug Abuse Treatment. *Inquiry* (March):29–47.

Gramlich, E.M. 1990. *A Guide to Benefit-Cost Analysis*, 2nd edn. Englewood Cliffs, N.J.: Prentice Hall.

Harwood, H.J., R.L. Hubbard, J.J. Collins, and J.V. Rachal. 1988. The Costs of Crime and the Benefits of Drug Abuse Treatment: A Cost-Benefit Analysis using TOPS Data. In *Compulsory Treatment of Drug Abuse: Research and Clinical Practice*. NIDA Research Monograph 86, ed. C.G. Leukefeld and F.M. Tims (209-35). Rockville, Md.: National Institute on Drug Abuse.

Horgan, C. 1991. Cost of Drug Treatment Programs: Preliminary Findings from the 1990 Drug Services Research Survey. Paper Presented at the NIDA National Conference on Drug Abuse Research and Practice, Washington, January.

Hser, Y.I., and M.D. Anglin. 1991. Cost-Effectiveness of Drug Abuse Treatment: Relevant Issues and Alternative Longitudinal Modeling Approaches. In *Economic Costs, Cost-Effectiveness, Financing, and Community-based Drug Treatment*. NIDA Research Monograph Series 113. Rockville, Md.: National Institute on Drug Abuse

Hser, Y.I., M.D. Anglin, and Y. Liu. 1990. A Survival Analysis of Gender and Ethnic Differences in Responsiveness to Methadone Maintenance Treatment. *International Journal of the Addictions* 25:1295–315.

Hu, T., N.S. McDonnell, and J. Swisher. 1991. The Application of Cost-Effectiveness Analysis to the Evaluation of Drug Abuse Prevention Programs: An Illustration. *Journal of Drug Issues* 11:125–38.

Hubbard, R.L., et al. 1983. An Overview of Client Characteristics, Treatment Services, and Treatment Outcomes for Outpatient Methadone Clinics in the Treatment Outcome Prospective Study (TOPS). In *Research on the Treatment of Narcotic Addiction – State of the Art*, ed. J.R. Cooper, F. Altman, B.S. Brown, and D. Czechowicz (714-47). Rockville, Md.: National Institute of Drug Abuse.

Hubbard, R.L. and M.T. French. 1991. New Perspectives on the Benefit-Cost and Cost-Effectiveness of Drug Abuse Treatment. In *Economic Costs, Cost-Effectiveness, Financing, and Community-based Drug Treatment*. NIDA Research Monograph Series 113 (94–113). Rockville, Md.: National Institute of Drug Abuse.

Hubbard, R.L., E.M. Marsden, J.V. Rachal, H.J. Harwood, E.R. Cavanaugh, and H.M. Ginzburg. 1989. *Drug Abuse Treatment: A National Study of Effectiveness*. Chapel Hill, N.C.: University of North Carolina Press.

Institute of Medicine Committee for the Substance Abuse Coverage Study. 1990. *Treating Drug Problems*, vol. 1. Washington: National Academy Press.

Joe, G.W., D.D. Simpson, and R.L. Hubbard. 1991. Treatment Predictors of Tenure in Methadone Maintenance. *Journal of Substance Abuse* 3:73–84.

Johnson, B.D., P. Goldstein, E. Preble et al. 1985. *Taking Care of Business: The Economics of Crime by Heroin Abusers.* Lexington, Mass.: Lexington Books.

Kamlet, M.S. 1992. *A Framework for Cost-Utility Analysis of Government Health Care Programs.* Washington: U.S. Department of Health and Human Services, Public Health Service.

Kosten, T.R., B.J. Rounsaville, and H.D. Kleber. 1987. Multidimensionality and Prediction of Treatment Outcome in Opioid Addicts: 2.5-year Follow-up. *Comprehensive Psychiatry* 28:3–13.

Little, I.M.D. 1958. *A Critique of Welfare Economics.* Oxford: Oxford University Press.

Maidlow, S.T. and H. Berman. 1972. The Economics of Heroin Treatment. *American Journal of Public Health* 62:1397–406.

McGlothlin W.H., and M.D. Anglin. 1981. Shutting off Methadone: Costs and Benefits. *Archives of General Psychiatry* 38:885–92.

McLachlan, J.F.C. and R.L. Stein. 1982. Evaluation of a Day Clinic for Alcoholics. *Journal of Studies on Alcohol* 43:261–72.

McLellan, A.T., L. Luborsky, G.E. Woody, et al. 1981. Are the "Addiction Related" Problems of Substance Abusers Really Related? *Journal of Nervous Mental Disorders* 169:232–9.

McLellan, A.T., L. Luborsky, C.P. O'Brien, et al. 1980. An Improved Diagnostic Evaluation Instrument for Substance Abuse Patients: The Addiction Severity Index. *Journal of Nervous Mental Disorders* 168:26–33.

McLellan, A.T., L. Luborsky, C.P. O'Brien, and G.E. Woody. 1991. The Addiction Severity Index, as adapted by the National Institute on Alcohol Abuse and Alcoholism and R.O.W. Sciences, Inc. Washington, January 28.

McLellan, A.T., L. Luborsky, C.P. O'Brien, G.E. Woody, and K.A. Druley. Is Treatment for Substance Abuse Effective? *Journal of the American Medical Association* 247:1423–28.

Metzger, D., G.E. Woody, D. De Philippis, A.T. McLellan, C.P. O'Brien, and J.J. Platt. 1991. Risk Factors for Needle Sharing among Methadone Treated Patients. *American Journal of Psychiatry* 148:636–40.

Miller, W.R., and R.K. Hester. 1986. Inpatient Alcoholism Treatment: Who Benefits? *American Psychologist* 41:794–805.

Mullahy, J., and W.G. Manning, Jr. 1995. Statistical Issues in Cost-effectiveness Analysis in *Valuing Health Care: Costs, Benefits, and Effectiveness of Pharmaceuticals and Other Medical Technology,* ed. Frank Sloan, 149–84. New York: Cambridge University Press.

National Institute on Drug Abuse. Drug Abuse Services Research Series (Background Papers on Drug Abuse Financing and Services Research). Washington: Department of Health and Human Services.

Newman, R.G. 1987. Methadone Treatment: Defining and Evaluating Success. *New England Journal of Medicine* 317:447–50.

Patrick, D.L. and P. Erickson. 1993. *Health Status and Health Policy: Allocating Resources to Health Care.* Oxford: Oxford University Press.

Peele, S. 1990. Research Issues in Assessing Addiction Treatment Efficacy:

How Cost-effective are Alcoholics Anonymous and Private Treatment Centers? *Drug and Alcohol Dependence* 25:179–82.

Rounsaville, B.J., T. Tierney, K. Crits-Christoph, et al. 1982. Predictors of Treatment Outcome in Opiate Addicts: Evidence for the Multidimensionality of Addicts' Problems. *Comprehensive Psychiatry* 23:462–78.

Rufener, B.L., J.V. Rachal, and A.M. Cruze. 1977. *Management Effectiveness Measures for NIDA Drug Abuse Treatment Programs, Volume I: Cost Benefit Analysis.* DHEW pub. no. (ADM) 77-423. Rockville, Md.: National Institute on Drug Abuse.

Shepard, D.S., and M. Thompson. 1979. First Principles of Cost-Effectiveness Analysis in Health. *Public Health Reports* 94:535–43.

Simpson, D.D., J. Savage, M. Lloyd et al. 1978. *Evaluation of Drug Abuse Treatments Based on First Year Follow-up.* NIDA Monograph Series 78 (701). Rockville, Md.: National Institute on Drug Abuse.

Sindelar, J.L. 1991. Economic Cost of Illicit Drug Studies: Critique and Research Agenda. In *Economic Costs, Cost-Effectiveness, Financing, and Community-Based Drug Treatment.* NIDA Research Monograph Series 113. Rockville, Md.: National Institute on Drug Abuse

Starrett, D.A. 1988. *Foundations of Public Economics.* Cambridge: Cambridge University Press.

Test, M.A., and L.I. Stein. 1980. Alternatives to Mental Hospital Treatment, III: Social Cost. *Archives of General Psychiatry* 37:407–12.

Tolley, G. D. Kenkel, and R. Fabian. 1994. *Valuing Health for Policy: An Economic Approach.* Chicago: University of Chicago.

Warner, K.E., and B.R. Luce. 1982. *Cost-Benefit and Cost-Effectiveness Analysis in Health Care: Principles, Practice, and Potential.* Ann Arbor, Mich.: Health Administration Press.

Weinstein, M.C., and W.B. Stason. 1977. Foundations of Cost-Effectiveness Analysis for Health and Medical Practices. *New England Journal of Medicine* 296:716–21.

Weisbrod, B.A., M.A. Test, and L.I. Stein. 1980. Alternatives to Mental Hospital Treatment: Economic Cost-Benefit Analysis. *Archives of General Psychiatry* 37:400–5.

8

Some Economics of Performance-Based Contracting for Substance-Abuse Services

Margaret Commons and Thomas G. McGuire

Introduction

In general, outcomes of substance-abuse treatment are monitored for two different, but overlapping purposes: treatment research and program evaluation.[1] Outcomes may be monitored as a means of researching the effectiveness of treatment in general or in specific modalities. Treatment research is intended to add to the general scientific knowledge of a treatment's effectiveness; it requires rigorous methodology, both in data collection and data analysis. Program evaluation, evaluating the outcome of treatment at specific program(s), is intended for the recipients of, or payers for, services. While scientific rigor would be the ideal in program evaluation as well, the need is for information which is more quickly accessible, in terms of both ease and expense of collection and analysis. Performance-based contracting (PBC) is built on program evaluation; the state monitors outcomes to assess the performance of the programs with which it contracts, helping the agency to allocate treatment resources efficiently.

PBC is intended to be a practical system with information collection and incentives designed to assist a state agency in overseeing treatment programs. Currently, PBC is used by the state substance-abuse agencies in Oregon and Maine. Numerous other states have expressed interest in PBC, and in at least one state, the Maine system is being studied as a way of meeting a legislative mandate requiring accountability. In this chapter, we review some of the practical issues associated with PBC from several perspectives. Our review proceeds using Maine's PBC system as a backdrop, so this system is briefly described first. We then review some of the basic economics of program budgeting, noting the inherent discrepancy between the conditions associated with economic efficiency and the information normally available for budgetary decisions. These inherent problems impose important limitations on PBC. Next, PBC raises the issue of how "performance" is to be defined in practice. The goals of treatment may not be agreed upon, and the ideal measures of performance may therefore not be obvious. Even if goals can be articulated and agreed upon, however, the next practical issue to be confronted is that attainment of these goals must be measured with accessible information. We illustrate the compromises necessary between validity and measurability discussing performance measures employed in Maine.

Performance-Based Contracting for Treatment Services in Maine

The Maine Office of Substance Abuse (OSA) is responsible for the planning, development, implementation, and coordination of all of the State's substance-abuse activities and services. OSA does not directly provide substance-abuse treatment services; it licenses, certifies, and contracts with private agencies which in turn provide services. On 1 July 1991, OSA introduced incentives and performance monitoring into its contracts with treatment providers.

Maine's performance monitoring system allows the State to observe outputs, measured in terms of treatment outcomes, and to pay providers on the basis of these outputs rather than inputs. Maine's contracts continue to require detailed income and expenditure budgets, which are used to determine the level of contracted services and payments. However, payments may not continue in following years if the outputs are not delivered; funding may be decreased or eliminated entirely. In addition, the Maine system attempts to dampen the incentive to treat the less disabled clients by requiring minimum levels of services to specified target populations.

OSA added performance standards to its FY 1992 contracts with treatment providers although no rewards or penalties were attached to performance ratings. OSA monitored performance and reported the results to the providers during the FY 1992 contract year, but the providers were "held harmless." As of 1 July 1992, the beginning of FY 1993, this hold-harmless provision was removed, and providers were held accountable for their performance. The contracting system was designed to reward a provider who met the performance standards within its contracted amount by allowing the provider to retain any surplus funds. A provider who did not meet standards would not be permitted to keep surplus funds, and furthermore, could lose all or part of its funding for the next year. Special conditions – adding/subtracting contract services or requiring that the provider take specific actions to improve performance – could also be attached to continued funding.

OSA receives an appropriation from the legislature, which it then allocates to different programs. Individual programs (or agencies with multiple programs) are notified of their allocations and requested to complete a standard contract, including detailed budget information for both the total program and the services contracted to OSA. The OSA allocation divided by total program income determines the percentage of total program service units purchased by OSA. The implied unit cost for services purchased by OSA is determined by dividing the OSA allocation by the number of service units. OSA, therefore, is purchasing a percentage of the total program and not services to specific individuals. Prior to the introduction of PBC, provider allocations were based on the amount of their funding in previous years, with decreases or increases in the legislative appropriation, spread, for the most part, evenly across all providers. Now, however, performance results may affect the total contract dollar amount used to determine the percentage of total units of service which OSA will purchase. The FY 1994 contracts specifically state "beginning in FY 1994, allocation of resources for the contract year may be affected by agency performance in the previous year."

The fact that OSA is a public-sector entity within a larger state government places constraints on the extent to which it is able to guarantee rewards for high performance. While a state agency may be able to commit contractually to allow retention of surplus, it has relatively little control over its budget. It is therefore possible that budget deappropriations could occur, requiring mid-contract cuts in provider funds. A program which has been allowed to retain its surplus funds but suffers decreases in its current allocation may not believe it has been rewarded. To date, OSA has not found it possible to reward good performers by allowing them to retain surplus funds, due to legislative deappropriations occurring as a result of Maine's current economic situation. However, good performers have been rewarded with additional block grant funds received as a result of the change in funding formula benefiting the rural states. OSA has recently formulated a recognition and reward system which defines levels of performance with associated incentives ranging from recognition from the OSA Director to possible financial rewards (including retention of surplus funds).

The majority of the data used to measure a program's performance come from OSA's standardized admissions and discharge data, the Maine Addiction Treatment System (MATS). This system, operating since October 1989, was designed to allow pre/post testing of potential performance indicators.

Performance is grouped into three areas: efficiency, effectiveness, and special populations. A program "meets standards" overall if it meets minimum levels of performance in each of these areas. For example, to meet overall performance standards, an outpatient program must deliver at least 90 percent of the contracted units of service (efficiency), meet 8 of the 12 effectiveness indicators and 5 of the 8 special population indicators. If a program does not meet minimum levels in each area, it does not meet standards overall. The contract includes separate performance standards for each type of service provided. Different modalities, while often sharing common indicators, have differing minimum standards and numbers of indicators which must be met.

Efficiency standards measure service utilization. In order to meet the efficiency standards, programs are required to deliver a modality-specific percentage of these units. Outpatient standards also specify how units of service are to be broken down into services to primary clients and to co-dependants/affected others.

Effectiveness standards measure treatment outcomes. The program's performance is the percentage of its clients experiencing "good" outcomes. The standards include self-report measures of drug use, employment and employability, lack of criminal involvement, and reduction in problems with family or employers. Effectiveness is measured at the time of a client's discharge from a program and is either a measure of the change in client status between the time of admission and the time of discharge (e.g., reduction in use) or a measure of the occurrence of an event (e.g., no arrest during treatment). The contract specifies a minimum standard, stated as a minimum percentage of clients who should experience the particular outcome, for each indicator and requires that program performance remain at or above the minimum level on a specified number of the total indicators. Table 8.1 lists this information for all program types. There are 12 effectiveness indicators specified for outpatient programs. For example, 60 percent of the program's clients must exhibit reduction of use of the primary substance-abuse problem in order for this indicator to be met. To comply with the effectiveness standards, the program must meet the minimal standard for 8 of the 12 indicators. If an outpatient program does not meet the minimum standard for at least 8 indicators, it is considered a low performer.

Special population standards measure service delivery to target populations, which include women, adolescents, the elderly, and poly-drug and IV drug users. Program performance in this area is based on admissions during the period under examination. Once again, the contract specifies a minimum standard and a required number of indicators which must be met for the program to be deemed in compliance; this information for all program types is contained in table 8.2. There are eight special populations indicators for an outpatient program. For example, 30 percent of an outpatient program's clients must be female. If an outpatient program does not meet the minimum standard on five of the eight indicators, it has not met the performance standards for special populations.

OSA does not directly adjust the performance measures for the possible differences in client severity among programs. The special population measures allow OSA to monitor trends in the type of clients being admitted to programs and therefore to observe whether a program is taking clients who may be easier to treat. Severity of the clients in treatment when performance is measured is not taken into account. In theory it would be possible to develop a severity score, based perhaps on the Addiction Severity Index (McLellan et al. 1986), with which to weight each program's performance. This is another example of the constraints faced by state agencies in implementing and maintaining a performance-based contracting system; to date, limits on OSA staff and financial resources have not allowed the Office to develop, test, and modify the data analysis to include adjustments for case-mix.

The contract between OSA and the provider does not contain explicit formulas equating performance level with funding or the

Table 8.1 Effectiveness indicators, 1993.

INDICATOR	OP	HH	RR	Detox	ES	ARR	NRR	EC	EmS	AOP
Abstinence/drug free 30 days prior to termination	70.0%	85.0%	85.0%	na	85.0%	85.0%	70.0%	80.0%	na	70.0%
Reduction of use of primary SA problem	60.0%	90.0%	85.0%	na	90.0%	95.0%	60.0%	85.0%	na	60.0%
Maintaining employment	90.0%	na	90.0%	na	na	na	90.0%	na	na	na
Employment improvement	30.0%	40.0%	5.0%	na	na	na	30.0%	5.0%	na	na
Employability	3.0%	5.0%	3.0%	na	na	na	3.0%	5.0%	na	na
Reduction in number of problems with employer	70.0%	na	na	na	na	na	70.0%	na	na	na
Reduction in absenteeism	50.0%	na	na	na	na	na	50.0%	na	na	50.0%
Not arrested for OUI offense during treatment	70.0%	na	na	na	na	na	70.0%	na	na	70.0%
Not arrested for any offense	95.0%	na	na	na	na	na	95.0%	na	na	95.0%
Participation in self help during treatment	40.0%	90.0%	80.0%	na	95.0%	90.0%	40.0%	55.0%	na	40.0%
Reduction of problems with spouse/significant other	65.0%	95.0%	60.0%	na	na	na	65.0%	na	na	na
Reduction of problems with other family members	65.0%	95.0%	60.0%	na	na	50.0%	na	na	na	65.0%
Reduction of problems in school	na	na	na	na	70.0%	50.0%	na	na	na	70.0%
Referral in continuum of care	na	40.0%	90.0%	45.0%	70.0%	40.0%	na	40.0%	40.0%	na
Referral to self help	na	na	na	20.0%	na	na	na	na	80.0%	na
Time in treatment	na	na	na	4 days	na	na	na	na	na	na
Number to be met:	8 of 12	5 of 8	5 of 9	2 of 3	3 of 4	4 of 6	8 of 11	4 of 6	2 of 2	5 of 8

Notes:
OP: Outpatient
RR: Residential rehabilitation
ARR: Adolescent residential rehabilitation
EC: Extended care
AOP: Adolescent outpatient

HH: Halfway house
ES: Extended shelter
NRR: Non-residential rehabilitation
EmS: Emergency shelter

na = not applicable

Table 8.2 Special population indicators, 1993.

MODALITY	Females	Age: 0–19	Age: 50+	POPULATION Corrections	Homeless	Concurrent psych problems	History of IV drug use	Poly-drug use	Number to be met
Outpatient	30.0%	10.0%	6.0%	25.0%	1.0%	8.0%	12.0%	35.0%	5 of 8
Halfway house	25.0%	na	5.0%	11.0%	4.0%	10.0%	25.0%	40.0%	4 of 7
Residential rehabilitation	40.0%	4.0%	5.0%	10.0%	1.0%	3.0%	15.0%	40.0%	5 of 8
Detoxification	14.0%	1.0%	12.0%	2.0%	20.0%	11.0%	27.0%	28.0%	5 of 8
Extended shelter	14.0%	1.0%	12.0%	2.0%	20.0%	11.0%	15.0%	40.0%	5 of 8
Adolescent residential rehabilitation	48.0%	na	na	18.0%	3.0%	12.0%	12.0%	75.0%	4 of 6
Non-residential rehabilitation	30.0%	10.0%	6.0%	25.0%	1.0%	8.0%	12.0%	35.0%	5 of 8
Extended care	10.0%	na	25.0%	1.0%	55.0%	12.0%	10.0%	15.0%	4 of 7
Emergency shelter	5.0%	1.0%	22.0%	na	59.0%	1.0%	na	6.0%	4 of 6

Note:
na = not applicable

procedures OSA will use to evaluate performance results. All indicators appear to be weighted equally; no indicator or group of indicators is considered to be more important to meet than others. Providers, therefore, do not have the incentive to focus on specific outcomes within the OSA performance-based contracting system. However, the incentive to focus on outcomes monitored by OSA to the exclusion of other possible outcomes remains.

OSA's Use of Performance Measures

OSA staff monitor the performance measures quarterly. They generate cumulative quarterly reports of each program's performance and submit copies to all programs, requesting their review and comment. Programs are given the opportunity to identify and correct any missing or incomplete MATS data. After corrections are made, OSA staff review the performance data and identify programs which are not meeting the standards in any of the three areas: efficiency, effectiveness, and special populations. These low performers are requested to submit a corrective action plan to OSA. The plan must identify the causes of the insufficient performance and the steps to be taken to meet the minimal standards. Programs are offered technical assistance which OSA will either arrange for or provide itself. Corrective action plans may include increased outreach, additional attention to admission and discharge interviews, re-examination of existing treatment policies to increase staff–client contact or similar activities.

The FY 1994 contract allocations are the first to be affected by performance data. In preparation for FY 1994 contracting decisions, OSA staff prepared summaries of the performance of all programs during the first six months of FY 1993[2] (no FY 1992 data could be considered due to the hold-harmless provision). A meeting was held to review the data and rank provider performance. Licensing and program-evaluation staff attended the meeting to add their input into the possible explanations for a program's performance. Each program which did not meet the performance criteria was asked to meet with OSA staff to review the performance data and additional data OSA had prepared (fiscal data – projected versus actual unit costs, recidivism and early dropout rates, time in treatment, and measures of client difficulty). OSA and program staff discussed possible actions to be taken to improve performance. OSA reiterated that FY 1993 performance would affect FY 1994 contracts.

OSA staff have indicated that the intent has been to assist programs in improving their performance and therefore few cuts in funding allocation for the FY 1994 contract year were made on the basis of performance scores. OSA has chosen to contract with certain low-efficiency performers on a fee-for-service basis, ensuring that OSA only pays for services that are actually delivered. Providers with low effectiveness or special population performance have special conditions which address specific indicators included in their 1994 contracts. For example, a program which has performed inadequately on the Age: 0–19 special population indicator might have conditions added to its new contract which require specific outreach activities aimed at this population. Finally, in the case of some low overall performers, OSA has only renewed the program's contract for a period of six months.

Providers have been rewarded for good performance. As mentioned above, additional block grant funds were awarded to certain providers for the provision of specialized group counseling services. In addition, performance data has allowed OSA to target specific agencies it wishes to assist in enhancing their continuum of services. For example, certain agencies offering shelter or residential treatment services have been encouraged to develop outpatient treatment services as well.

Efficient Allocation of Contract Funds

The purpose of PBC is to improve the efficiency of contract fund allocation. It will be helpful in evaluating the potential of PBC to describe efficient fund allocation as a benchmark.

Conditions for efficiency and the goals of PBC

Consider the case of one outcome or output. This output could be an amalgam of a number of outcomes, and include results for the client as well as for society. To enable comparison with cost, measure the value of the output in dollars. Assume further that for any individual who may receive treatment, at least at some point, there are diminishing returns to treatment. For a single potential client, the relationship between funds allocated to that client and output or outcome can be described as in figure 8.1, with cost of treatment the client receives on the horizontal axis, and the value of output in dollars and total cost on the vertical axis. Cost is tracked by a 45° line beginning at the origin. Output or outcome is produced according to the curved line OA. When the client receives no treatment, no outcome is produced. As treatment resources devoted to the client increase, the outcome produced increases, but at a decreasing rate.[3] The efficient expenditure to allocate to this client is E*. At E*, the marginal value of the treatment is just equal to the marginal cost of that treatment, and the difference between benefits and costs is maximized. A better or higher outcome could be achieved for this client if more resources were devoted to his treatment, but the cost of these treatment resources exceed their value, so it is efficient to treat only at level E*.

Each client is characterized by a unique OA schedule. Some respond quickly to treatment, some slowly. The limit on achievable outcome will differ across clients. For any potential client, however, efficiency will be characterized by the same equality between marginal value of output and marginal cost of treatment. Note that this implies that different treatment levels are efficient for each client, and different outcomes will be achieved in efficiency, depending on the shape of the OA schedule.

To sum up, the condition for economic efficiency in fund allocation is that the marginal value of treatment for every potential client is equal to the marginal cost of treatment.

In practice, no decision-maker is in a position to consider allocation of funds for treatment across all potential clients in a state. The decision about resource allocation is made in stages. The legislature decides the level of funding for substance-abuse services, the state agency (OSA) allocates funds to contracts (within legislative restrictions), and personnel at the agency use contract funds to treat clients. It is useful therefore to translate the efficiency condition stated above into what it means for each stage of decision-making.

Efficiency in fund allocation is achieved when:

1   The legislature allocates the right amount of money to OSA to equalize the marginal value of funds to substance-abuse treatment with other social purposes;
2   OSA allocates funds so as to equalize the marginal return across contracts;
3   With contracted funds, the agency allocates funds so as to equalize the marginal return across clients treated;
4   Funds allocated to a client are used to maximize output.

If all four of these conditions are met by the decisions of the legislature, OSA, agencies, and their personnel, social efficiency in contracting for substance-abuse services is achieved.[4]

The four conditions form a natural hierarchy of decisions about funding for substance-abuse programs. While all are necessary for full efficiency to be achieved, conditions lower down the list should still be met for a kind of constrained efficiency, even if higher-level criteria are unmet. In other words, whatever level of funding is available to treat this client, agency personnel should use that money to produce the greatest return (Condition 4 should be met even if 3 and above are not). Whatever level of funds are available in a contract, an agency should allocate that among potential clients to equalize marginal return (Condition 3 should be met even if 2 and above are not). And whatever level of funds OSA has available for contracts, these funds should be allocated among contracts to equalize marginal returns across contracts (Condition 2 should be met, even if Condition 1 is not).

The policy problem addressed in connection with PBC is concerned with Conditions 2–4. Given a budget, can PBC improve efficiency of fund allocation? The basic mechanism, in these terms, is to provide incentives to agencies to do better on 3 and 4. This improves efficiency by itself, of course, and then given this, OSA can do better on 2.

Marginals and averages

An important observation prompted by the production and cost conditions for efficiency just laid out is the distinction between conditions for efficiency and the nature of the information typically reported back to the state contracting agency. Efficiency has to do with marginal conditions, whereas totals or averages are observable and reportable. Consider the client depicted in figure 8.1. The agency responsible for treating the client may be able to report the funds spent on the client, E, and the outcome Q, but the marginal change in output with a change in funds is not observable or reportable. A fundamental problem in PBC or related policies is that OSA does not see the information necessary to make an allocation based on relative marginal productivities.

Figure 8.2 shows cost and productivity curves for two clients, which could be regarded as two clients typical of those receiving treatment in two different contracts. As before, the efficient level of funding for each client is E_1^* and E_2^*, with the efficient outcome designated Q_1^* and Q_2^*, respectively, for the two clients. Figure 8.2 illustrates the difficulty of judging relative efficiency with reports on totals. The behaviors (E_1^*, Q_1^*) and (E_2^*, Q_2^*) are efficient in the sense that the marginal benefit is equated to marginal cost for each client. It is impossible to reallocate treatment funds and improve

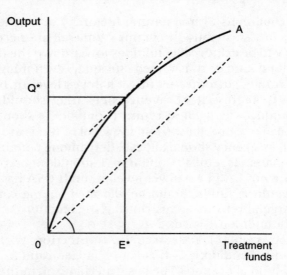

Figure 8.1   Efficient level of treatment.

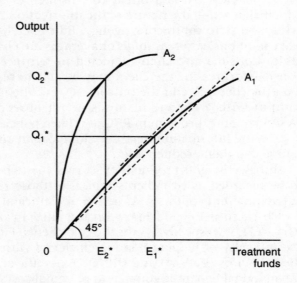

Figure 8.2   Efficient level of treatment two clients.

net social product. And yet, $E_1^* > E_2^*$ and $Q_1^* < Q_2^*$. Contract 2 appears to be conducted more efficiently than Contract 1, whereas in fact they are both as efficient as possible. The cause of the problem is partly an unobserved case mix issue – the state contracting agency may not know that Contract 1's clients are more difficult to treat. Over and above this problem, however, is the problem that the state agency does not in general know where on the productivity curve a program is operating. By seeing just total cost and total output, even assuming as here that these can be perfectly observed, the marginal/total distinction introduces limitations of PBC.

Incentives Under Performance-Based Conditions

In PBC, performance is usually rated by some version of average performance for clients in treatment. An example of such a statistic might be the percentage of clients in an outpatient program who were abstinent for thirty days prior to discharge. In this section, we note some of the basic problems with creating incentives on performance defined in this way. This discussion is informal, but brings out some of the main points. In our ongoing research we are developing more formal theoretical models to study incentives, and will test these with data from the Maine OSA system.

The intended incentives in PBC are to encourage agencies to do better with respect to Conditions 3 and 4 above: to treat the right clients, and to maximize the output for those that are treated. PBC can introduce perverse incentives as well.[5]

Taking clients to look good
The easiest way to attain a high performance in terms of clients abstinent at discharge is to recruit clients who don't use drugs. If you want clients to look healthy at discharge, the best thing is to make sure they are healthy at intake. One version of this selection problem is a levels/change issue. Output of treatment should be considered to be the change in performance caused by treatment. If measured performance is instead the level of performance at discharge, the agency has an incentive under PBC to seek clients who are already rated high in terms of performance. Figure 8.3 illustrates this distinction. Here the level of performance is on the vertical axis, and clients may start at different levels (instead of all being normalized at zero as in previous figures). Client 1 starts at a low initial level, but is

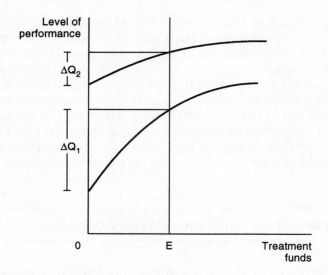

Figure 8.3   Levels and change in performance.

highly responsive to treatment. Client 2 is healthier to start with, and responds less. Clearly, money is better spent on Client 1. This is illustrated by comparing the change in performance, DQ1 for Client 1 and the DQ2 for Client 2 attainable for the same treatment funds E. However, if the agency is rated by the level and not the change, the agency looks better by choosing to treat client 2, since the final performance level is higher.

Taking too few clients
The total/marginal distinction builds in an incentive to take too few clients. Suppose there are a large number of identical clients eligible for treatment and all respond to treatment according to a function $Q(E)$ describing the form of productivity relation depicted in the previous figures. The key feature of $Q(E)$ is that the first derivate, $Q'(E)$ is positive and decreasing. Give the agency a budget, B, and ask what incentives the agency has to take more or fewer clients, given that it will be judged on the average performance, Q, of the clients it treats. Given a budget, how does performance vary by the number of clients treated? And what is the actual total output of the program, and how does that vary with the number of clients treated given a budget? If the agency has a budget B, the funds available per client are B/N, where N is the number of clients.

Total output is number of clients treated times output per client, or NC(B/N). Measured performance is output for the average client or simply Q(B/N). It is straightforward to show that Q(B/N) falls with N, and NCQ(B/N) rises with N. Thus, and very perversely, with positive but diminishing marginal product, economic efficiency implies the agency should spread its treatment resources widely among clients, but the incentive from PBC based on average performance drives the agency in exactly the opposite direction.

Other incentive problems related to PBC have been recognized. Hanushek (1994) discusses Pennsylvania's experience with outcome-based education. Proponents of the system believe improvements will occur as schools focus on student achievement rather than the provision of government-specified course work, allowing teachers and administrators the flexibility to develop new methods and curricula. Opponents argue that the outcomes are poorly defined and the measurement tools are too subjective. They believe top students will suffer as less effort will be required of them to meet the standardized outcomes. Hanushek questions the effectiveness of the entire system since, for the most part, the incentives are undefined.

In a review of the same book, Passell (1994), in comparing two experiments in market socialism in Yugoslavia and Hungary, states that the losers' ability to avoid the consequences of poor performance jeopardizes the entire system. Murnane, cited in Passell, believes it is not easy to create appropriate incentives. The risk is that teachers will "teach to the tests" (Gramlich and Koshel 1975).

One can imagine analogies in the substance-abuse field. As we discuss below, defining and correctly measuring performance is not straightforward; compromises may need to be made between data accuracy and accessibility. Providers may "treat to outcomes" and state agencies, subject to legislative pressures, may not be able to reward the good performers or sanction the bad. Further, as Campbell (1979) warned, "The more any quantitative social indicator is used for social decision-making, the more subject it will be to corruption pressures and the more apt it will be to destroy and corrupt the social processes it is intended to monitor." In other words, improvements in reported performance may be due to induced changes in reporting as well as to "true" improvements. In our continuing research, we will be examining "teaching to the test" type phenomena, as well as changes in reporting practice, and will continue to monitor how the state uses the system.

We close this section by noting that our discussion of incentives is incomplete, focusing as it does only on the unintended incentives created by performance contracting. A more complete treatment would attempt to integrate these considerations with the intended influences on accountability and efficiency.

Up to this point, we have essentially assumed that the state agency is able to measure "performance" and have examined the allocation and incentive issues of the system which is built on this measurement. In the section which follows we discuss some of the issues which face the agency as it defines and measures performance.

Measurement Issues

By definition, performance-based contracting requires that the state define performance and how it will be measured. At a basic level, what the state considers the goals of treatment must be agreed upon. This is not as straightforward as it seems as the treatment field has yet to come to an agreement. One opinion is that substance abuse is a disease which can only be controlled by permanent abstinence; this group might therefore argue that a treatment program should be judged only on the number of clients who are abstinent after treatment. The group at the other end of the spectrum would argue that life functioning outcomes must be measured since substance abuse is a reflection of psychosocial dysfunction and can only be treated by addressing the client's underlying problems. (A detailed discussion of this issue can be found in Longabaugh and Clifford 1992.) The Institute of Medicine, in *Treating Drug Problems*, describes abstinence as "the central goal of drug treatment" but not the only goal. Other goals, "assigned overtly or implicitly by public policy or private payers," include reducing crime, increasing employment, and improving the abusers' physical and mental health (Institute of Medicine 1990, p. 8). A state agency like OSA, with jurisdiction over thousands of abusers in numerous different programs, would design a PBC system to encompass all these goals. However, defining measurable treatment outcomes which confirm that the treatment goals are being met necessarily involves compromises. The state is constrained by the financial and staff resources available (both to the state and to the programs) to collect and analyze the data, the necessity of collecting standardized data, and by factors outside the treatment system. We discuss these problems in relation to certain measures employed in the OSA system.

Self-report issues

In collecting the data with which to measure performance, a state is constrained by both time and funds. The theoretical ideal would be to have the behavior of each client observed 24 hours a day from the time he initiates treatment through discharge and even into a multi-year follow-up period. This is clearly not possible. For many outcome measures, the state must depend on client self-report. Even with measures which are theoretically verifiable, the verification cost and time burden may be prohibitive.

We would expect abstinence to be a treatment outcome measured in any program evaluation system. On face value, abstinence appears to be easily measured; either the client abused his substance(s) of choice during the specified period or not. In order to measure abstinence, a state could either require periodic blood or urine testing or rely on the client's report of substance use.[6] It is hard to imagine a state agency which would have the funds required to test all clients as often as would be required for each substance.[7] If such funds were available to the state agency, they could also be used to finance additional treatment services. Therefore, expending funds to test for abstinence would not necessarily be an efficient allocation of treatment resources by the state.

The state agency, however, must recognize that reliance on client self-report is problematic. The client may not report truthfully for a number of reasons. He may not consider using once or twice to be an issue and may consider himself essentially abstinent and so report. He may be reluctant to admit use of any, or a particular, substance. He may adopt what Aiken (1986) terms "impression management," believing that claiming abstinence will gain him access to treatment or get him out of treatment he does not want. Further, the state agency should recognize that the degree of accuracy across programs may vary with the client population in particular programs, the type and pattern of use, and the conditions and procedures under which the self-report data is collected (Magura et al. 1987).

Magura et al. examined 13 studies on the validity of self-reported drug use in high-risk populations, comparing them using Cohen's (1960) kappa and conditional kappa (attributed to Bishop et al. 1975) as validity coefficients. These coefficients measure the degree of agreement between two variables beyond that expected solely as a result of chance.[8] In their review, Magura et al. found heroin and other narcotics to be more accurately reported than nonopiate drugs. However, the mean of conditional kappa for opiates for all studies reviewed was .48, just under half of the maximum possible agreement score. In their own study, self-reports of drug use by 248 clients of four methadone maintenance clinics in New York City were compared with results of urinalysis. Kappa scores were considerably higher than the mean of the earlier studies reviewed: .61 for opiates, .78 for cocaine, and .74 for benzodiazepines.

The study explored whether selected demographic, behavioral, or treatment-related differences existed between underreporters and those reporting accurately. They found five variables to be associated with underreporting:[9] clinic where enrolled;[10] type of interviewer; client's age; number of medication pickup days; and denial of current criminal activities. For example, clients over the age of 30 were more likely to underreport than those under 30 (50 percent vs. 31 percent). Fifty-three percent of the clients interviewed by professionals underreported drug use, while only 28 percent of those interviewed by paraprofessionals did so. Magura et al. hypothesize that the higher degree of accuracy when questioned by paraprofessionals may be due to better rapport, better detection of inaccuracy, or better interviewing techniques. Whatever the reason, the clinician or other data collector can, intentionally or unintentionally, affect the accuracy of the client's response. This is particularly troublesome for a state which is allocating resources to the program, at least in part, on the basis of response to clinicians' questions.

Another drawback of reliance on self-report concerns the period of time under question. There are two time period issues: recall and immediacy. A client may not remember if an event occurred or the frequency with which it occurred in the applicable time period. For example, if the outcome under question were reduction in use, measured by the response to "How often did you use in the past 30 days?", a client might not remember every time he used and either under or overestimate, reporting truthfully, in his mind, but nonetheless inaccurately, thereby causing mismeasurement of reduction in use. Magura et al. did not ask about use on the days immediately preceding the interview, stating that previous research indicates that "clients' willingness to admit drug use apparently decreases the closer the question relates to the present" (Magura et al., p. 737). They cite a Marsden and Hubbard (1984) study reporting that subjects were more willing to admit drug use in the two weeks preceding the interview than in the three days before the interview.

OSA collects information on a client's primary, secondary, and tertiary substances of abuse. A client is considered abstinent at discharge if he has not used any of the three identified substances during the month prior to discharge. Reduction in use compares frequency of the primary substance between admission and discharge. OSA does not require that programs test for evidence of substance abuse; the clinician's response to the frequency of use question is based on his or her own observation of the client and on the client's report. While recognizing the potential inaccuracy of the data, in order to institute a system which is affordable and practical, OSA must rely on client self-report. Financing testing, even periodic testing, is not feasible. Removing the interviewing from the clinicians is neither feasible nor practical, and may not be in the best interests of the clients.[11]

Data standardization issues

Even if we could assume that self-reports were always completely accurate, outcome data could be flawed due to the requirement that data be standardized. We discuss issues of standardized definitions and of loss of detailed information.

OSA's performance measurement requires that services be targeted to specific populations; one such population is the homeless. People in different areas of the state may have different definitions of what it means to be homeless. In the very rural sections, people might live in camps without running water or reliable heating, but consider themselves to have a "home." However, people living under these conditions in Augusta or Portland would most probably be considered homeless. Individuals often move in and out of homelessness; should a person who is temporarily homeless but in a shelter be placed in the same category as one who lives on the street? Homelessness may also be seasonal, especially in New England. Finally, one individual's definition of homelessness may be different from another's; living temporarily with family or friends may be considered having a roof over one's head and therefore a home, or may be considered not having one's own home and therefore homeless. A state would need a very exact definition of "homeless" to ensure complete standardization across all clients in all programs. Just as it is not possible for a state's contract to cover all contingencies, it may not be possible for a state to define a measure which covers all possible interpretations.

Furthermore, it may not be possible to gather the level of detail necessary to measure an outcome accurately and completely. McAuliffe (1989) contends that the degree of unemployment among active abusers is overestimated, noting that a third of heroin addicts are employed and continue to be mostly employed even while heavily addicted. When measuring employment outcome for clients employed at admission, improvement is more subtle and subjective. Suppose we are measuring improvement in employment status for two individuals. Both are employed, but the substance-abuse problems of one have forced his employer to move him to a job with less responsibility, while the abstinence of the other has enabled his employer to move him to a job with more responsibility. Data standardization requirements – the level of detail necessary to capture the changes described could not easily be standardized or quantified – require that the state utilize much broader measures, such as changes between full-time and part-time status, or simply employed to unemployed. The state is not able to get the full picture.

OSA collects data on employment status at admission and discharge. Six responses are possible: full-time, part-time, irregular (less than 17 hours a week), unemployed but sought work, unemployed but did not seek work, and not in the labor force. Each category is further explained in the OSA manual; for example, full time is defined as 35 hours a week, including part-time jobs totalling at least 35 hours a week, or not working due to illness, strikes, or similar reasons. Two employment outcomes are monitored: maintained employment, and employment improvement.[12] A client is said to have maintained employment if he is employed full time, part time, or irregularly at both admission and discharge. No differentiation is currently made between a client who is full time at admission and discharge and one who is full time at admission but part time at discharge. Both clients are considered employed at both points in time and therefore their "maintained employment" outcome is "good." Employment improvement is measured as a change from unemployed to employed. Again, the finer distinction between a client who is employed irregularly at admission and full time at discharge and one who is employed irregularly at both times is not made. Both clients were employed at admission, and therefore no improvement in employment status has occurred.

External factors

Events outside the control of both treatment programs and clients may affect outcomes. An individual, employed when he entered treatment, becomes and remains abstinent due to the treatment he receives, but loses his job because the local factory closed. The treatment he received was effective but his employment outcome is "bad." In certain areas of Maine, employment fluctuates with the season, where employment rises during potato-picking and wreath-making seasons, but falls at other times. Employment-outcome measures may be artificially inflated or deflated depending on the time of admission and discharge. As another example, the state police in one area of the state begin to strictly enforce drunk driving laws, hiring additional policemen and setting up additional road blocks. Naturally, a larger percentage of the clients of the programs in that area have "bad" criminal involvement outcomes than do the clients of the programs in other areas. This is not, however, a reflection of treatment effectiveness, but of influences outside of the treatment program, and in fact, outside the entire treatment system. Longabaugh and Clifford (1992) suggest a different type of external influence: luck. In their example, one person may drink and drive numerous times without incident while another is in an accident his first time. Treatment of the latter person may have been effective for the most part; he just had a minor relapse but luck was against him and, in terms of program performance measures, against the program as well.

Other measurement issues

When to measure outcomes. Data must be collected at client admission to provide a baseline against which to measure the effectiveness of treatment. Research has shown, however, that data collected at entry or early in treatment are particularly susceptible to self-report inaccuracy. Maisto et al. (1990) found that underreporting of at least certain types of drug use and related events occurred more frequently when the interview took place close to the time of admission. Aiken (1986) found that the clients' initial reports of illicit behavior, sources of income, and life satisfaction were more positive than when they were questioned about the same time period later in treatment or at follow-up. She contends that clients presented a better picture of themselves in order to gain access to treatment. Underreporting at admission may negatively bias outcome measures; treatment gains would be measured against a distorted, higher baseline.

The state would want to collect data at the time of discharge. Longabaugh and Clifford (1992) argue that "for the average patient, treatment's maximum impact will be at completion" (p. 244). Changes in certain outcomes, however, may not be entirely measurable for quite some time after discharge. Consider employment measures. An individual may be employed when he seeks treatment and continue to be employed when he is discharged for noncompliance with the program's abstinence requirement. The treatment he received was not effective. It may take many more months for his employer to fire him, if ever. Nevertheless, this client's employment outcome is "good." Another outcome measure where time to event plays an even more striking part is criminal involvement. An abuser, while in treatment, may support himself through criminal activities for years before being arrested. Treatment has not been effective for these individuals, but their criminal involvement outcomes are "good." Longabaugh and Clifford (1992) argue that follow-up periods of 5 to 10 years may be required to measure health problems adequately but acknowledge that "such feedback would no longer be useful to ongoing programs. . . ." State agencies which are making allocation decisions based on program performance would also find such information of no use.

Due to resource constraints, OSA collects data at admission and at discharge but does not require programs to follow clients beyond the end of treatment. It is recognized that some treatment outcomes may not be measured but to keep PBC practical and manageable, this compromise is necessary.

Attributing effectiveness to a treatment episode. Substance-abuse treatment usually involves multiple treatment episodes in various programs and modalities. The Institute of Medicine (1990) found that the populations treated in different modalities had distinct demographic and drug-use profiles and warns against comparing performance in different modalities "as if their client populations were interchangeable" (p. 134). Recognizing this, the OSA contracting system tailors the indicators and standards to the modality and compares programs within modality rather than across the entire treatment system.

However, PBC does attribute good outcomes to the treatment episode during which the outcome is evidenced in the data, and in this case, ignores the "career" aspect of an individual's treatment. Treatment in a previous program may have laid the foundation for successful treatment later in the course of treatment. Research evidence suggests that the effects of treatment may be delayed and cumulative; it may, therefore, be inaccurate to attribute the effects appearing during a particular treatment episode entirely to that episode (Institute of Medicine 1990, p. 134). This is a compromise which any state agency must make, however, as it is not possible to determine which episode contributed to which effect. As the OSA system has numerous indicators for each modality, it may tie effects to a particular episode, or at least credit programs with effects, as accurately as possible. For example, a program may have laid the foundation for a client's abstinence but during this episode only succeed in reducing use; the program's performance data would at least reflect this success.

Setting standards. In setting the standards which must be met to indicate that a particular indicator or outcome is "good," a state might attempt to employ a norm which is widely accepted by those in the treatment field. Unfortunately, there is little consensus in the treatment field as to what should be considered a "good" outcome or, more specifically, what should be considered a "good" outcome for particular treatments or particular client populations. Treatment is not standardized enough to define rules or formulas converting specific types and numbers of treatment units into specific outcomes. When employing average outcomes during a baseline period to determine standards, the state agency should take into account the affect of outliers. The measurement issues discussed above will affect the baseline data. Perhaps, due to some underlying population difference or external factor, clients treated in specific areas or programs may exhibit a large proportion of good outcomes. The danger is that this might skew the baseline average to a higher level than is accurate, causing the state agency to set standards higher than is reasonable.

When PBC was being instituted by OSA, a committee of agency staff and providers met to review baseline data and discuss standards. This process allowed discussion of and modification of possibly misleading averages.

Level of detail of information reviewed by decision-makers. Ideally all decision-makers would have available to them all details regarding the effectiveness of the treatment received by all clients at all programs. The data would be weighted by the severity of each client's substance abuse, and all noise from external events would be removed. And, of course, the decision-makers would have ample time to review all this information prior to allocating funds. It is not reasonable to believe that a state agency could afford to dedicate this amount of staff time; even if it were possible, it could be argued that it would not be an efficient allocation of resources as the funds supporting the staff salaries could instead be supporting treatment services. There is a loss of information due to the fact that data must be summarized and results aggregated to be presented in a manageable form to decision-makers. Therefore, not only is it an issue of what cannot be observed (as seen above in the discussion of marginal versus average outcome), but it is also an issue of what it is feasible for the decision-maker to review.

Maine has a relatively small population and therefore a relatively small number of abusers and treatment services (for example, consider the treatment system in New York City alone). Therefore, it is possible for the fiscal staff and agency director to be aware of the issues facing specific providers and take into consideration a greater level of detail than might be possible in other areas. Nevertheless, it is not feasible for all involved in the allocation process to know how each program performed on every indicator and what might have affected this performance.

In order to allocate funds to providers on the basis of their performance in terms of treatment outcomes, a state agency must define the desired outcomes and the indicators it will use to measure the outcomes. In this section we have illustrated some of the measurement issues facing the agency. Any PBC system will be the result of compromises between completely accurate outcome measurement on the one hand and practicality, manageability, and affordability on the other.

Conclusion

As Jencks (1994) puts it in his recent book *The Homeless*, "the idea behind performance contracting is simple: service providers should be paid more when they do a good job." The arguments for PBC include the basic one that it would improve accountability, along with a political one stressed by Jencks: if providers were paid only for success, "even Republicans might support their request for more money."

As we have discussed here, PBC is a potentially promising but also a problematic policy. "Doing a good job" must be made concrete in terms of measures that can be supplied to the funding agency in a timely fashion to be used within budgetary cycles. Our detailed review of the Maine system for funding substance-abuse treatment shows that many gaps are introduced between the way "doing a good job" is defined in practice, and the real thing.

This is unavoidable in a real system. The test of PBC is not against some theoretical ideal of performance financing, but must be defined in empirical terms. Has PBC improved the performance of provider agencies? To conduct such research, the empirical investigator must remain aware of the distinction between performance as defined by and reported to the funding agency, and true measures of performance.

Notes
This chapter was supported by Grants 1 R01 DA08715-01 and 271-89-8516 from the National Institute on Drug Abuse, and K05-MH01263 from the National Institute of Mental Health. We are grateful to Jereal Holley and Marlene McMullen-Pelsor of the Office of Substance Abuse in Maine, and Michael Riordan of Boston

University, for assistance in the research reported here. Two reviewers made many helpful suggestions. The views expressed here are the authors' alone.

1 There is, of course, a natural flow of information and results between treatment research and program evaluation. Results from program evaluation may cause researchers to initiate scientific studies, while results from treatment research may bring about changes in treatment methods and therefore the evaluation of programs.

2 The performance of programs with only a few clients was noted. In these programs, the treatment outcome of one unusual client could skew the program's performance. In addition, performance of that provider over time could be subject to large random variation.

3 The assumption of universal diminishing marginal productivity is made for simplicity. It is possible, as is sometimes alleged, that treatment only becomes effective after some point, implying an increasing marginal return. Eventually, however, diminishing returns must set in.

4 The conditions here are slightly more general. Condition 1 allows for the shadow price on public funds to be different than $1. The reason usually given for this is that collection of taxes creates a welfare loss, and therefore one dollar spent on a public program should have a social value exceeding one dollar. Also, Condition 4 is implicit in the earlier discussion, and made explicit here. In the discussion above we assumed the agency was on the production possibility schedule OA. Condition 4 states this explicitly as necessary for full efficiency.

5 Experience with performance contracting in primary education bears this out. Gramlich and Koshel (1975) discuss the experience with government-funded experiments in PBC in education in the late 1960s and early 1970s.

6 We note that the state could also question a spouse or other family member concerning the client's use of substances. This, while not *client* self-report, is nonetheless a "report" and is subject to many of the same drawbacks as client self-report. In fact, Maisto et al., in a review of 14 studies on the validity of self-reported data, found that when discrepancies between self-report and the report of a collateral informant existed, the subjects usually reported more use than did the other source (Maisto et al. 1990).

7 Different substances pass through the body at different rates. It appears then that to ensure accuracy, different testing schedules would need to be established for different substances. This becomes even more complicated in the case of poly-drug users, a growing population in all programs. Barnum and Gleason (1990) show that the accuracy of drug tests falls as the number of drugs tested simultaneously increases. This seems to imply that poly-drug users would have to be tested at separate times for each drug to ensure as much accuracy as possible. The burden and expense for both the client and the state or program makes this unrealistic.

8 Kappa equal to 0 indicates agreement resulting from chance alone, while kappa equal to 1 indicates maximum possible agreement. Less than chance agreement appears as negative kappa (Bishop, Fienberg and Holland 1975, as cited in Magura et al. 1987). If the time periods covered by the self-report and the criterion are similar, kappa is the appropriate measure. However, if, as is often the case in studies of substance abusers, the time period covered by the self-report is longer than that measured by the criterion (e.g., urinalysis), conditional kappa is a more appropriate measure of agreement.

9 In addition, they found no statistically significant difference on sex, ethnicity, marital status, education, employment, age at first use of the three drugs, length of time on the program, daily methadone dosage, previous arrests, psychiatric diagnosis, or current court involvement.

10 In more detailed analysis, Magura et al. 1987 report that the type of interviewer at the clinic directly affected the underreporting, rather than the clinic per se.

11 Aiken (1986) reports that many programs will not allow outside researchers to collect information from clients at admission, stating that "intake is a difficult period for clients, and programs may not want outside evaluators disturbing clients at this time" (p. 785).

12 Employability is also monitored. This measures whether the client is employable, not whether the client is actually employed. A good employability outcome is defined as a change from "unable to work for physical or psychological reasons" to "employable or working now."

References

Aiken, L.S. 1986. Retrospective Self-Reports by Clients Differ from Original Reports: Implications for the Evaluation of Drug Treatment Programs. *International Journal of the Addictions* 21(7):767–88.

Barnum, D.T., and J.M. Gleason. 1990. Determining Transit Drug Test Accuracy: The Multi-Drug Case. Paper prepared for Transportation Research Board 70th Annual Meeting, Washington, January 1991.

Campbell, D.T. 1979. Assessing the Impact of Planned Social Change. *Evaluation and Program Planning* 2:85.

Gramlich, E.M., and P.P. Koshel. 1975. *Educational Performance Contracting: An Evaluation of an Experiment.* Washington: The Brookings Institution.

Hanushek, E.A. 1994. *Making Schools Work.* Washington: The Brookings Institution.

Institute of Medicine. 1990. *Treating Drug Problems.* Washington: National Academy Press.

Jencks, C. 1994. *The Homeless.* Cambridge, Mass.: Harvard University Press.

Longabaugh, R., and P.R. Clifford. 1992. Program Evaluation and Treatment Outcome. *Annual Review of Addictions Research and Treatment* 17:223–47.

Magura, S., D. Goldsmith, C. Casriel, P.J. Goldstein, and D.S. Lipton. 1987. The Validity of Methadone Clients' Self-Reported Drug Use. *International Journal of the Addictions* 22(8):727–49.

Maisto, S.A., J.R. McKay, and G.J. Connors. 1990. Self-Report Issues in Substance Abuse: State of the Art and Future Directions. *Behavioral Assessment* 12:117–34.

Marsden, M.E., and R.L. Hubbard. 1984. *Assessing the drug-crime relationship: A comparison of results with alternative methods.* Paper presented at the American Society of Criminology. Cincinnati, Ohio.

McAuliffe, Wm. 1989. From Theory to Practice: The Planned Treatment of Drug Users. *International Journal of the Addictions* 24(6):527–608.

McLellan, A.T., L. Luborsky, F. Griffith, and F. Evans. 1986. Predictions and Measurement of Outcome in Substance Abuse Treatment Using the Addiction Severity Index. *American Journal of Drug and Alcohol Abuse* 12:101–20.

Passell, P. 1994. After Years of Trying to Fix Education, Why Isn't It Fixed? *New York Times* (October 13):D2.

Part III

Special Issues in Drug-Abuse Treatment

9

The Development of Effective Drug-Abuse Services for Youth

Scott W. Henggeler

The overriding purpose of this chapter is to recommend directions in the development of more effective drug-abuse prevention and treatment programs for youth. To accomplish this purpose, several pertinent research literatures are examined and their respective findings are integrated. These literatures pertain to (a) the correlates of drug use and abuse in adolescents, (b) findings from the prevention and treatment literatures, (c) lessons learned from the ongoing national reform of mental health services for children, adolescents, and their families, and (d) lessons learned from the treatment of drug abuse and dependence in adults.

Assuming that prevention and treatment programs should focus on the empirically-determined correlates/predictors of drug use and abuse, such correlates are examined, with special emphasis on findings from well-designed causal modeling studies. The correlational literature presents a clear and consistent picture: Drug use and abuse in youth are multidetermined, with contributing factors pertaining to youth cognitive structures, family relations, peer associations, school performance, and neighborhood context.

In light of the multidetermined nature of adolescent drug use and abuse, broad-based prevention and treatment strategies designed to address multiple aspects of the youth's cognitive processes and ecology are needed to maximize the probability of favorable outcome. Yet, with rare exception, prevention efforts have been narrowly focused, and consequently have obtained minimal success with those youth at high risk of drug abuse. Likewise, treatment approaches for adolescent drug abusers have usually addressed only a limited number of the multiple determinants of drug abuse and have often provided services that have little bearing upon the youth's natural environment (e.g., hospitalization, traditional outpatient services).

The more mature field of mental health services for children has experienced difficulties similar to those reported in the literature on drug-abuse services for adolescents (e.g., reliance on expensive and restrictive treatments with little proven effectiveness, lack of service integration, and coordination). In response to such difficulties, several major reform and research initiatives have been funded by the federal government and private foundations. Following Stroul and Friedman's (1986) guidelines for the reform of children's mental health services, these initiatives have advocated the development of service systems that are family-centered, community-based, child-focused, individualized, comprehensive, less restrictive, and accountable for client outcome and satisfaction. The present chapter argues for the adoption of the Stroul and Friedman (1994) guidelines in the development of more effective prevention and treatment programs for youth drug use and abuse. Furthermore, findings regarding the treatment of drug abuse and dependence in adults support the viability of services that are individualized, comprehensive, and community-based.

Predictors of Adolescent Drug Use and Abuse

The empirical literature strongly supports a social-ecological (Bronfenbrenner 1979) view of behavior, in which drug use and abuse are multidetermined by the reciprocal interplay of characteristics of the individual youth and the key social systems in which youth are embedded (i.e., family, peer, school, neighborhood). Evidence of the multidetermined and social-ecological nature of adolescent drug use and abuse is derived from studies examining the cross-sectional correlates and longitudinal predictors of adolescent drug use, problem drug use, and drug-use patterns following treatment (i.e., relapse). This section briefly examines consistent findings regarding univariate correlates of drug use and abuse, and then integrates results from several complex and well-designed causal modeling studies that vividly illustrate the multidetermined nature of drug use and abuse.

Correlates of drug use and abuse

Based on conclusions of several recent reviews (e.g., Hawkins, Catalano, and Miller 1992; Kumpfer 1989; Office of Technology Assistance 1991), the correlates of adolescent drug use and abuse demonstrated most consistently are as follows.

- *Individual:* other antisocial behaviors, low self-esteem, low social conformity, psychiatric symptomatology, positive expectancies for drug effects, genetic loadings.
- *Family:* ineffective management and discipline, low warmth and high conflict, parental drug abuse.
- *Peer:* association with drug-using peers, low association with prosocial peers.
- *School:* low intelligence, achievement, and commitment to achievement.
- *Neighborhood:* disorganization, high crime.

Causal modeling studies. In light of the numerous correlates of drug use and abuse and the covariation among these correlates, several research groups have developed multidimensional causal models that specify the interrelations among pertinent correlates. Figures 9.1–9.4 present the results of four of the most comprehensive causal modeling studies (Brook, Nomura, and Cohen 1989; Dishion, Reid, and Patterson 1988; Elliott, Huizinga, and Ageton 1985; Oetting and Beauvais 1987). All four studies modeled the roles of family and peers in adolescent drug use, and three considered school-related factors.

The findings of these studies are relatively clear and consistent: (a) Association with drug-using peers was always a powerful and direct predictor of adolescent drug use. (b) Family relations either predicted drug use directly (contributing unique variance) or indirectly by predicting association with drug-using peers. (c) School difficulties predicted association with drug-using peers. Thus, in the most sophisticated studies to date, investigators have demonstrated that adolescent drug use is linked directly or indirectly with the key systems in which youth are embedded – family, peers, and school.

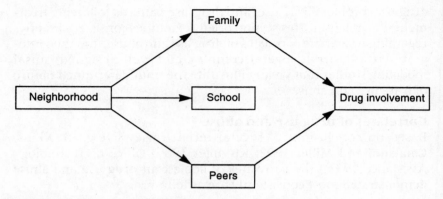

Figure 9.1   Adolescent drug involvement over time.
Source: from Brook, Nomura, and Cohen, 1989.

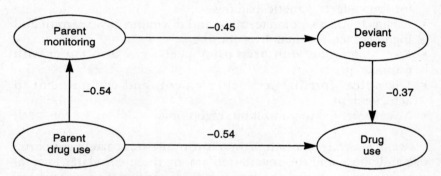

Figure 9.2   Drug sampling in middle childhood.
Source: from Dishion, Reid, and Patterson 1988.

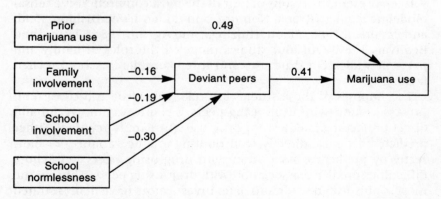

Figure 9.3   Integrated model.
Source: from Elliott, Huizinga, and Ageton 1985.

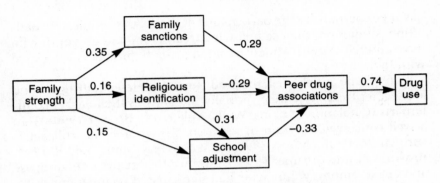

Figure 9.4 Socialization characteristics and adolescent drug use.
Source: from Oettings and Beauvais 1987.

Findings from the broader causal modeling literature (including studies that used related statistical procedures such as hierarchical regression analyses) suggest that several additional variables are linked with drug use and abuse. As presented in figure 9.1, living in a stable neighborhood contributed to adolescent functioning with family, peers, and school (Brook et al. 1989). In addition, several studies have demonstrated the sometimes unique and sometimes indirect contributions of cognitive/emotional variables, though each of these studies omitted critical constructs (i.e., either family relations or peer associations) from their measurement methods. Stein, Newcomb, and Bentler (1987) showed that low social conformity (i.e., not religious, conservative, or law abiding) predicted several important future outcomes including drug abuse. Likewise, White, Pandina, and LaGrange (1987) found that several personality variables contributed unique variance to drug abuse, and Rhodes and Jason (1990) reported that low assertion contributed directly to adolescent drug use. Swaim, Oetting, Edwards, and Beauvais (1989) found that adolescent anger predicted association with drug-using peers, which, in turn, predicted drug use. Finally, Needle et al. (1986) reported that drug using older siblings can contribute to adolescent drug use above and beyond the effects of parents and peers.

Correlates of drug use following treatment. Studies of drug-abusing adolescents' resumption of drug use or abuse following treatment (i.e., relapse) have many of the same methodological features (i.e., similar dependent and independent measures and statistical analyses), as do studies of the initiation of drug use and the development of drug abuse. The primary distinction between the groups of studies pertains to the participants of the relapse studies. By definition, studies of drug use following treatment focus on youth who have entered drug-treatment programs due to problems associated with their drug use.

As might be anticipated, the predictors of adolescent drug use and abuse after treatment are essentially the same as their earlier counterparts (Catalano, Hawkins, Wells, Miller, and Brewer 1990–1). In a well-conceived program of research, Brown and her colleagues (Brown, Mott, and Myers 1990; Brown, Myers, Mott, and Vik 1994; Brown, Vik, and Creamer 1989) examined the predictors of drug use and abuse among youth who had participated in inpatient drug-treatment programs. The initial return to drug use almost always occurred in social contexts, most frequently while associating with pretreatment friends; and youth usually considered the possibility of using drugs prior to initiation. Similarly, Brown and her colleagues have linked favorable posttreatment outcome with high support from parents, less lifetime exposure to drug-abusing family members, increased association with prosocial peers, decreased association with drug-using peers, improved emotional functioning (e.g., anxiety, depression), a more flexible coping repertoire, and improved functioning in school and recreational settings.

Barrett, Simpson, and Lehman (1988) used causal modeling

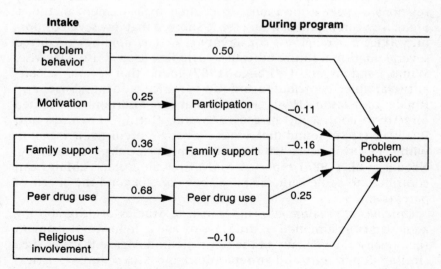

Figure 9.5 Changes during treatment.
Source: from Barrett, Simpson, and Lehman 1988.

procedures to examine the predictors of problem behavior of adolescents during the first three months of drug-abuse treatment. As shown in figure 9.5, high problem behavior (a composite variable reflecting drug use, school, and legal problems) was directly predicted by prior problem behavior, low religious involvement, low family support, high peer drug use, and low participation in treatment. Note the similarity between these results and previously reported findings supporting the multidetermined nature of adolescent drug use and abuse (see figures 9.1–9.4).

Conclusion. In spite of considerable variation in research methods and measurement, similar findings have been obtained from the most sophisticated investigations of the correlates of adolescent drug use and abuse. Key individual, family, peer, school, and neighborhood factors contribute directly or indirectly to adolescent drug use and abuse.

Prevention and Treatment

An understanding of the determinants of adolescent drug use and drug abuse is necessary for the development of interventions that effectively prevent or treat drug abuse. As described above, overwhelming evidence supports the view that drug use and abuse are multidetermined – that is, linked with key characteristics of adolescents and the systems in which they are embedded. Hence, if a primary goal of intervention is to attenuate the probability of drug abuse, prevention efforts should focus on attenuating the impact of risk factors while enhancing protective factors (e.g., family and extrafamilial support; Hawkins et al. 1992). Similarly, treatment programs should address the known determinants of drug abuse and its related problems (Henggeler 1993) while promoting the strengths of the adolescents and the systems in which they are embedded (e.g., Henggeler and Borduin 1990). This premise is a guiding assumption of the present review.

Prevention
Several reviews examining the drug-abuse prevention literature have been published during the past few years (e.g., Botvin, Schinke, and Orlandi 1989; Felner, Silverman, and Adix 1991; Hawkins et al. 1992; Kumpfer 1989; Office of Technology Assessment 1991; Newcomb and Bentler 1989). An impediment to reviewing this literature, however, is that most prevention projects

"mix and match" interventions so that the theoretical orientations and corresponding thrusts of the projects are difficult to classify. Such difficulty in categorization restricts the reviewer's ability to discern the relative effectiveness of the diverse approaches. Nevertheless, moderate convergence of opinion is apparent regarding several important issues.

Demand-side approaches. As summarized by the OTA Report (1991), "it is clear that most demand side prevention programs targeted at individuals have yet to make a compelling case for their effectiveness." Thus, although several prevention approaches aimed at decreasing youth "demand" for drugs have enjoyed widespread dissemination and/or federal support, the need remains for the development and validation of well-conceived innovative approaches that reduce the desire of youth to experiment with and continue to use drugs.

Information/affective education. Approaches that seek to prevent drug abuse by presenting factual information and/or through affective education (i.e., designed to enhance self-esteem and social growth) are ineffective. The failure of such approaches probably reflects the relatively small roles that variables such as knowledge and self-esteem play in the etiology of drug abuse, especially when compared with the impact of family relations, peer associations, school performance, and neighborhood culture.

Life-skills training. Qualified success has been achieved by school-based prevention programs aimed at developing the life skills (social skills) of youth. These programs generally use cognitive behavioral strategies to enhance skills pertaining to problem-solving, self-control, adaptive coping, and assertion. Although such programs have demonstrated modest success in reducing the onset and prevalence of cigarette smoking, effects with other drugs have been less apparent. Moreover, youth at high risk of drug abuse (e.g., dropouts, incarcerated youth) are often not included in these school-based studies or have high rates of study attrition.

The qualified success of the life-skills model is exemplified in a well-designed study conducted by Botvin and his colleagues (Botvin, Baker, Dusenbury, Tortu, and Botvin 1990) using a randomized design. Results at a three-year follow-up showed that life-skills training significantly reduced cigarette smoking and marijuana use. Importantly, the investigators also showed that hypothesized mediators of drug use (i.e., drug-use attitudes, normative expectations, social skills) were influenced by life-skills training. On the other hand, effect sizes for the significant results were quite small (with $N = 3,684$, clinically insignificant changes can readily attain statistical significance due to high power), and high attrition was observed among high-risk youth. Thus, the actual impact of the life-skills program was quite small and did not pertain to those youth in greatest need of preventive services.

Multidimensional, comprehensive approaches. In light of existing knowledge that adolescent drug abuse is multidetermined, reviewers have logically called for the development of comprehensive prevention approaches that address multiple risk factors in an integrated fashion. Although few such approaches have been rigorously evaluated, findings from at least one well-designed study are encouraging. Johnson et al. (1990) contrasted a comprehensive prevention program that integrated individual, family, peer, school, and community-wide components versus a program that included only the community-wide component. Follow-up findings indicated that the comprehensive integrated approach was significantly more effective at attenuating tobacco and marijuana use than was the community-wide component alone. Importantly, the comprehensive approach was as successful with high-risk youth as with low-risk youth.

Focus on high-risk youth. Several reviewers (Felner et al. 1991; Hawkins et al. 1992; Kumpfer 1989) have argued that prevention efforts should focus on high-risk youth. As cogently noted by Newcomb and Bentler (1989), "It is misleading to bask in the success of some peer programs that have reduced the number of youngsters who experiment with drugs (but would probably never have become regular users, let alone abusers) and ignore the tougher problems of those youngsters who are at high risk for drug abuse as well as other serious difficulties" (p. 246). Clearly, a high priority should be given to the development of effective interventions for those youth who are most likely to present grave economic, criminal, and social problems linked with drug abuse. Also, because the determinants of drug abuse are generally the same as the determinants of delinquency, school dropout, and unprotected sexual activity (Henggeler, Melton, and Rodrigue 1992; Jessor and Jessor 1977), the development of effective comprehensive prevention programs can have many additional benefits to participants and society.

Early prevention. Several reviewers (Felner et al. 1991; Hawkins et al. 1992; Kumpfer 1989) have urged drug-abuse prevention researchers to address risk factors that occur in early and middle childhood, before the initiation of drug use. Several types of interventions have already demonstrated effectiveness regarding the attenuation of established risk factors and the development of protective factors. Viable childhood programs include early childhood and family-support programs, parenting programs, and programs that promote academic achievement through tutoring and restructuring school environments. Note that a common element of these diverse programs is that interventions are directly targeted at modifying the child's natural environment (Kumpfer 1989).

Treatment

In spite of the enormous personal, family, and societal costs of adolescent drug abuse as well as the billions of dollars spent annually on treatment, a central contention of this chapter is that no treatment of adolescent drug abuse has demonstrated superiority over any other treatment or no services. In support of this contention, recent reviews have concluded that the state of knowledge regarding the treatment of adolescent drug abuse is highly unsatisfactory (IOM 1990) and that such lack of knowledge is seriously hampering the development of public policy (OTA 1991). On the other hand, several well-respected reviewers (e.g., Brown et al. 1994; Catalano et al. 1990–1; De Leon 1993; Liddle and Dakof 1994) have recently concluded, in effect, that several treatments of adolescent drug abuse are effective. For example, certain of the family therapies are regarded as having clearly demonstrated effectiveness, and treatment in general has been considered better than no treatment, based on findings regarding adolescents in the DARP (Sells and Simpson 1979) and TOPS (Hubbard et al. 1983) studies.

The question of whether or not effective treatments for adolescent drug abuse exist has extremely important implications for the development of policy. If, for example, traditional drug-abuse services or more recently developed services such as the family therapies are effective, policy efforts might aim at increasing the accessibility and affordability of such services. If, on the other hand, existing services are largely ineffective, priority should be placed on the development and validation of new and innovative treatments as well as on the reform of drug-abuse service systems. As discussed later in this chapter, the field of mental health services for children and adolescents is currently undergoing considerable scrutiny and reform in light of the acknowledged failures of traditional mental health treatments and service systems. Moreover, it will be shown that lessons learned from the children's mental health services literature are directly applicable to the topic at hand.

In light of the central importance of the issue, the existing treatment literature regarding adolescent drug abuse is critiqued. A basic assumption of the critique is that treatment effectiveness is best established in the context of well-designed and well-implemented clinical trials including methodological features such as randomized assignment to experimental conditions, use of valid measures, and follow-up evaluations. The state of the literature is reflected in the fact that few studies of adolescent drug-abuse treatment include these relatively basic methodological criteria, much less other features needed to establish the internal validity of findings (e.g., attrition analyses, treatment specificity, evaluations of treatment integrity, multimethod and multidomain measurement evaluations, specified subject selection criteria).

The following conclusions should inform policy regarding the treatment of adolescent drug abusers.

Quasi-experimental studies and one-group pre–post designs. Findings from most quasi-experimental studies and one-group pre–post designs can not demonstrate that treatment is better than no treatment. In the absence of an equivalent comparison condition (e.g., no treatment, usual services, alternative treatment), pre–post changes in the treatment condition can result from several factors unrelated to the effects of the treatment delivered (e.g., Borkovec 1993): (1) Statistical regression effects are likely with youth who enter treatment at a time of crisis, when drug-related problems have peaked. (2) Differential attrition can give a false sense of treatment effectiveness. For example, the often cited finding that treatment duration is linked with outcome may simply reflect the fact that individuals with more serious problems and lower motivation are more likely to terminate treatment prematurely. (3) Especially important for adolescents are the effects of history and maturation. As Brown and her colleagues reported for adolescent drug abusers (Brown et al. 1994) and as the Institute of Medicine (1990) concluded for adult drug abusers, rates of individual drug use show wide normal variation over time. Additional support for the view that treatment effects in uncontrolled studies may be spurious are findings from the drug-abuse treatment and delinquency treatment literatures. (4) Regarding the former, youth in no treatment or minimal treatment control conditions have shown substantial decreases in drug use at posttest or follow-up (see e.g., Joanning et al. 1992; Sells and Simpson 1979; Amini et al. 1982). (5) The delinquency treatment literature has a long history of interventions that seem successful in uncontrolled studies, but that fail to demonstrate favorable outcome when submitted to controlled clinical trials (Henggeler 1989).

Experimental studies. Randomized trials have provided minimal support for the effectiveness of any treatment of adolescent drug abuse. Several relatively well-designed experimental studies have compared two treatment modalities for adolescent drug abuse: (Amini et al. 1982) inpatient vs. outpatient; (Friedman 1989) family therapy vs. parent training; (Lewis et al. 1990) family therapy vs. parent training; (Szapocznik et al. 1983, 1986) conjoint vs. one-person family therapy. Across studies, findings generally revealed that adolescent drug use decreased equally in both treatment conditions, and authors concluded that both treatments were effective. Such conclusions may be in error because these studies and their results present the same difficulties in interpretation and significant threats to internal validity as noted above for single-group designs. That is, history, maturation, and regression may have accounted for the similar decreases in drug use across treatment conditions. Indeed, preliminary findings from a randomized trial that we are currently conducting with substance-abusing/dependent delinquents (Henggeler et al. 1994) shows that youth in the usual services condition evidenced large decreases in behavior problems at five months postreferral even though the vast majority had received zero hours of substance-abuse or mental health services.

Other randomized trials with adolescent drug abusers have produced minimal results or highly qualified outcomes. Joanning et al. (1992) reported that family therapy was more effective than social-skills group therapy and family drug education at ameliorating drug problems, but results are mitigated by the fact that the sample excluded serious drug users (included a mix of occasional users and regular users), the key criterion measure was of dubious validity, family therapy had no observed effect on family relations (the assumed causal mechanism for apparent treatment gains), and no follow-up was included. Similarly, studies comparing cognitive-behavioral (Friedman and Utada 1992) and group-home (Braukmann et al. 1985) approaches with high risk youth have had minimal success.

Traditional treatments. The least is known regarding the effectiveness of the most widely used treatments for adolescent drug abuse. Controlled trials have not been conducted for specialized inpatient treatments or for 12-step-based programs, to which drug-abusing youth are often referred. Based on the causal modeling literature and findings regarding the correlates of relapse, however, treatments that *increase* association with problem peers and do not attend directly to family and school issues would not be expected to attain desired goals. Findings in the highly similar delinquency treatment literature strongly support this contention (Henggeler 1989). Likewise, it seems unrealistic to expect treatment programs (e.g., boot camps, wilderness training) that are not family- and community-based and do not address the multiple determinants of drug abuse, to be effective, and such a view is supported by findings in the adult drug-abuse (Institute of Medicine 1990) and delinquency (Henggeler and Schoenwald 1994) treatment literatures.

Conclusion

Research consistently supports the view that adolescent drug use and abuse are multidetermined, linked directly or indirectly with cognitive/emotional characteristics of youth and key aspects of the family, peer, school, and neighborhood systems in which youth are embedded. Yet, with rare exception, preventive and treatment programs address only a limited portion of the factors contributing to adolescent drug abuse. Also, treatment efforts typically provide services outside of the youth's natural environment, thereby further decreasing the probability of effecting positive change (Henggeler, Schoenwald, and Pickrel forthcoming). Thus, in light of the failure to provide comprehensive services with ecological validity, the lack of established effectiveness for most current prevention and treatment strategies is not surprising. As discussed next, reform efforts in the field of children's mental health services may inform similar efforts in the prevention and treatment of adolescent drug abuse.

Lessons from the Reform of Mental Health Services for Children, Adolescents, and their Families

Several important commonalities in the treatment of youth with serious emotional disturbances (SED) and of drug-abusing youth (Henggeler 1993) suggest that lessons learned regarding the reform of children's mental health services may apply to the development of more effective services for adolescent drug abusers. (Note that by current federal definition [Section 1912c of the Public Health Service Act, as amended 42 U.S.C. 29Off et seq.] a youth with SED has a DSM-III-R diagnosis, *excluding substance-use disorders*, "V" codes, and developmental disorders; and has service needs involving at least two community agencies.) First, the identified risk factors and correlates for drug abuse and SED are largely the same.

Second, little empirical support is evident for the treatment of drug abuse or SED. Third, the delivery of services to youth with SED and drug-abusing youth share several obstacles (e.g., fragmentation of services; gap between need and service system capability; reliance on expensive, restrictive, and unproven services). In light of such commonalities, this chapter argues that several key systems-level and clinical-level changes are required to create services that meet the needs of drug-abusing youth. The rationale and conclusions that follow are based largely on papers developed for a recent Task Force Report (Henggeler 1994) and edited volume (Henggeler and Santos forthcoming) that pertain to innovative services for difficult-to-treat clinical populations and how such services fit with health-care reform.

Systems-level changes

In 1986, Stroul and Friedman published a monograph, "Guiding Principles for the System of Care," which has become the philosophical blueprint for the national reform of mental health services for children, adolescents, and their families. This monograph has served as the basis of major initiatives from the Center for Mental Health Services (RFA No. SM 94-01), the Annie E. Casey Foundation (Maloy 1991), and the Robert Wood Johnson Foundation (England and Cole 1992). Recently, and quite justifiably, this monograph has been revised (Stroul and Friedman 1994) to, in part, address the reform of services for treating drug abuse. The recommended systems-level changes that follow are consistent with the Stroul and Friedman (1994) principles for a system of care (see table 9.1).

Reduce the use of restrictive services. A grossly disproportionate percentage of treatment dollars for adolescent drug abuse are spent on expensive and restrictive services. Although such services might be justified if they were clinically effective, no experimental evidence supports such effectiveness. Moreover, the deleterious effects of restrictive services such as hospitalization and residential treatment for adolescents has been well documented (for review see Weithorn 1988).

Increase the availability of home- and community-based services. In mental health, reviewers have consistently argued for the development of services that address problems in children's natural environments, including their homes (Borduin 1994; Nelson 1994), schools (Duchnowski 1994), and neighborhoods (Friedman 1994; Rodrigue 1994). Regarding drug abuse, findings from the reviewed causal-modeling, prevention, and treatments literatures

Table 9.1 Values and principles for the system of care (Stroul and Friedman 1994).

CORE VALUES

1 The system of care should be child centered and family focused, with the needs of the child and family dictating the types and mix of services provided.
2 The system of care should be community based, with the locus of services as well as management and decision-making responsibility resting at the community level.
3 The system of care should be culturally competent, with agencies, programs, and services that are responsive to the cultural, racial, and ethnic differences of the populations they serve.

GUIDING PRINCIPLES

1 Children with emotional disturbances (and youth who abuse drugs) should have access to a comprehensive array of services that address the child's physical, emotional, social, and educational needs.
2 Children with emotional disturbances (and youth who abuse drugs) should receive individualized services in accordance with the unique needs and potentials of each child and guided by an individualized service plan.
3 Children with emotional disturbances (and youth who abuse drugs) should receive services within the least restrictive, most normative environment that is clinically appropriate.
4 The families and surrogate families of children with emotional disturbances (and youth who abuse drugs) should be full participants in all aspects of the planning and delivery of services.
5 Children with emotional disturbances (and youth who abuse drugs) should receive services that are integrated, with linkages between child-serving agencies and programs and mechanisms for planning, developing, and coordinating services.
6 Children with emotional disturbances (and youth who abuse drugs) should be provided with case management or similar mechanisms to ensure that multiple services are delivered in a coordinated and therapeutic manner and that they can move through the system of services in accordance with their changing needs.
7 Early identification and intervention for children with emotional disturbances (and youth who abuse drugs) should be promoted by the system of care in order to enhance the likelihood of positive outcomes.
8 Children with emotional disturbances (and youth who abuse drugs) should be ensured smooth transitions to the adult service system as they reach maturity.
9 The rights of children with emotional disturbances (and youth who abuse drugs) should be protected, and effective advocacy efforts for children and youth with emotional disturbances should be promoted.
10 Children with emotional disturbances (and youth who abuse drugs) should receive services without regard to race, religion, national origin, sex, physical disability, or other characteristics, and services should be sensitive and responsive to cultural differences and special needs.

Note: Clauses in parentheses were added.

strongly suggest that interventions should directly address key aspects of these same natural contexts (i.e., family, school, neighborhood).

Increase provider accountability. Drug-abuse treatment providers (and mental health service providers) have virtually no accountability for client outcome or consumer satisfaction. An important aspect of President Clinton's Health Security Plan (The White House Domestic Policy Council 1993) and a strong recommendation of the Institute of Medicine (1990) report is to track client-level outcomes. If linked with reimbursement rates, tracking of client outcome and satisfaction may have high potential for enhancing standards of care.

Increase service integration. Drug-abusing youth are being treated in a fragmented and uncoordinated fashion across all the child service systems (i.e., education, mental health, primary care, social welfare, and juvenile justice), often by professionals with little knowledge of drug abuse. In mental health, evidence is accumulating that integrating systems of care for youth with SED can reduce the use of restrictive and expensive services (Rosenblatt and Attkisson 1993).

Reform mechanisms for financing services. Restrictive services are usually reimbursed at higher rates than community-based services, thereby providing a financial incentive for removing youth from their families and communities. Curbing this incentive will facilitate the development of community-based programs. Moreover, several excellent options for funding innovative services have recently become available (Meyers, forthcoming).

Train providers in the delivery of clinically effective and cost-effective services. Friedman (1993) and Hanley (forthcoming) have noted that traditional training in the mental health professions bears little relation to the types of clinical practices needed in community settings. The office-based 50-minute hour is not sufficient to address the multiple and complex problems presented by most real-world clinical cases. For example, little good can come from individually-oriented therapy with a youth who has learning problems, an alcoholic parent, criminal friends, and who lives in a crime-ridden neighborhood. Clearly, more intensive and ecologically-oriented interventions are needed to have a reasonable chance of attaining and maintaining treatment gains.

Clinical-level changes

Although system-level changes are needed to increase the availability, accessibility, and affordability of drug-abuse services, clinical-level changes are needed to increase the probability that services will have their intended effect on adolescent behavior. As noted previously, empirical support for the effectiveness of any treatment of adolescent drug abuse is almost non-existent. Similarly, reviewers (Weisz and Weiss 1993) have recently concluded that the child psychotherapies in the mental health arena have limited efficacy as practiced in real-world settings (e.g., community mental health centers vs. university research laboratories) with clinical populations. In addition, only recently has a treatment of serious antisocial behavior in adolescents (i.e., violent and chronic criminal offending) shown favorable long-term effects (i.e., multisystemic therapy: Borduin et al. forthcoming; Henggeler, Melton, and Smith 1992; Henggeler et al. 1993). Importantly, in these two clinical trials multisystemic therapy also decreased self-reported drug use at posttreatment, and drug-related arrests at long-term follow-up (Henggeler et al. 1991). The following recommendations are based on previous conclusions concerning the drug-abuse causal modeling, prevention, and treatment literatures, as well as the views of advocates for the reform of children's mental health services and empirical findings from recently completed and ongoing clinical trials of multisystemic therapy.

Services should be flexible and individualized. Individualization of services means that treatment is tailored to the particular strengths and weaknesses of the youth and of the key systems in which the youth is embedded. In other words, interventions are designed and often modified as needed to fit the individualized needs and changing circumstances of the youth and family. Such individualization contrasts sharply with many existing drug-abuse programs that provide the same treatment to virtually all youth. Moreover, the individualization of services requires that interventions be flexible regarding intensity, foci, and duration; and with the overriding purpose being the attainment of desired treatment goals.

Services should be comprehensive. Few drug-abusing youth and youth with SED present singular or straightforward problems, and the interrelations of problem behavior in youth are well-documented (Jessor and Jessor 1977). A high percentage of youth with SED are involved with drugs, and a high percentage of drug-abusing youth present emotional and/or behavioral problems. In addition, adolescent drug abusers and youth with SED typically present difficulties in family, peer, and school functioning. In light of such comorbidity and in consideration of the determinants of drug abuse and SED, it follows logically that effective treatments must have the capacity to intervene successfully in multiple contexts – including youth cognitive processes, the family system, the peer network, the school/vocational arena, and even the neighborhood.

Moreover, before treatment is even delivered, providers may first need to address a range of logistic, cultural, and environmental barriers. Unfortunately, few treatments of drug abuse, antisocial behavior, or SED provide the comprehensiveness (and ecological validity) needed to attain positive outcomes.

Services should empower families. In many traditional mental health and drug-abuse services, parents (especially parents with problems) are viewed as barriers to therapeutic change rather than as vehicles to change. As demonstrated in the relapse literature, advocated in the Stroul and Friedman (1994) principles, and validated in clinical trials (Henggeler et al. 1994), parental efforts and support are often critical to favorable therapeutic outcome for youth. Thus, families should be viewed as active collaborators in all aspects of treatment (i.e., assessment, goal setting, service delivery, evaluation, etc.).

In summary, the recommended systems-level and clinical-level changes in adolescent drug-abuse service systems are based on extant knowledge in the field of drug abuse and on current systems- and clinical-level changes concerning children's mental health services. As described next, such recommendations are also consistent with findings in the adult drug-abuse and dependence literature.

Lessons from the Treatment of Drug Abuse and Dependence in Adults

In the concluding chapter of a recent NIDA Monograph (Onken, Blaine, and Boren 1993) on state-of-the-art empirically-based treatments of drug abuse and dependence, Miller (1993a) noted that contributors to the monograph uniformly suggested that "drug abusers are fundamentally like other people except that they use drugs and suffer the consequences" (p. 304). Such a view contrasts with the disease-model assumption that drug abusers are qualitatively different from normal human beings. Supporting the view that drug abuse is not fundamentally a biological/characterological problem, use of drugs by individuals in methadone treatment has been influenced by relatively simple clinic contingencies (Grabowski et al. 1993; Stitzer et al. 1993), and the development of active coping strategies has been modestly successful with cocaine abusers (Childress et al. 1993). Moreover, considerable decrease in drug use is possible when interventions are integrated into the natural ecologies of cocaine-dependent individuals (Higgins and Budney 1993).

Important implications derive from the view that drug abuse in adolescents is fundamentally similar to other types of serious anti-social behavior presented by teenagers. First, interventions should aim at modifying those cognitive characteristics and environmental contingencies (e.g., family, neighborhood) that are supporting drug use. Second, emphasis should be placed on developing youth relations in natural prosocial peer contexts (e.g., church youth groups, athletics, school-based activities), rather than on developing peer-group affiliations with other youth presenting serious problems. Third, interventions should address problems in their natural contexts, rather than removing youth from family, neighborhood, school, and community to treat them in environments that bear little relation to the real world.

The implications for viewing drug-abusing youth as "fundamentally like other people except that they use drugs and suffer the consequences" are essentially the same as those discussed previously for findings in the causal-modeling/prevention/treatment literature and the children's mental health services literature. Moreover, as described next, the conclusions and recommendations drawn from these literatures are buttressed even further by findings regarding services for drug-abusing and drug-dependent adults (Institute of Medicine 1990; Onken et al. 1993).

Reduce the use of restrictive services

Little is known about the effectiveness of hospital-based drug-treatment programs, which are the most expensive treatments of drug abuse in adults (Institute of Medicine 1990). Moreover, in spite of their high cost, residential and inpatient treatments have demonstrated no benefit over outpatient treatments (Miller 1993a).

Increase the availability of community-based services

In light of the lack of demonstrated effectiveness for costly drug-treatment services, less expensive and potentially more effective community-based services should be developed. For example, through restructuring the natural environments of drug users (especially involving nondrug-using family/friends in treatment), the Community Reinforcement Approach (Higgins and Budney 1993) has demonstrated very favorable results. Similarly, the Institute of Medicine (1990) report has argued for aggressive outreach to address the needs of difficult-to-reach populations of drug abusers (e.g., young mothers who abuse drugs).

Increase provider accountability

Consistent with the Health Security Plan (The White House Domestic Policy Council 1993), authors (Institute of Medicine 1990; Miller 1993a; Schuster and Silverman 1993) have urged funding sources to demand increased program (and therapist) accountability for client outcome. Indeed, mandating such accountability can provide strong incentive and motivation to develop innovative, community-based services that are clinically effective and attractive to consumers.

Reform mechanisms for financing services

Regarding public coverage, the Institute of Medicine (1990) report recommended several significant changes from the current federal response. In general, these changes aim to: (a) develop and enhance information systems that will eventually guide funding decisions; (b) provide technical assistance aimed at improving the quality of services; (c) enhance local and state accountability for the use of federal dollars; (d) reimburse hospital and non-hospital services at the same rate; and (e) consolidate drug treatment with the mainstream of health care. Regarding private coverage, the report recommended several similar changes aimed at curbing costs and promoting accountability among providers.

Train providers in the delivery of clinically effective and cost-effective services

Human-resource development and annual training for treatment providers are core features of the Institute of Medicine's (1990) recommendations for improving current service systems. As noted by Miller (1993b) and Schuster and Silverman (1993), many current practitioners are wedded to treatment models with little established efficacy. Mandating program accountability for client outcome, however, can only be effective if providers have access to the resources (expert training, consultation, and technical assistance) needed to optimize clinical outcomes.

Services should be flexible and individualized

"Harm reduction" (Marlatt and Tapert 1993) and the Community Reinforcement Approach (Higgins and Budney 1993) are two treatment models that exemplify the value of providing flexible and individualized services for adult drug abusers. Rather than fitting individual clients to specific interventions a priori, these treatment models have attained relatively strong outcomes by setting therapeutic goals and designing interventions based on the particular strengths and weaknesses of each client and his/her social network.

Services should be comprehensive

Drug-abusing and drug-dependent adults frequently present a wide range of difficulties including emotional, relationship, legal, vocational, housing, medical, and financial. In light of the interrelations among these problems, the provision of a broad array of integrated services seems most likely to produce desired outcomes (Higgins and Budney 1993; Institute of Medicine 1990; Marlatt, Somers, and Tapert 1993).

Conclusion

Although much is known about the correlates and predictors of drug use and abuse in youth, such knowledge has not been used effectively by prevention and treatment programs. This lack of knowledge utilization paired with the tendency of programs to provide services divorced from the natural environments of youth may account for the generally poor results obtained when interventions are rigorously evaluated. In light of the lack of knowledge regarding the necessary components of effective prevention and treatment for drug use and abuse in youth, policymakers and investigators should attend to parallel developments in the more mature fields of mental health services for children, and drug abuse and dependence treatment for adults. Such developments suggest that the more promising services are those that are individualized, comprehensive, family-based, community-based, and integrated. Reforming financing mechanisms and mandating provider accountability (with commensurate training and technical assistance) are critical to the development of more responsive services.

Note

Preparation of this chapter was supported by the National Institute on Drug Abuse, Grant DA-08029; and Center for Mental Health Services, SAMHSA, Grant MH48136.

Correspondence should be addressed to Scott W. Henggeler, Family Services Research Center, Department of Psychiatry and Behavioral Sciences, Medical University of South Carolina, 171 Ashley Avenue, Charleston, South Carolina 29425-0742.

References

Amini, F., N.J. Zilberg, E.L. Burke, and S. Salasnek. 1982. A Controlled Study of Inpatient vs. Outpatient Treatment of Delinquent Drug Abusing Adolescents: One Year Results. *Comprehensive Psychiatry* 23:436–44.

Barrett, M.E., D.D. Simpson, and W.E.K. Lehman. 1988. Behavioral Changes of Adolescents in Drug Abuse Intervention Programs. *Journal of Clinical Psychology* 44:461–73.

Borduin, C.M. 1994. Innovative Models of Treatment and Service Delivery in the Juvenile Justice System. *Journal of Clinical Child Psychology* 23 (Suppl.):19–25.

Borduin, C.M., B.J. Mann, L. Cone, et al. Forthcoming. Multisystemic Treatment of Serious Juvenile Offenders: Long-Term Prevention of Criminality and Violent Offending. *Journal of Consulting and Clinical Psychology* (in press).

Borkovec, T.D. 1993. Between-Groups Therapy Outcome Research: Design and Methodology. In *Behavioral Treatments for Drug Abuse and Dependence.* NIDA Research Monograph no. 137, ed. L.S. Onken, J.D. Blaine, and J.J. Boren (249-89). Rockville, Md.: National Institute on Drug Abuse.

Botvin, G.J., E. Baker, L. Dusenbury, S. Tortu, and E.M. Botvin. 1990. Preventing Adolescent Drug Abuse through a Multimodal Cognitive-Behavioral Approach: Results of a 3-year Study. *Journal of Consulting and Clinical Psychology* 58:437–46.

Botvin, G.J., S.P. Schinke, and M.A. Orlandi. 1989. Psychosocial Approaches to Drug Abuse Prevention: Theoretical Foundations and Empirical Findings. *Crisis* 10:62–77.

Braukmann, C.J., M.M. Bedlington, B.D. Belden, et al. 1985. Effects of Community-Based Group-Home Treatment Programs on Male Juvenile Offenders' Use and Abuse of Drugs and Alcohol. *American Journal on Drug and Alcohol Abuse* 11:249–78.

Bronfenbrenner, U. 1979. *The Ecology of Human Development: Experiments by Design and Nature.* Cambridge, Mass.: Harvard University Press.

Brook, J.S., C. Nomura, and P. Cohen. 1989. A Network of Influences on Adolescent Drug Involvement: Neighborhood, School, Peer, and Family. *Genetic, Social, and General Psychology Monographs* 115:125–45.

Brown, S.A., M.A. Mott, and M.G. Myers. 1990. Adolescent Drug and Alcohol Treatment Outcome. In *Prevention and Treatment of Drug and Alcohol Abuse*, ed. R.R. Watson (373–403). Clifton, N.J.: Humana Press.

Brown, S.A., M.G. Myers, M.A. Mott, and P.W. Vik. 1994. Correlates of Success Following Treatment for Adolescent Substance Abuse. *Applied and Preventive Psychology* 3:61–73.

Brown, S.A., P.W. Vik, and V.A. Creamer. 1989. Characteristics of Relapse Following Adolescent Substance Abuse Treatment. *Addictive Behaviors* 14:291–300.

Catalano, R.F., J.D. Hawkins, E.A. Wells, J. Miller, and D. Brewer. 1990–1. Evaluation of the Effectiveness of Adolescent Drug Abuse Treatment,

Assessment of Risks for Relapse, and Promising Approaches for Relapse Prevention. *International Journal of the Addictions* 25:1085–140.

Childress, A.R., A.V. Hole, R.N. Ehrman, S.J. Robbins, A.T. McLellan, and C.P. O'Brien. 1993. In *Behavioral Treatments for Drug Abuse and Dependence.* NIDA Research Monograph No. 137, ed. L.S. Onken, J.D. Blaine, and J.J. Boren (73-95). Rockville, Md.: National Institute on Drug Abuse.

De Leon, G. 1993. What Psychologists Can Learn from Addiction Treatment Research. *Psychology of Addictive Behavior* 7:103–9.

Dishion, T.J., J.B. Reid, and G.R. Patterson. 1988. Empirical Guidelines for a Family Intervention for Adolescent Drug Use. *Journal of Chemical Dependency* 2:189–224.

Duchnowski, A.J. 1994. Innovative Service Models: Education. *Journal of Clinical Child Psychology* 23 (Suppl.):13–18.

Elliott, D.S., D. Huizinga, and S.S. Ageton. 1985. *Explaining Delinquency and Drug Use.* Beverly Hills: Sage.

England, M.J., and R.F. Cole. 1992. Building Systems of Care for Youth with Serious Mental Illness. *Hospital and Community Psychiatry* 43:630–3.

Felner, R.D., M.M. Silverman, and R. Adix. 1991. Prevention of Substance Abuse and Related Disorders in Childhood and Adolescence: A Developmentally Based, Comprehensive Ecological Approach. *Family and Community Health* 14:12–22.

Friedman, A.S. 1989. Family Therapy vs. Parent Groups: Effects on Adolescent Drug Abusers. *American Journal of Family Therapy* 17:335–47.

Friedman, A.S., and A.T. Utada. 1992. Effects of Two Group Interaction Models on Substance-Using Adjudicated Adolescent Males. *Journal of Community Psychology* (OSAP Special Issue):106–17.

Friedman, R.M. 1993. Preparation of Students to Work with Children and Families, Is It Meeting the Need? *Administration and Policy in Mental Health* 20:297–310.

Friedman, R.M. 1994. Restructuring of Systems to Emphasize Prevention and Family Support. *Journal of Clinical Child Psychology* 23 (Suppl.):40–7.

Grabowski, J., H. Rhoades, R. Elk, J. Schmitz, and D. Creson. 1993. Clinicwide and Individualized Behavioral Interventions in Drug Dependence Treatment. In *Behavioral Treatments for Drug Abuse and Dependence.* NIDA Research Monograph no. 137, ed. L.S. Onken, J.D. Blaine, and J.J. Boren (5–17). Rockville, Md.: National Institute on Drug Abuse.

Hanley, J.H. 1994. Use of Bachelor Level Psychology Majors in the Provision of Mental Health Services to Children, Adolescents, and Their Families. *Journal of Clinical Child Psychology* 23 (Suppl.):55–8.

Hawkins, J.D., R.F. Catalano, and J.Y. Miller. 1992. Risk and Protective Factors for Alcohol and Other Drug Problems in Adolescence and Early Adulthood: Implications for Substance Abuse Prevention. *Psychological Bulletin* 112:64–105.

Henggeler, S.W. 1989. *Delinquency in Adolescence.* Newbury Park, Calif.: Sage.

———. 1993. Multisystemic Treatment of Serious Juvenile Offenders: Implications for the Treatment of Substance Abusing Youths. In *Behavioral Treatments for Drug Abuse and Dependence*. NIDA Research Monograph No. 137, ed. L.S. Onken, J.D. Blaine, and J.J. Boren (181–99). Rockville, Md.: National Institute on Drug Abuse.

———. (Ed.) 1994. American Psychological Association Task Force Report on Innovative Models of Mental Health Services for Children, Adolescents, and Their Families. *Journal of Clinical Child Psychology* 23 (Suppl.).

Henggeler, S.W., and C.M Borduin. 1990. *Family Therapy and Beyond: A Multisystemic Approach to Treating the Behavior Problems of Children and Adolescents*. Pacific Grove, Calif.: Brooks/Cole.

Henggeler, S.W., C.M. Borduin, G.B. Melton, et al. 1991. Effects of Multisystemic Therapy on Drug Use and Abuse in Serious Juvenile Offenders: A Progress Report from Two Outcome Studies. *Family Dynamics of Addiction Quarterly* 1:40–51.

Henggeler, S.W., G.B. Melton, and J.R. Rodrigue. 1992. *Pediatric and Adolescent AIDS: Research Findings from the Social Sciences*. Newbury Park, Calif.: Sage.

Henggeler, S.W., G.B. Melton, and L.A. Smith. 1992. Family Preservation Using Multisystemic Therapy: An Effective Alternative to Incarcerating Serious Juvenile Offenders. *Journal of Consulting and Clinical Psychology* 60:953–61.

Henggeler, S.W., G.B. Melton, L.A. Smith, S.K. Schoenwald, and J.H. Hanley. 1993. Family Preservation Using Multisystemic Treatment: Long-Term Follow-Up to a Clinical Trial with Serious Juvenile Offenders. *Journal of Child and Family Studies* 2:283–93.

Henggeler, S.W., S.G. Pickrel, S.K. Schoenwald, and P.B. Cunningham. 1994. Multisystemic Family Preservation Therapy with Substance Abusing Delinquent Adolescents. Symposium at the 102nd Annual Convention of the American Psychological Association, Los Angeles, August.

Henggeler, S.W., and A.B. Santos (eds). Forthcoming. *Innovative Services for "Difficult to Treat" Populations*. Washington: American Psychiatric Press.

Henggeler, S.W. and Schoenwald, S.K. 1994. Boot Camps for Juvenile Offenders: Just Say "No." *Journal of Child and Family Studies* 3:243–8.

Henggeler, S.W., S.K. Schoenwald, and S.G. Pickrel. Forthcoming. Multisystemic Therapy: Bridging the Gap between University- and Community-Based Treatment. *Journal of Consulting and Clinical Psychology* (in press).

Henggeler, S.W., S.K. Schoenwald, S.G. Pickrel, M.D. Rowland, and A.B. Santos. 1994. The Contribution of Treatment Research to the Reform of Children's Mental Health Services: Multisystemic Family Preservation as an Example. *Journal of Mental Health Administration* 21:229–39.

Higgins, S.T., and A.J. Budney. 1993. Treatment of Cocaine Dependence through the Principles of Behavior Analysis and Behavioral Pharmacology. In *Behavioral Treatments for Drug Abuse and Dependence*.

NIDA Research Monograph no. 137, ed. L.S. Onken, J.D. Blaine, and J.J. Boren (97-121). Rockville, Md.: National Institute on Drug Abuse.

Hubbard, R.L., E.R. Cavanaugh, S.G. Craddock, and J.V. Rachal. 1983. *Characteristics, Behaviors, and Outcomes for Youth in the TOPS Study.* Report submitted to the National Institute on Drug Abuse, Contract No. 271-79-3611. Research Triangle Park, N.C.: Research Triangle Institute.

Institute of Medicine. 1990. *A Study of the Evolution, Effectiveness, and Financing of Public and Private Drug Treatment Systems* (Treating Drug Problems, vol. 1.). Washington: National Academy Press.

Jessor, R., and S.L. Jessor. 1977. *Problem Behavior and Psychosocial Development: A Longitudinal Study of Youth.* New York: Academic Press.

Joanning, H., W. Quinn, F. Thomas, and R. Mullen. 1992. Treating Adolescent Drug Abuse: A Comparison of Family Systems Therapy, Group Therapy, and Family Drug Education. *Journal of Marital and Family Therapy* 18:345–56.

Johnson, C.A., M.A. Pentz, M.D. Weber et al. 1990. Relative Effectiveness of Comprehensive Community Programming for Drug Abuse Prevention with High-Risk and Low-Risk Adolescents. *Journal of Consulting and Clinical Psychology* 58:447–56.

Kumpfer, K.L. 1989. Prevention of Alcohol and Drug Abuse: A Critical Review of Risk Factors and Prevention Strategies. In *Prevention of Mental Disorders, Alcohol and Other Drug Use in Children and Adolescents.* OSAP Prevention Monograph-2, ed. D. Shaffer, I. Philips, and N.B. Enzer (309-71). Rockville, Md.: Office for Substance Abuse Prevention, DHHS.

Lewis, R.A., F.P. Piercy, D.H. Sprenkle, and T.S. Trepper. 1990. Family-Based Interventions for Helping Drug-Abusing Adolescents. *Journal of Adolescent Research* 5:82–95.

Liddle, H.A., and G.A. Dakof. 1994. Family-Based Treatment for Adolescent Drug Use: State of the Science. In *Adolescent Drug Abuse: Assessment and Treatment,* ed. E. Rahdert et al. Rockville, Md.: National Institute on Drug Abuse Research Monograph.

Maloy, K.A. 1991. *Mental Health for Children: Can We Get There From Here?* Washington: Mental Health Policy Resource Center.

Marlatt, G.A., and S.F. Tapert. 1993. Harm Reduction: Reducing the Risks of Addictive Behaviors. In *Addictive Behaviors Across the Lifespan: Prevention, Treatment, and Policy Issues,* ed. J.S. Baer, G.A. Marlatt, and R.J. McMahon. Newbury Park, Calif.: Sage.

Marlatt, G.A., J.M. Somers, and S.F. Tapert. 1993. Harm Reduction: Application to Alcohol Abuse Problems. In *Behavioral Treatments for Drug Abuse and Dependence.* NIDA Research Monograph No. 137, ed. L.S. Onken, J.D. Blaine, and J.J. Boren (147-66). Rockville, Md.: National Institute on Drug Abuse.

Meyers, J.C. 1994. Financing Strategies to Support Innovations in Service Delivery to Children. *Journal of Clinical Child Psychology* 23 (Suppl.):48–54.

Miller, W.R. 1993a. Behavioral Treatments for Drug Problems: Where Do We Go from Here? In *Behavioral Treatments for Drug Abuse and Dependence.*

NIDA Research Monograph no. 137, ed. L.S. Onken, J.D. Blaine, and J.J. Boren (303-320). Rockville, Md.: National Institute on Drug Abuse.

——. 1993b. Behavioral Treatments for Drug Problems: Lessons from the Alcohol Treatment Outcome Literature. In *Behavioral Treatments for Drug Abuse and Dependence*. NIDA Research Monograph no. 137, ed. L.S. Onken, J.D. Blaine, and J.J. Boren (167-80). Rockville, Md.: National Institute on Drug Abuse.

Needle, R., H. McCubbin, M. Wilson, R. Reineck, A. Lazar, and H. Mederer. 1986. Interpersonal Influences in Adolescent Drug Use: The Role of Older Siblings, Parents, and Peers. *International Journal of the Addictions* 21:739–66.

Nelson, K.E. 1994. Innovative Delivery Models in Social Services. *Journal of Clinical Child Psychology* 23 (Suppl.):26–31.

Newcomb, M.C. and P.M. Bentler. 1987. The Impact of Late Adolescent Substance Use on Young Adult Health Status and Utilization of Health Services: A Structural Equation Model over Four Years. *Social Science and Medicine* 24:71–82.

——. 1989. Substance Use and Abuse among Children and Teenagers. *American Psychologist* 44:242–8.

Oetting, E.R., and F. Beauvais. 1987. Peer Cluster Theory, Socialization Characteristics, and Adolescent Drug Use: A Path Analysis. *Journal of Counseling Psychology* 34:205–13.

Office of Technology Assessment, U.S. Congress. 1991. *Background and the Effectiveness of Selected Prevention and Treatment Services*. Adolescent Health – Volume II: OTA-H-466 (499–578). Washington: U.S. Government Printing Office.

Onken, L.S., J.D. Blaine, and J.J. Boren (eds). 1993. *Behavioral Treatments for Drug Abuse and Dependence*. NIDA Research Monograph No. 137). Rockville, Md.: National Institute on Drug Abuse.

Rhodes, J.E., and L.A. Jason. 1990. A Social Stress Model of Substance Abuse. *Journal of Consulting and Clinical Psychology* 58:395–401.

Rodrigue, J.R. 1994. Beyond the Individual Child: Innovative Systems Approaches to Service Delivery in Pediatric Psychology. *Journal of Clinical Child Psychology* 23 (Suppl.):32–9.

Rosenblatt, A. and C.C. Attkisson. 1993. Integrating Systems of Care in California for Youth with Severe Emotional Disturbance III: Answers that Lead to Questions about Out-of-Home Placements and the AB377 Evaluation Project. *Journal of Child and Family Studies* 2:119–41.

Schuster, C.R., and K. Silverman. 1993. Advancing the Application of Behavioral Treatment Approaches for Drug Dependence. In *Behavioral Treatments for Drug Abuse and Dependence*. NIDA Research Monograph no. 137, ed. L.S. Onken, J.D. Blaine, and J.J. Boren (5–17). Rockville, Md.: National Institute on Drug Abuse.

Sells, S.B., and D.D. Simpson. 1979. Evaluation of Treatment Outcome for Youths in the Drug Abuse Reporting Program (DARP): A Follow-Up study. In *Youth Drug Abuse: Problems, Issues and Treatment*, ed. G.M.

Beschner and A.S. Friedman (571–628). Lexington, Mass.: Lexington Books.

Stein, J.A., M.D. Newcomb, and P.M. Bentler. 1987. An 8-Year Study of Multiple Influences on Drug Use and Drug Use Consequences. *Journal of Personality and Social Psychology* 53:1094–105.

Stitzer, M.L., M.Y. Iguchi, M. Kidorf, and G.E. Bigelow. 1993. Contingency Management in Methadone Treatment: The Case for Positive Incentives. In *Behavioral Treatments for Drug Abuse and Dependence*. NIDA Research Monograph no. 137, ed. L.S. Onken, J.D. Blaine, and J.J. Boren (19–36). Rockville, Md.: National Institute on Drug Abuse.

Stroul, B.A., and R.M. Friedman. 1986. *A System of Care of Severely Emotionally Disturbed Children and Youth*. Washington: Georgetown University Child Development Center.

———. 1994. *A System of Care for Children and Youth with Severe Emotional Disturbance*. Washington: Georgetown University Child Development Center.

Swaim, R.C., E.R. Oetting, R.W. Edwards, and F. Beauvais. 1989. Links from Emotional Distress to Adolescent Drug Use: A Path Model. *Journal of Consulting and Clinical Psychology* 57:227–31.

Szapocznik, J., W.M. Kurtines, F. Foote, A. Perez-Vidal, and O. Hervis. 1983. Conjoint versus One-Person Family Therapy: Some Evidence for the Effectiveness of Conducting Family Therapy through One Person with Drug-Abusing Adolescents. *Journal of Consulting and Clinical Psychology* 51:889–99.

———. 1986. Conjoint versus One-Person Family Therapy: Further Evidence for the Effectiveness of Conducting Family Therapy through One Person with Drug-Abusing Adolescents. *Journal of Consulting and Clinical Psychology* 54:395–7.

Weisz, J.R., and B. Weiss. 1993. *Effects of Psychotherapy with Children and Adolescents*. Newbury Park, Calif.: Sage.

Weithorn, L.A. 1988. Mental Hospitalization of Troublesome Youth: An Analysis of Skyrocketing Admission Rates. *Stanford Law Review* 40:773–837.

White, H.R., R.J. Pandina, and R.L. LaGrange. 1987. Longitudinal Predictors of Serious Substance Use and Delinquency. *Criminology* 25:715–40.

White House Domestic Policy Council. 1993. The President's Health Security Plan. Washington, September 7.

10

Casualties of the Drug War: An Equality-Based Argument for Drug Treatment

David Cole and Barry Littman

Introduction

Allen James was an on-again, off-again heroin addict for seventeen years. An African-American man with a high-school diploma, nearly two years of college education, and an honorable discharge from the Army, Mr. James first became addicted to heroin in the summer of 1968, at age 22. He tried at the time to wean himself from the drug, entered various detoxification programs, and even bought illegal methadone on the streets, all to no avail.[1]

The addiction continued, and in the summer of 1972, Mr. James left his wife and child and took up drug dealing. In August of that year, he was arrested for attempted homicide, reckless endangerment, and possession of a weapon. He spent ten months in detention awaiting trial, eventually pleading guilty to attempted possession of a weapon. He was sentenced to one to three years in a New York

State prison. He served 14 months in maximum security state prisons, and was never offered any drug treatment.

Released in the fall of 1974, Mr. James went to live with a friend in Colorado, where he attended college and worked full-time for IBM and part-time as a counselor. He returned to New York City to be with his family in the winter of 1976 and worked there as a computer technician while studying theater arts. In 1978, however, he relapsed into heroin addiction. Once again, he left his family and resorted to crime to support his habit. During this period, he was arrested between five and seven times for misdemeanors, three or four of which resulted in convictions. Later that year, he was arrested for the burglary of an insurance office, convicted, and sentenced to one year in the Westchester County Penitentiary.

Ever resourceful, Mr. James began to write scripts for a local theater company while serving his one-year sentence. The theater company hired him upon his release, and from 1979 to 1981 he worked and performed in the theater, taught theater and creative writing, and completed two non-fiction books published in the United States and Europe.

Even this success, however, was not enough to keep him off heroin. In 1981, Mr. James again relapsed into drug abuse and abandoned his career. He was arrested six or seven times and convicted of at least five additional misdemeanors over the next two years. He served a short sentence in a New York City jail in 1983, but managed upon release to find work with a health care center in New York as Director of Communications and Audio-Visual Services.

Mr. James suffered his third drug-abuse relapse in 1985. His addiction was costing him $200–500 per day, and he again resorted to crime to support his habit. In 1985, he was arrested for stealing a car, and served about 45 days in pre-trial detention. While there, he sought admission to several drug-treatment programs. Project Return Foundation, Inc. agreed to take him in, and the judge gave him the option of a 90-day jail sentence or one year probation with the stipulation that he complete drug treatment in Project Return. He took the probation and treatment. He later explained, "I had no idea of how to break the pattern of relapse into drugs and crime that had persisted over so many years. My decision was to ask for help in doing something I had given up any hope of doing alone."

Mr. James entered Project Return in August 1985 and remained in treatment for 18 months. During the last six months of treatment, the Project hired him as Assistant to a Program Director. In June 1987, he went to work for the Fortune Society, an organization that provides services for ex-offenders. By 1989, he had risen to the position of Director of Career Development and Adult Counseling.

Mr. James's talents and resourcefulness are quite extraordinary; yet notwithstanding those gifts, his addiction repeatedly led him out of work, onto the streets, into a life of crime, and ultimately into prison. He was arrested over 15 times, convicted a dozen times, and incarcerated on four separate occasions. It was not until he received serious, long-term drug treatment that he was freed from the cycle of drugs, crime, and incarceration.

The cycle in which Mr. James was trapped for 17 years is not unusual. What is unusual is that he was able to find treatment and escape. All too often, the story ends not with a promotion to Director of Career Development, but with an extended prison sentence for a serious crime. That end is increasingly likely today, as Congress and many states have enacted "three strikes and you're out" provisions, which mandate life sentences without the possibility of parole for a third drug-related felony.

As a society, we have always spent far more on law enforcement responses to drug abuse than on treatment and prevention. This trend was exacerbated during the Reagan–Bush era by the so-called "War on Drugs," in which ever-escalating government resources were directed towards arresting, prosecuting, and imprisoning drug users. The war had little recognizable effect on the drug problem, but has had a devastating impact on the African-American community in particular.

Many arguments have been made against the law enforcement approach to our nation's drug problem. Some have argued that it is immoral, because we are essentially punishing individuals for a disease or a status offense.[2] Others have contended that it is inefficient; a Rand Corporation study recently concluded that a dollar spent on drug treatment reduces cocaine consumption by the same amount as seven dollars spent on the most successful law enforcement efforts.[3] Still others have pointed to Prohibition and speculated that much drug-related crime would be reduced if drugs were legalized and regulated by government.[4]

But the particular impact that the criminalization of drug use and possession has had on the black community provides another, perhaps even more compelling, rationale for reconsidering our response to the drug problem. Drug law enforcement has devastated the black community, consigning a remarkably high proportion of young African-American men to long prison sentences that will further restrict their already limited opportunities to become productive members of society. By effectively incapacitating a large segment of the black community, drug law enforcement thereby contributes to the subordinate social status of the black community. As Michael Tonry has written:

> Many disadvantaged black males start out with bleak life chances, and disadvantaged young men ensnared in the criminal justice system have even bleaker prospects. No solution to problems of the urban underclass, or more broadly, of black poverty can succeed if young men are not part of it . . . Unless America can devise ways to make its crime control policies less destructive of poor black males and poor black communities, there can be no solution to the problem of the black underclass.[5]

While there are many different causes of drug addiction, there is little doubt that one factor is the absence of other life opportunities, such as good education and employment prospects.[6] It is not surprising, therefore, that urban, poor, minority communities are hardest hit by the drug problem. If we respond to the drug problem principally by incarcerating drug addicts, we have chosen a solution that is likely to exacerbate the inequalities that led to the drug problem in the first place. While we do not believe that this was the intent of the drug war, the effects cannot be ignored, and demand a response. Several responses have been suggested – from decriminalization to increasing the educational and employment opportunities of those who grow up in urban poverty, where the drug problem is at its worst. We believe that the drug problem's concentration in the poorest communities underscores the need to redress the socioeconomic roots of the problem, namely the inequitable provision of education, housing, and job opportunities that characterizes these communities. Recognizing the formidable political and economic obstacles to such solutions, however, we advocate here a more moderate response: drug treatment. And because individuals' drug problems are first publicly revealed through the criminal justice system, we focus specifically on the issue of treatment within the criminal justice system.

Unlike decriminalization, drug treatment does not present the danger of condoning drug abuse. Rather, it addresses drug abuse as a medical, psychological, and social problem. Drug treatment can give more people the chance that Allen James eventually got – the chance to escape the downward spiral of drugs, crime, and incarceration. Treatment should be widely available in the communities hardest hit by drugs, so that individuals can address the problem before they enter the criminal justice system. But even if treatment were widely available, it is likely that many persons would not consider it seriously until they were caught. It is therefore especially critical to offer treatment *after* an individual is arrested – as an alternative to punishment, while in prison, or as a condition of parole. The important point is to ensure that drug abuse, once revealed, is treated, not merely punished. Otherwise, we are allowing a systemic problem – drug abuse among the urban poor, and particularly among minorities – to become yet another building block in the structure of subordination.

I   The War on Drugs

In the 1980s, as the Cold War was winding down, the United States embarked on a new conflict on the domestic front: the war on drugs. Over the decade, the federal drug enforcement budget increased by nine times, to nearly $13 billion a year.[7] President Ronald Reagan declared a war on drugs in 1982.[8] The war had two principal components: (1) escalation of government resources directed toward drug law enforcement measures; and (2) redirection of enforcement efforts on users rather than suppliers of drugs. Prior to 1984, drug reduction measures concentrated on suppliers, focusing on impeding international import and targeting large-scale traffickers.[9] Laws such as the Racketeer-Influenced and Corrupt Organizations (RICO) and Continuing Criminal Enterprise (CCE) of 1970 were primarily directed at such large-scale traffickers. The international supply side was also a priority, and the United States undertook several cooperative efforts with other nations to reduce the supply of narcotics.[10]

The Reagan–Bush era saw the enactment of four new federal antidrug bills, greatly expanding the reach of federal drug laws and increasing penalties for offenses. The 1984 Crime Control Act expanded drug forfeiture laws, increased federal penalties for drug offenses, and introduced determinate sentencing through the "sentencing guidelines." The 1986 Anti-Drug Abuse Act restored mandatory prison sentences for large-scale distribution,[11] and created a drug law enforcement grant program to assist state and local authorities. The 1988 Anti-Drug Abuse Act again increased penalties for drug offenses, and specifically endorsed the use of sanctions targeted at drug users to reduce the demand for drugs.[12] And the Crime Control Act of 1990 allocated still more grants to state and local authorities for drug law enforcement. While some money was also directed at prevention and treatment, 70 percent of the federal drug budget authorized by these Acts went to increased law enforcement efforts – more police, more prosecutors, and more prisons.[13]

The "War on Drugs" was prompted at least in part by the visibility of drug use and the threat of drug-related crime and violence, which led the American public to rate drug abuse as "the nation's most important domestic and foreign policy problem."[14] In response, enforcement efforts were often focused on the most visible manifestations of the problem: those who lived in poor urban areas and did their business on the streets.[15] From an elected official's perspective, the fastest way to show that the problem is being addressed is to reduce the most visible symptoms – the pushers and users on the streets.[16] In New York City, for example, the two biggest drug law enforcement initiatives of the 1980s focused on neighborhoods beset by open drug dealing – Manhattan's Lower East Side, Washington Heights, and Harlem, Brooklyn's East New York section, and the South Bronx.[17]

2   Effects of the War on Drugs

General impact of the war on drugs

The results of the "War on Drugs" are startling. It has severely strained law enforcement resources, from police to prosecutors to public defenders to courts to prisons. From 1980 to 1993, state and federal prison populations increased 188 percent, to a total of 948,881 prisoners.[18] Almost half the growth in new court commitments since 1980 is due to drug offenses.[19] Today, the number of federal prison inmates serving time for drug offenses alone exceeds the entire federal prison population in 1980.[20]

The percentage of drug convictions relative to convictions for other serious crimes has risen dramatically since 1980 (table 10.1). While the absolute numbers of commitments for all types of crime have risen, new commitments for drug offenses increased by more than eleven times from 1980 to 1992. In 1980, new commitments for drug crimes (8,900) were far below new commitments for property offenses (55,000) and violent crimes (62,000). As table 10.1 indicates, by 1992, drug commitments had overtaken violent crime and nearly matched property offenses as the leading cause of new commitments.[21]

These numbers have had a profound impact on all aspects of the

Table 10.1   New court commitments.

| | Number of new court commitments for most prevalent crimes | |
	1980	1992
Drugs	8,900	102,000
Property	55,000	104,000
Violent Crimes	62,000	95,000
Public Order	1,000	29,000
	Percentage of new court commitments	
	1980	1992
Drugs	6.8%	30.5%
Property	41.1%	31.2%
Violent Crimes	48.2%	28.5%
Public Order	4.0%	8.8%

Source: Bureau of Justice Statistics, June 1994. Prisoners in 1993 at 7, 10, figures 1, 2; appendix tables 1, 2.

criminal justice system.[22] At the close of 1993, the federal prison system was operating at 36 percent over capacity, and state prisons were estimated to be operating at 118 percent of capacity.[23] Among industrialized nations, only Russia incarcerates more citizens per capita than the United States. We imprison 519 of every 100,000 citizens, while Canada, our neighbor to the north, imprisons only 116 per 100,000.[24]

The courts are also overwhelmed. Narcotics prosecutions in the federal courts have increased 229 percent in the past decade, and drug cases currently account for 40–65 percent of all criminal trials. The backlog of drug cases in federal courts increased six times between 1989 and 1991.[25] The large numbers of drug-related cases cause delays in the prosecution of other criminal cases and even further delays for civil cases, which have lower priority.[26]

Judges and commentators have argued that the drug war has undermined the constitutional protections afforded to all, as courts pressured to uphold drug convictions have watered down constitutional constraints on police action. Judge Harry Edwards, for example, now Chief Judge of the United States Court of Appeals for the District of Columbia, has expressed his "growing concern about the degree to which individual rights and liberties appear to be falling victim to the Government's 'War on Drugs.'"[27] He warned that "when the war is over, we [will] find that departures from constitutional norms, legitimized by the courts, have lasting and wide-ranging effects."[28]

There is little evidence that these efforts have paid off. While self-reported drug use is down,[29] the self-reports are based on interviews with senior high-school students and persons in their homes, and thus miss those parts of the population most at risk of drug addiction – those in the criminal justice system, the homeless, and high-school drop-outs.[30] Other studies show an increasing drug problem over the course of the 1980s.[31]

Meanwhile, the cost of cocaine has decreased, not increased, suggesting that supply has not been significantly reduced.[32] Domestic production of marijuana has increased.[33] And those responsible for the front lines report that the war is not being won. The New York Police Department's Assistant Police Chief Francis C. Hall, who directed the Narcotics Division, has stated that

> Drug enforcement . . . is like the Vietnam War. In Vietnam, we under-estimated the number of Vietcong and their will to fight. We appear to be doing the same thing with street-level drug traffickers . . . We lost the Vietnam War with a half-million men. We're doing the same thing with drugs.[34]

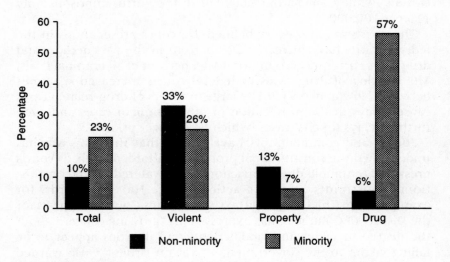

Figure 10.1   Change in arrests by type of crime and race, 1986–90

Racial impact of the war on drugs

While the general effects of the "War on Drugs" are troubling in themselves, the effects on African-Americans are even more stark. African-Americans account for approximately 12 percent of the general population, yet as of the end of 1992, 50.2 percent of sentenced state and federal prisoners were black.[35] Much of this disparity can be attributed to enforcement of the drug laws. Between 1986 and 1991, overall minority arrests increased more than non-minority arrests (23 percent minority increase, 10 percent non-minority). Yet *drug offenses are the only area in which minority arrests actually increased more than non-minority arrests* (figure 10.1).[36]

While minorities account for fewer than one-third of arrests,[37] they make up increasing percentages of the correctional population. In 1990, minorities accounted for half of all jail inmates and more than half of the prisoners, probationers, and parolees. The increase in jail inmates from 1986 to 1990 was more than twice as great for minorities as non-minorities, and almost as disparate for prisoners and parolees as well (figure 10.2).[38]

Between 1980 and 1992, the number of prisoners in state and federal prisons increased by 531,000, or more than 150 percent. Over that same period the number of black men in prison increased by 186 percent. When black females are included, black prisoners made up over half of the prison population expansion from 1980 to 1992 (278,600 out of 531,000).[39]

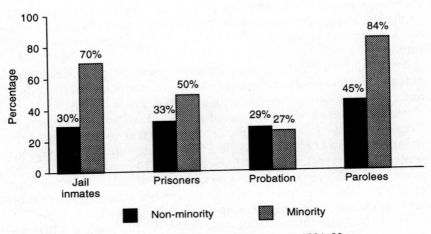

Figure 10.2 Increase in correctional supervision by race, 1986–90

Much of this expansion is attributable to the drug laws: 59.1 percent of all black males in federal prisons in 1992 were there for drug violations.[40] From 1983 to 1989, the percentage of persons in local jails charged with drug offenses who were black increased from 35 percent to 48 percent, while the white percentage dropped from 44 percent to 25 percent.[41] In 1986, only 7.2 percent of African-Americans in state prisons had drug offenses as their most serious offense; by 1991, that figure was up to 25 percent.[42] In New York State, more than 90 percent of those imprisoned for drug felonies in 1988 were black or Hispanic.[43]

A substantial number of those serving time for drug offenses have no prior or current violence on their records, no involvement in sophisticated criminal activity, and no prior commitment. Such "low-level drug offenders" make up 36.1 percent of all drug-law offenders in the prison system and 21.2 percent of federal prisoners. Approximately one-third of these low-level offenders are black. Yet because of the drug war, these offenders serve sentences nearly as long as those convicted of violent crimes. The average federal sentence for a low-level drug offense is 81.5 months, while the average sentence for a violent offense is 90.6 months.[44]

Once arrested, black defendants charged with drug offenses fare worse in the criminal justice system than white defendants. In federal district courts in 1989, for example, black drug offenders were incarcerated 94 percent of the time, while white drug offenders were incarcerated 88 percent of the time.[45] More significantly, the average sentence for a black drug offender in federal court was 89.4 months, while the average sentence for a white offender was 70 months, a disparity of nearly two years.[46] For all offenders sentenced under the federal guidelines from 20 January 1989 to 30 June 1990, black offenders received sentences 41 percent longer than white offenders.[47]

Much of the sentencing disparity in the federal system is attributable to a distinction in the sentences imposed for possession of crack and powder cocaine. Possession of a gram of crack cocaine receives the same sentence as possession of 100 grams of powder cocaine.[48] Because of this differential, the average federal sentence for trafficking in powder cocaine was 79 months, while the average sentence for trafficking in crack cocaine was 141 months.[49] Over 90 percent of those sentenced for crack-related offenses are black and only 3 percent are white, while 32 percent of those sentenced for powder cocaine offenses are white, and only 27 percent are black.[50]

As of 1992, the incarceration rate for black males in state prisons was seven times that for white males (2,678 per 100,000 for black males, 372 per 100,000 for white males). Nearly three out of every 100 black males were incarcerated in state prisons in 1992; less than four out of every *1000* white males were so incarcerated.[51] When one includes federal prisons, state and local jails, and probation and parole, the numbers soar even higher. Nationwide, in 1989 one in four black men between the ages of 20 and 29 was under some type of correctional supervision.[52] In 1986, the number of young black men under correctional supervision was greater than the total number of all black men enrolled in college.[53] In urban areas, the numbers are still worse: in Baltimore 56 percent of young black men are either in prison or jail, or on probation or parole on any given day; in the District of Columbia the figure approaches 40 percent.[54]

Racial disparities are also pervasive in the juvenile justice system's treatment of drug offenders. Between 1986 and 1991, arrests for all crimes increased by 25 percent for minority juveniles and by only 5 percent for non-minorities. Yet *for drug offenses, minority arrests increased by 78 percent, while non-minority arrests decreased by 34 percent.*[55]

Once in the juvenile justice system, black youth are on average treated far more severely than white youth. In 1991, white juveniles were involved in 50 percent of all drug-related cases, while black juveniles accounted for 48 percent.[56] Black juveniles, however, were detained for drug violations at nearly twice the rate of whites (13,800 drug cases detained for blacks; 7,400 for whites);[57] Eighty-two percent of drug cases involving black juveniles, and only 53 percent of cases involving whites, were handled formally, or petitioned.[58] Once petitioned, 5.7 percent of black juvenile drug cases were transferred to criminal courts for adult prosecution, as compared with 1.4 percent of white cases.[59] From 1987 to 1991, the number of black youth placed outside the home for drug offenses *increased* by 28.5 percent, while placement for whites *decreased* 30 percent.[60]

We do not suggest that the drug war was intentionally designed to incarcerate massive numbers of black citizens – that just happens to be its result.[61] The result is so dramatic, however, that it cries out for a response. Several courts, influenced by the significant racial disparities caused by punishing possession of crack cocaine far more severely than possession of powder cocaine, have invalidated such laws.[62] We do not address the constitutional arguments here, but argue instead that the disparate racial impact of the "War on Drugs" provides, at a minimum, compelling moral and policy arguments for providing treatment, as either an alternative or a supplement to punishment for drug crimes.

If one in four young *white* men were under the supervision of the correctional system, primarily for drug-law violations, we think it likely that the nation would demand treatment. Indeed, when large numbers of white middle-class youth were arrested for marijuana possession in the late 1960s and early 1970s, public complaints led Congress and 11 states to decriminalize or to reduce substantially the penalties for marijuana possession.[63] While there are undoubtedly differences between marijuana and cocaine, this historical example suggests that selective indifference to the plight of a minority community may well play a part in the continuation of a get-tough response to the drug problem.[64]

Unconscious racism is not the only racial disparity demonstrated above. Black citizens may simply violate the drug laws more frequently than white citizens. Indeed, some have argued that disparities such as those created by the crack/cocaine differential should be seen as the result of providing equal protection of laws to the black community. If drug abuse is more prevalent in the black community, there should be more arrests, convictions, and incarcerations of black defendants; anything less would deny equal protection to the law-abiding members of the black community, who are threatened by the crime and violence associated with drug abuse in their community.[65]

In our view, this argument misses a fundamental point. Even if drug abuse is more prevalent in the black community, and even if the disparate results described above are the result of equal application of the criminal laws, a strong argument for changing our mode of response remains. If the black community is more susceptible to drug addiction, it seems likely that this is at least in part attributable to the vestiges of past race discrimination and current inequalities.

Studies have consistently found a strong link between the prevalence of drug use in a community and its socioeconomic status.[66] This is true across racial lines, and even internationally.[67] The African-American urban community is disproportionately poor: 33.3 percent of African-Americans live in poverty, as compared with 11.6 percent of whites, and the median net worth of white households is more than ten times that of black households.[68] Black children are routinely denied equal educational opportunities.[69] And the black unemployment rate is twice that in the white community.[70] Drugs and the drug trade fill the gaps, providing a psychological escape and fiscal opportunities. In turn, the drug problem creates still more obstacles to success for those born into the black community. If as a society we respond to the drug problem principally by imposing long prison sentences, we take a problem that is both partially caused by and partially a cause of social subordination, and exacerbate its subordinating effects by hobbling the community's young black men.

As Elliott Currie has stated, "we will not begin to comprehend America's drug problem, much less resolve it, until we understand that drugs and inequality are closely and multiply linked . . . our national willingness to tolerate unusually severe levels of social deprivation and marginality goes a long way toward explaining why we lead the world in drug abuse."[71] We agree with Currie that the solution to the drug problem ultimately lies in redressing the inequalities that feed the problem in the first place. But we also recognize the political difficulties presented by such a solution.

Accordingly, we propose that if we are to both respond to the drug problem in the black community and not exacerbate the structural and social problems that contribute to it, we should consider treatment alternatives. Treatment acknowledges that drug addiction itself is a serious problem, but does not merely take the drug war's victims and lock them up for long periods of time. Admittedly, treatment – within or without the criminal justice system – is only a partial solution, but it is a necessary (and feasible) step in the right direction.

3 Treating the Problem

Numerous studies have demonstrated that compulsory treatment for drug-dependent persons works, and is a viable alternative to incarceration.[72] Unlike legalization, moreover, there is substantial support for compulsory drug treatment, both as an alternative to incarceration for low-level offenders, and as a complement to incarceration for more serious drug-dependent offenders. Several jurisdictions have begun to experiment with "drug courts" that divert persons charged with drug possession to mandatory treatment programs, using the stick of incarceration as an incentive to participation.

Drug treatment can come at three different points: (1) before arrest; (2) after arrest, as an alternative to incarceration; and (3) after conviction, while the defendant is in prison or on probation. We believe that treatment at all three points is important, but in this chapter we focus on treatment in connection with the criminal justice system.

Treatment as an alternative to incarceration

Several jurisdictions, from the District of Columbia to Oakland, California, have begun to run specialized "drug courts" designed to oversee compulsory treatment programs for low-level drug offenders as an alternative to incarceration. Rather than exhaustively review these programs, we will briefly describe one such drug court, in Dade County, Florida, and note the preliminary assessments of its effectiveness.

Dade County's criminal justice system has experienced trends similar to those of the nation as a whole. Drug offenses make up an increasing proportion of the courts' already overburdened dockets.[73] In response to these demands, Dade County created the Diversion and Treatment Program, which channels almost all nonviolent defendants facing drug possession charges into a court-supervised rehabilitation program as an alternative to prosecution.

Only those arrested for possession or purchase of drugs are eligible for the program. A history of violent crime, an arrest for drug trafficking, or more than two previous non-drug felony convictions are disqualifying. In addition, the State Attorney must approve the diversion. Defendants are eligible regardless of whether it is their first drug offense, and with the exception of marijuana, possession of any controlled substance qualifies for consideration.

All new participants are brought before the Drug Court judge. He explains the program to each defendant individually, making it clear that they should expect a year of treatment, that success will be difficult, and that they will be provided with all the assistance they need. He tells them that they will be drug-tested frequently and that if progress is unsatisfactory, the criminal prosecution can be resumed. Once the defendant consents to the program (almost all do), the judge remands him to the custody of the program for at least one year.

The treatment program generally consists of three distinct phases – detoxification, stabilization, and aftercare – but may be tailored to each individual. Detoxification takes place at the county's main treatment clinic. The client's primary counselor, a licensed addiction treatment professional, oversees daily urine testing, provides individual and group counseling, and works with the client to prepare a treatment plan. Acupuncture is also offered, as it is said to reduce cravings, mitigate withdrawal symptoms, and ease the anxiety associated with the period immediately after drug use ceases. Phase I can last from two to six weeks.

Other Phase I treatment options include group and individual counseling, fellowship meetings such as the 12-step programs and, if deemed necessary, inpatient treatment at a county facility. Clients who are having particular trouble may ask to be removed temporarily and incarcerated for two weeks to use one of the jail treatment beds reserved for Drug Court participants. Approximately 60 percent of the clients who graduate from the program spend at least two weeks in jail. Once detoxification is completed, they may ask to be returned to the program.

When the Drug Court judge concludes that the client can function in a less structured environment, he is moved into Phase II. Through the use of individual and group counseling sessions and attendance at local fellowship meetings, Phase II seeks to maintain the client's abstinence and to help him accept the idea of drug-free living. As long as the client's samples remain clean and he shows up for all required treatment and court sessions, he is allowed to decide which treatment methods he prefers. Although Phase II is scheduled to last 14 to 16 weeks, clients can remain in this Phase for longer or shorter periods depending on their progress. Clients may also be returned to Phase I if they have difficulty remaining drug-free.

In Phase III, the treatment site changes to a local community college, and the focus shifts from maintaining abstinence to preparing the client academically and occupationally for the future. Clients still return to court regularly, urine samples are still monitored, and counseling is still available, but the focus of this stage is to give clients the tools they need to become productive members of society. Clients may get literacy education, GED courses, vocational training, and job-search assistance. Phase III is scheduled to last from 8 to 12 months.

When monitoring is no longer deemed necessary, the counselor recommends the client's discharge to the court. If the judge agrees, he releases the client from the program and from ongoing court supervision. One year later, the court seals the arrest record of any client with no previous felony conviction who has not been rearrested.

It is too early to determine conclusively the success of Miami's program, since it has been in existence for just over four years, but the statistical evidence thus far is encouraging. Between June 1989 and March 1993, approximately 4,500 defendants entered the Diversion and Treatment Program, or 20 percent of all county arrestees charged with drug-related offenses. Approximately 60 percent of those diverted are either still in the program or have successfully graduated. A study comparing Drug Court defendants with similar defendants not in the Program found that Drug Court defendants have less frequent rearrests;[74] 67 percent of Drug Court defendants had no rearrests during the 18-month observation period, while less than 50 percent of similar defendants processed through the traditional criminal justice system had no rearrests.[75] Moreover, of those rearrested, the median time to first rearrest of drug treatment participants was three to four times longer than for drug defendants in the traditional criminal justice system.[76] Recidivism rates for general prison populations range up to 60 percent, yet only 11 percent of those who successfully completed the drug court program were rearrested in the year following graduation.[77]

The Program's $1.8 million budget for fiscal year 1992 works out to roughly $800 per client per year, about the same as the cost of jailing an offender for nine days. Funding for the program was raised through redistribution of traffic fines, so that no taxes were increased. Clients who can pay are required to do so, although this does not amount to much: total monthly income from clients ranges from $11,000 to $23,000.

If the treatment program works even for a few clients, it is probably a sound investment. A study of 573 substance abusers in Miami found that in a one-year period they committed more than 84,000 assorted, non-drug-related crimes. At approximately 200 crimes per person per year, the crime reduction potential is great if even a small portion of these people become drug-free and employed. By addressing the drug problem with a little extra cost on the front end, long-term benefits should appear in the form of lower recidivism rates (which will save resources for both the prisons and the courts), a reduced demand for drugs, and the re-entry into society of productive individuals who might otherwise have been a lifelong burden on the taxpayers.[78]

These types of programs hold great promise for the overburdened court systems, for the demand-reduction side of the war on drugs, and also for the black communities that have been devastated by the long-term incarceration of a generation of young males. According to the Criminal Justice Sourcebook, 25 percent of the 321,217 blacks in State prisons in 1991 had as their most serious offense a non-violent drug crime. With more expansive treatment alternatives, it is reasonable to expect that a significant portion of those 80,000 prisoners could be diverted from the prison system, rehabilitated, and prepared for a future with more to offer than just another trip to the courtroom.

Treatment in prisons and jails

Substance-abuse problems are obviously not limited to those arrested for low-level non-violent drug offenses, and who might therefore be eligible for treatment as an alternative to incarceration. Many of those serving time for crimes not involving drugs are substance abusers: 79.4 percent of the 710,798 state prison inmates in 1991 reported that they had used drugs at some point; 49.4 percent said they had used drugs in the month before committing their offense; 36 percent had used drugs daily in the month before their offense; and 30.9 percent were under the influence of drugs at the time of their offense.[79] A 1989 report based on studies by the Bureau of Justice Statistics estimated that 62 percent of the total prison population used drugs regularly prior to their arrest.[80] More than 13 percent of all convicted inmates said that they committed their offense for money to buy drugs; 24.4 percent of all property offenses were assertedly committed for drug money.[81]

Dr. Douglas S. Lipton, Director of the Research Institute of Narcotic and Drug Research, Inc., estimates that 60 to 75 percent of untreated parolees with histories of heroin and/or cocaine use return to drug use within three months after release, and then become reinvolved in criminal activity.[82] Compared with nondrug-using inmates, heroin-addicted inmates in California prisons have committed fifteen times as many robberies, twenty times as many burglaries, and ten times as many thefts.[83]

Yet we do not provide nearly enough treatment in prisons and jails. The General Accounting Office has estimated that while nearly three-quarters of all state prisoners need substance-abuse treatment, only about 15 percent were actually receiving treatment.[84] And much of the treatment that is provided in prisons and jails is not likely to be successful, because it consists of low-cost but also minimally effective group counseling.[85]

Thus, the prison and jail setting provides a population very much in need of drug treatment, and even moderately successful treatment programs might produce significant reductions in criminality. Moreover, the evidence suggests that appropriate treatment can lead to reduced recidivism.[86] Treatment in prisons, however, raises a number of difficult issues. As Allen James explained in Congressional testimony:

> Social values in prisons are largely negative; offenders convicted of the most serious crimes often occupy the upper portion of the inmate social hierarchy. Social mechanisms are skewed to make violence an acceptable method of conflict resolution. An inmate who attempts to

confront his troubling emotions or to explore some early emotional experience through talk or show of such emotions in the prison culture is viewed as weak and is likely to become extremely vulnerable. Pursuit of higher positive values is not encouraged in the prison culture and behavior change is accomplished by negative reinforcement. Prisons tend to provide opposites to the principles of addiction treatment and rehabilitation.[87]

Since the prison and jail setting is not itself conducive to effective drug treatment, treatment programs that isolate inmates in a separate setting are most promising. Several such "therapeutic community" programs exist in prisons, such as the Stay 'N Out program in New York and the Key Program in Delaware. They remove eligible prisoners from the prison environment and house them in a community of prisoners isolated for treatment. Therapeutic communities generally contemplate an 18-month treatment program.[88]

Douglas Anglin and Thomas Maugh have set forth a number of useful guidelines for effective in-prison drug treatment.[89] They suggest:

1   Prisoners with chronic cocaine and heroin use should be identified for treatment, enrolled in treatment about 9 to 12 months prior to release, and segregated from the main population;
2   Prisoners should be kept under supervision for an extended period of time, no less than five years, including regular drug testing;
3   The corrections-based program should be linked to a follow-up community-based program, so that supervision and treatment can continue with the transition to freedom;
4   Incentives should be developed to reward progress in treatment, and sanctions for relapses should be flexible;
5   Successful patients should be hired as staff, and staff should be rewarded for successful results.

The kind of intensive drug treatment that is required in a prison setting will plainly not be cheap. Compared with the basic cost of housing a prisoner, however, the cost of treatment is marginal, and if it is more successful in keeping people away from crime and out of prison, it will more than pay for itself in the long run.

Conclusion

The drug war has left the African-American community seriously wounded. Young black men routinely face mandatory long-term sentences for nonviolent, low-level drug offenses. There is little hard evidence that such get-tough tactics have decreased the demand for drugs, but one thing is beyond dispute: the drug war has left a large proportion of young black men without meaningful opportunities to live a productive life. Even if one believes that drug abuse itself, rather than drug law enforcement, is the root of the problem, the law enforcement response exacerbates the problem by effectively depriving a significant portion of the black community of a reasonable chance to succeed. If the drug abuse is itself at least in part a manifestation of the diminished opportunities available to those who grow up in urban poverty, a law enforcement response is particularly troubling, since it further diminishes opportunities, and thereby contributes to the cycle of poverty, unemployment, and drugs.

Compulsory treatment as an alternative or supplement to incarceration, while by no means fully adequate to address this serious and ongoing problem of racial subordination, at least offers the promise of improving the situation. Serious treatment programs of a year or more, which not only treat the drug dependency but also address the underlying conditions that lead to such dependency through education and employment training, have been shown to lead to significantly less recidivist behavior than traditional law enforcement responses to drug crimes. While treatment may be more costly at the outset, studies suggest that it is more cost-effective in the long term. Perhaps most importantly, drug treatment provides the hope that some of the thousands of young black men now serving long prison terms, with nothing to look forward to, could return to their communities as productive citizens and role models.

Treatment plainly cannot be seen as an end in itself. Curing an individual's dependency and giving him or her vocational skills will not solve the problem. If there are few or no jobs available, the drug trade becomes an attractive alternative to unemployment. In the late 1980s, when the national unemployment rate reached highs of 8 percent, the unemployment rate in inner cities hovered around 20 percent, and in some instances reached 50 to 60 percent for young black males.[90] It is therefore critical to recognize the need for

efforts in other areas in conjunction with alternatives to incarceration – education, increased employment opportunities, enhanced
treatment opportunities for those who need it and are not under the
control of the criminal justice system, community programs that
provide adolescents with alternative activities, such as sports or arts
– are all important elements of an attempt to get beyond the drug
problem. Without improvement in other areas, the system may
simply be sending these "rehabilitated" individuals back into the
same circumstances that led them to drugs in the first place. But
while treatment is not an end in itself, it is an important beginning
to a more socially responsible and equitable response to the problem
of drug abuse.

Notes

1   The following account is based on Allen James's testimony at S. Hrg.
    101-646, *Incarceration and Alternative Sanctions for Drug Offenders, Hearing
    before the Committee on the Judiciary*, United States Senate, 101st Cong.,
    1st Sess. 44–52 (25 July 1989).

2   See, e.g., Thomas Szasz, *Our Right to Drugs: The Case for a Free Market*
    (1992); David Elkins, *Drug Legalization: Cost Effective and Morally
    Permissible*, 32 B.C.L. Rev. 575 (1991); James Ostrowski, *The Moral and
    Practical Case for Drug Legalization*, 18 Hofstra L. Rev. 607 (1990).

3   Peter C. Rydell, Rand Corporation, *Controlling Cocaine: Supply vs. Demand*
    (1994); Steven B. Duke and Albert C. Gross, *America's Longest War:
    Rethinking Our Tragic Crusade Against Drugs* (1993).

4   See, e.g., David R. Henderson, *A Humane Economist's Case for Drug
    Legalization*, 24 U.C. Davis L. Rev. 655 (1991); Steven Wisotsky,
    Exposing the War on Cocaine: The Futility and Destructiveness of Prohibition,
    1983 Wis. L. Rev. 1305 (1983); Doug Bandow, *War on Drugs or War on
    America?*, 3 Stan. L. & Pol'y Rev. 242 (1991).

5   Michael Tonry, *Malign Neglect: Race, Crime and Punishment in America* 8
    (1985).

6   Tonry, *supra* note 5 at 131–34.

7   In 1991, state and local governments devoted approximately
    $10 billion to drug law enforcement measures. Richard J. Dennis,
    The Economics of Legalizing Drugs, Atlantic Monthly, Nov. 1990, at 126,
    129.

8   President's Radio Address to the Nation, 18 Weekly Comp. Pres. Doc.
    1249 (Oct. 2, 1982); President's Message Announcing Federal
    Initiatives Against Drug Trafficking and Organized Crime, 18 Weekly
    Comp. Pres. Doc. 1311 (14 Oct. 1982).

9   *U.S.* v. *Clary*, 846 F. Supp. 768 (E.D. Mo. 1994), rev'd, 1994 U.S. App.
    LEXIS 24500 (8th Cir. 1994).

10 Bureau of Justice Statistics, *Drugs, Crime, and the Justice System* 78–89
    (1992) (timeline of drug laws and initiatives).

11 The Act imposed a ten-year mandatory minimum sentence for posses-
    sion with intent to distribute of 11 pounds of cocaine, 2.2 pounds of
    heroin, or 1.7 pounds of crack. John A. Powell and Eileen B.
    Hershenov, *Hostage to the Drug War: The National Purse, the Constitution,
    and the Black Community*, 24 U.C. Davis L. Rev. 557, 577 n. 78 (1991).

12 For example, the 1988 Act established a mandatory five-year
    minimum sentence for simple possession of 5 grams of crack. 21 U.S.C.
    §§841(b)(1)(B), 844(a).

13 Bureau of Justice Statistics, *Drugs, Crime, and the Justice System* 128
    (1992); *see also* National Association of Criminal Defense Lawyers, *The
    Black Community and the Cost of the "War on Drugs,"* The Champion, Nov.
    1990, at 18, 19.

14 Mathea Falco, *Winning the Drug War: A National Strategy* 1 (1989). In a
    1989 Gallup Poll, 58 percent of respondents felt that drugs were the
    major cause of crime in the United States, up from 13 percent in 1981.
    The Gallup Report 285 (June 1989).

15 Tonry, *supra* note 5 at 105–07.

16 Police officials have admitted that it is cheaper and more efficient to
    target the black community for drug law enforcement. Sam Meddis, *Is
    the Drug War Racist?*, USA Today (23 July 1993) at 1A. While a typical
    conspiracy investigation against upper- or middle-class whites may last
    six months and yield fewer than six arrests, an inner-city sweep can
    lead to large numbers of arrests without warrants, and visible evidence
    of success. *Id.*

17 Michael Z. Letwin, *Report From the Front Line: The Bennett Plan, Street-
    Level Drug Enforcement in New York City and the Legalization Debate*, 18
    Hofstra L. Rev. 795, 799, 802 n. 51 (1990).
    In hearings before the Senate Judiciary Committee, Benjamin Ward,
    Police Commissioner of New York City, explained that he felt it impor-
    tant from a public standpoint to target the most open and obvious areas
    of drug trade for massive sweeps:

    > On the Lower East Side . . . [w]e did not have a drug store; we had
    > a drug bazaar in a place called Alphabet City . . . People were liter-
    > ally lined up by the hundreds at this time, starting very early in the
    > morning and running to quite late at night . . . We felt that although
    > we were making thousands of arrests in that area, the public did not
    > know about it. There were so many people to replace the ones that
    > we were arresting that it did not seem to have any effect. What
    > seemed to be needed was a concentrated infusion of uniformed per-
    > sonnel into that area so that we could get the cooperation of the
    > public . . . and people would know what was going on. You had to
    > stop worrying about what the courts did about the case, stop worry-
    > ing about what the district attorney's problems were with all the
    > thousands of cases he had, but keep arresting these people over and
    > over again and then retaking those streets with a large commitment
    > of uniformed police.

Drug Enforcement: Hearing Before the Senate Committee on the Judiciary, 100th Cong., 2d Sess. 12-14 (testimony of Benjamin Ward) (June 14, 1988).

18 Bureau of Justice Statistics, *Prisoners in 1993* 1 (June, 1994).

19 Prisoners in 1993, *supra* at 7.

20 *Id.*

21 Adult arrests for drug offenses jumped 108 percent between 1980 and 1992, from 471,200 in 1980 to 980,700 in 1992. The incarceration rate for drug offenses increased about 450 percent, from 19 per 1000 arrests in 1980 to 104 per 1000 arrests in 1992. *Prisoners in 1993* at 8 – tables 11, 12. Within the federal system, the story is similar. Between the years 1984 and 1992, the number of arrests for drug offenses more than doubled (from 9191 to 19,168); the percentage of convictions increased from 81 percent to 89 percent; and the average prison sentence increased by almost two years (from 65.7 months to 87.5 months). Bureau of Justice Statistics, *Sourcebook of Criminal Justice Statistics* (1993) – table 5.31.

22 The effects are not limited to the criminal justice system. As we have devoted more and more resources to arrest, prosecution, and incarceration of drug offenders, we have had less and less resources available for basic social services. One of every five California state employees, for example, works in its prison system. Dan Baum, *Tunnel Vision: The War on Drugs, 12 Years Later*, ABA Journal 70, 71 (March 1993).

23 *Prisoners in 1993.*

24 Joseph A. Califano, *It's Drugs, Stupid*, New York Times Magazine, 29 Jan 1995, at 41.

25 Elliott Currie, *Reckoning: Drugs, the Cities, and the American Future* 15 (1993).

26 Lawrence O. Gostin, *Compulsory Treatment for Drug-dependent Persons: Justifications for a Public Health Approach to Drug Dependency*, 69 Milbank Quarterly 561, 575 (1991).

27 *Hartness* v. *Bush*, 919 F.2d 170, 174 (D.C. Cir. 1990) (Edwards, J. dissenting); *see also Skinner* v. *Railway Labor Executives Ass'n*, 489 U.S. 602, 641 (1989) (Marshall, J., dissenting) (criticizing majority for creating a "drug exception" to the Fourth Amendment); Saltzburg, *Another Victim of Illegal Narcotics: The Fourth Amendment (As Illustrated by the Open Fields Doctrine)*, 48 U.Pitt.L.Rev. 1 (1986); Wisotsky, *Crackdown: The Emerging "Drug Exception" to the Bill of Rights*, 38 Hastings L.J. 889 (1987); Powell and Hershenov, *supra* note 11 at 580–99.

28 919 F.2d at 175.

29 Substance Abuse and Mental Health Services Administration, Dept. of Health and Human Services, *Preliminary Estimates from the 1993 National Household Survey on Drug Abuse (Advance Report Number 7)* (1994).

30 Currie, *Reckoning, supra* note 26 at 23–24.

31 *Id.* at 25–29.

32 Powell and Hershenov, *supra* note 11 at 566.

33 *Id.*

34 Massing, *Crack's Destructive Sprint Across America*, New York Times, Oct. 1, 1989, §6 (Magazine), at 62; *see generally* Letwin, *supra* note 17 (describing failure of massive street-level enforcement initiatives to reduce drug problem in New York); *see also* Office on Technology Assessment, *The Border War on Drugs* 1 (1987) (reporting that "the quantity of drugs smuggled into the United States is greater than ever").

35 *Prisoners in 1993* at 9.

36 State of Criminal Justice at 9.

37 State of Criminal Justice at 9.

38 State of Criminal Justice at 10.

39 *Prisoners in 1993* at 9 – table 13.

40 Sourcebook of Criminal Justice Statistics – table 6.85. In 1986, 19 percent of all black defendants convicted in Federal court were convicted of drug trafficking. By the first half of 1990, that percentage had more than doubled, to 46 percent. Over the same period, the number of white defendants convicted for drug trafficking increased from 26 percent to 35 percent. Bureau of Justice Statistics, *Sentencing in Federal Courts: Does Race Matter?* 10 (1993).

41 Bureau of Justice Statistics, Survey of State Prison Inmates, 1991 (March 1993).

42 Sourcebook – table 6.70.

43 New York State Coalition for Criminal Justice, *Update* 6 (Feb. 1990).

44 Sourcebook, Table 5.21; U.S. Department of Justice, *An Analysis of Non-Violent Drug Offenders with Minimal Criminal Histories* (1994) – pp. 2, 3 and table 2.

45 Sourcebook, table 5.18.

46 *Id.* at table 5.21.

47 Bureau of Justice Statistics, *Sentencing in the Federal Courts: Does Race Matter?* 1–4 (Summary) (1993).

48 *Id.*

49 *Id.* at 13.

50 Sourcebook of Criminal Justice Statistics, table 5.47.

51 *Prisoners in 1993* at 9 – table 14.

52 Marc Mauer, *Young Black Men and the Criminal Justice System: A Growing National Problem* 3 (The Sentencing Project, Feb. 1990). For white men in the same age group, one in 16 is under correctional supervision of some kind.

53 *Id.* at 9, table 2.

54 National Center on Institutions and Alternatives, Hobbling a Generation: Young African Males in Washington, D.C.'s Criminal Justice System (1992).

55 State of Criminal Justice at 11.

56 Office of Juvenile Justice and Delinquency Programs, *Juvenile Court Statistics 1991* at p. 25, Table 35, p. 71, Table 114 (May 1994). In this source, Hispanic youth were included in the "white" racial category.

57 *Id.* at p. 74, table 118, p.28, Table 39.

58 A petition is a document filed in juvenile court alleging that a juvenile is a delinquent, status offender, or dependant, and asking that the court either assume jurisdiction over the juvenile or transfer the case to criminal court for prosecution as an adult.

59 *Id.* at 29, Table 40.

60 When the 1991 figures are compared with 1984, the change is even more dramatic. In 1984, 1.73 out of 1000 white juveniles were charged with drug possession or use, while 1.37 of 1000 non-white juveniles were so charged. By 1991, the figures for white juveniles was down to 1.4 of 1000, while for black youth the number had jumped four-fold to 7.3 of 1000. Office of Juvenile Justice and Delinquency Programs, U.S. Dept. of Justice, *Juvenile Court Statistics 1984* (Aug. 1987), at p. 64, Table 43; Office of Juvenile Justice and Delinquency Programs, U.S. Dept. of Justice, *Juvenile Court Statistics 1991* at p. 25, Table 37.

61 For an argument that this result was foreseeable, see Tonry, *supra* note 5 at 104–16.

62 *United States* v. *Clary*, 846 F. Supp. 768 (E.D. Mo. 1994) (holding differential under federal sentencing guidelines violates equal protection clause because of "unconscious racism"), rev'd, 1994 U.S. App. LEXIS 24500 (8th Cir. 1994); *United States* v. *Walls*, 841 F. Supp. 24 (D.D.C. 1994) (holding differential under federal sentencing guidelines violates Eighth Amendment prohibition on cruel and unusual punishment); *State* v. *Russell*, 477 N.W.2d 886 (1991) (declaring unconstitutional under Minnesota Constitution's equal protection clause a state mandatory minimum statute creating similar differential); *see also United Statees* v. *Majied*, 1993 WL 315987 (D.Neb. 1993) (justifying downward departure under federal sentencing guidelines because of racially disparate impact of differential).

   Many courts, however, have rejected equal protection challenges to the differential in the federal sentencing guidelines, noting that there is no evidence that it was created with the intent to harm black defendants. *See, e.g., United States* v. *Thompson*, 27 F.3d 671, 678 (D.C. Cir. 1994); *United States* v. *Stevens*, 19 F.3d 93, 97 (2d Cir. 1994); *United States* v. *Williams*, 982 F.2d 1209, 1213 (8th Cir. 1992). The Supreme Court has long held that a facially neutral practice or law will only violate equal protection where it is intentionally adopted to harm an identifiable group. *Washington* v. *Davis*, 426 U.S. 229 (1976).

63 Bureau of Justice Statistics, *Drugs, Crime and the Justice System* 84–85 (1992).

64 *See generally* Charles Lawrence, *The Id, the Ego, and Equal Protection: Reckoning with Unconscious Racism*, 39 Stan. L. Rev. 317 (1987) (discussing unconscious racism and selective indifference).

65 *See* Randall Kennedy, *The State, Criminal Law, and Racial Discrimination: A Comment*, 107 Harv. L. Rev. 1255 (1994); Kate Stith, "The Government Interest in Criminal Law: Whose Interest Is It, Anyway?," in Stephen E. Gottlieb, (ed.), *Public Values in Constitutional Law* 137, 153 (1993).

66 Currie, *Reckoning, supra* note 26 at 77–91 (reviewing studies linking illicit drug use to low socioeconomic status and high unemployment); Substance Abuse and Mental Health Services Administration, *National Household Survey on Drug Abuse: Race/Ethnicity, Socioeconomic Status, and Drug Abuse 1991* (finding that most of the differences in drug use between black, Hispanic, and white adults aged 18 to 49 years were largely or entirely attributable to differences in various socio-demographic characteristics).

67 *Id.* at 83–85 (reviewing studies of illicit drug use and class in Holland, England, and Scotland).

68 National Urban League, *The State of Black America 1994* 217 (1994). The median net worth of black households in 1988 was $4,169; the median net worth of white households was $43,279. *Id.* at 20.

The situation is even more stark in the cities: 80 percent of New York City's 1.7 million poor people and 85 percent of the city's 700,000 poor children are African-American and Latino. Over 44 percent of all African-American children in New York City are poor. The Correctional Association of N.Y. and N.Y. State Coalition for Criminal Justice, *Imprisoned Generation: Young Men Under Criminal Justice Custody in New York State* 6 (1990).

69 Jonathan Kozol, *Savage Inequalities: Children in America's Schools* (1991).

70 *The State of Black America 1994* at 223.

71 Currie, *Reckoning, supra* note 26 at 77–78.

72 Gostin, *supra* note 27; *see also* M. Douglas Anglin and Thomas H. Maugh II, *Ensuring Successful Interventions with Drug-Using Offenders*, Annals, AAPSS, May 1992, at 76–78 (and studies cited therein).

73 Much of the following description is drawn from National Institute of Justice, *Miami's "Drug Court": A Different Approach* (June 1993).

74 John S. Goldkamp and Doris Weiland, National Institute of Justice, *Assessing the Impact of Dade County's Felony Drug Court* (December 1993).

75 *Id.* at p.6, Exhibit 5.

76 *Id.* at p. 7, Exhibit 6.

77 National Institute of Justice, *Miami's "Drug Court": A Different Approach* at 13.

78 Studies also show that similar programs, such as Treatment Alternatives to Street Crime (TASC), have been successful in rehabilitating criminal drug users. Established as a small experimental program in 1972, by 1988 18 states were operating TASC programs. Gostin, *Compulsory Treatment for Drug Dependent Persons*, at 580-581. The goals of TASC are to identify drug users who come into contact with the criminal justice system, get them treatment, monitor their progress, and return violators to the criminal justice system. Strategies employed include deferred prosecution, community sentencing, diversion to voluntary treatment systems, and pretrial intervention to help funnel drug users into treatment. Evaluations have found the program to be effective in reducing drug abuse and criminal activity, as well as in

increasing employment and social coping skills. National Criminal Justice Association, *Treatment Options for Drug Dependent Offenders: A Review of the Literature for State and Local Decisionmakers* (1990). *See also* Anglin and Maugh, *supra* note 73 at 78–81.

79 Sourcebook of Criminal Justice Statistics, table 6.74, p. 627.

80 Robert Frohling, National Conference of State Legislatures, *Promising Approaches to Drug Treatment in Correctional Settings* 1 (August 1989).

81 Sourcebook of Criminal Justice Statistics, table 6.74, p. 627.

82 *Drug Treatment in Prisons: Hearing Before the Select Committee on Narcotics Abuse and Control, House of Representatives,* 102d Cong., 1st Sess. 76 (1991).

83 Frohling, *supra* note 81 (citing Graham, Mary G. *Controlling Drug Abuse and Crime: A Research Update" National Institute of Justice Reports* 1 (March–April 1987)).

84 U.S. General Accounting Office, *Drug Treatment: State Prisons Face Challenges in Providing Services* (GA)/HRD-91-128 Sept. 20, 1991).

85 For a comprehensive review of drug treatment programs in jails and prisons nationwide, see Roger H. Peters, *Substance Abuse Services in Jails and Prisons,* 17 L. & Psych. Rev. 85 (1993) (describing broad variance in treatment programs provided to inmates).

86 Anglin and Maugh, *supra* note 73 at 79–82.

87 *Incarceration and Alternative Sanctions for Drug Offenders,* Hearing Before the Senate Judiciary Committee 50 (25 July 1989) (testimony of Allen James).

88 For a general description of the Key Program, see *Incarceration and Alternative Sanctions for Drug Offenders, supra* note 1 at 56–73 (testimony of Bruce Wald, Director of Key Program).

89 The following guidelines are drawn from Anglin & Maugh, *supra* note 73 at 84–86.

90 The Urban League, *The State of Black America 1994* (1994).

References

Anglin, M.D. and Maugh, T.H., II. 1992. Ensuring Successful Interventions with Drug-Using Offenders, *Annals of the American Academy of Political and Social Science* (May):76–8.

Bandow, D. 1991. War on Drugs or War on America? *Stanford Law and Policy Review* 3:242.

Baum, D. 1993. Tunnel Vision: The War on Drugs, 12 Years Later. *ABA Journal* (March):70–1.

Bureau of Justice Statistics. 1992. *Drugs, Crime, and the Justice System* (timeline of drug laws and initiatives). Washington: Department of Justice.

Bureau of Justice Statistics. 1993. *Sourcebook on Criminal Justice Statistics.* Washington: Department of Justice.

Bureau of Justice Statistics. 1994. *Prisoners in 1993.* Washington: Department of Justice. June.

Bureau of Justice Statistics. 1993. *Sentencing in Federal Courts: Does Race Matter?* Washington: Department of Justice.

Bureau of Justice Statistics. 1993. Survey of State Prison Inmates 1991 (March). Washington: Department of Justice

Califano, J.A. 1995. It's Drugs, Stupid. *New York Times Magazine* 41. January 29.

The Correctional Association of New York & New York State Coalition for Criminal Justice. 1990. Imprisoned Generation: Young Men Under Criminal Justice Custody in New York State. Albany, N.Y.

Currie, E. 1993. *Reckoning: Drugs, the Cities, and the American Future.* New York: Hill and Wang.

Dennis, R. J. 1990. The Economics of Legalizing Drugs. *Atlantic Monthly* (November):126–9.

Duke, S.C. and A.C. Gross. 1993. *America's Longest War: Rethinking our Tragic Crusade Against Drugs.* New York: Putnam.

Elkins, D. 1991. Drug Legalization: Cost Effective and Morally Permissible. *Boston College Law Review* 32:575

Falco, M. 1989. *Winning the Drug War: A National Strategy.* New York: Priority Press Publications.

Frohling, R. 1989. Promising Approaches to Drug Treatment in Correctional Settings. Boulder, Colo.: National Conference of State Legislatures. August.

Gallup Organization. 1989. *The Gallup Report.* Princeton, N.J. June.

Gostin, L.O. 1991. Compulsory Treatment for Drug-dependent Persons: Justifications for a Public Health Approach to Drug Dependency. *Milbank Quarterly* 69:561–75.

Henderson, D.R. 1991. A Humane Economist's Case for Drug Legalization. University of California – Davis Law Review 24:655

James, A. 1989. Testimony before the Senate Judiciary Committee Hearing on Incarceration and Alternatives Sanctions for Drug Offenders (101st Congress, 1st Sess. 44-52). Washington. July 25.

Kennedy, R. 1994. The State, Criminal Law, and Racial Discrimination: A Comment. *Harvard Law Review* 107:1255.

Kozol, J. 1991. *Savage Inequalities: Children in America's Schools.* New York: Crown Publishers

Lawrence, C. 1987. The Id, the Ego, and Equal Protection: Reckoning with Unconscious Racism. *Stanford Law Review* 39:317

Letwin, M.Z. 1990. Report From the Front Line: The Bennett Plan, Street-Level Drug Enforcement in New York City and the Legalization Debate. *Hofstra Law Review* 18(51):795–802

Massing, M. 1989. Crack's Destructive Sprint Across America. *New York Times Magazine,* p. 62. October 1.

Mauer, M. 1990. Young Black Men and the Criminal Justice System: A Growing National Problem. Washington: The Sentencing Project. February.

Meddis, S. 1993. Is the Drug War Racist? *USA Today,* 1A. July 23.

National Association of Criminal Defense Lawyers. 1990. The Black Community and the Cost of the "War on Drugs." *The Champion* (November):18–19.

National Center on Institutions and Alternatives. 1992. Hobbling a Generation: Young African Males in Washington D.C.'s Criminal Justice System. Washington.

National Criminal Justice Association. 1990. Treatment Options for Drug Dependent Offenders: A Review of the Literature for State and Local Decisionmakers. Washington.

National Institute of Justice. 1993. Miami's "Drug Court": A Different Approach. Washington: Department of Justice. June.

National Institute of Justice. 1993. Assessing the Impact of Dade County's Felony Drug Court. Washington: Department of Justice. December.

National Urban League. 1994. *The State of Black America 1994.* Washington.

New York State Coalition for Criminal Justice. 1990. Update 6 (February). Albany, N.Y.

Office of Juvenile Justice and Delinquency Programs. 1994. Juvenile Court Statistics 1991, 25–71. Washington: Department of Justice. May.

Office of Juvenile Justice and Delinquency Programs. 1987. Juvenile Court Statistics 1984, 64. Washington: Department of Justice. August.

Ostrowski, J. 1990. The Moral and Practical Legal Case for Drug Legalization. *Hofstra Law Review* 18:607.

Peters, R.H. 1993. Substance Abuse Services in Jails and Prisons. *Law and Psychiatric Review* 17:85.

Powell, J.A. and E.B. Hershenov. 1991. Hostage to the Drug War: The National Purse, the Constitution, and the Black Community. *University of California – Davis Law Review* 24(78):557–77.

Reagan, R. 1982a. President's Radio Address to the Nation (18 Weekly Comp. Pres. Doc. 1249) Washington: The White House. October 2.

———. 1982b. President's Message Announcing Federal Initiatives Against Drug Trafficking and Organized Crime (18 Weekly Comp. Pres. Doc. 1311). Washington: The White House. October 14.

Rydell, P.C. 1994. *Controlling Cocaine: Supply vs. Demand Programs.* Santa Monica, Cal.: Rand Corporation.

Saltzburg, S.A. 1986. Another Victim of Illegal Narcotics: The Fourth Amendment (As Illustrated by the Open Fields Doctrine). *University of Pittsburgh Law Review* 48:1

Stith, K. 1993. The Government Interest in Criminal Law: Whose Interest Is It, Anyway?. In *Public Values in Constitutional Law,* ed. Stephen E. Gottlieb, 137–53. Ann Arbor: University of Michigan Press.

Substance Abuse and Mental Health Services Administration. 1992. *National Household Survey on Drug Abuse: Race/Ethnicity, Socioeconomic Status, and Drug Abuse 1991.* Washington: Department of Health and Human Services.

Substance Abuse and Mental Health Services Administration. 1994. Preliminary Estimates from the 1993 National Household Survey on Drug Abuse (Advance Report Number 7). Washington: Department of Health and Human Services.

Szasz, T. 1992. *Our Right to Drugs: The Case for a Free Market.* New York: Praeger.

Tonry, M. 1985. *Malign Neglect: Race, Crime and Punishment in America.* New York: Oxford University Press.

U.S. Congress Office on Technology Assessment. 1987. *The Border War on Drugs.* Washington.

U.S. Department of Justice. 1994. An Analysis of Non-Violent Drug Offenders with Minimal Criminal Histories. Washington.

U.S. General Accounting Office. 1991. Drug Treatment: State Prisons Face Challenges in Providing Services Report (GA)/HRD-91-128. Washington. Sept. 20.

Ward, B. 1988. Testimony before the Senate Committee on the Judiciary Hearing on Drug Enforcement (100th Cong., 2d Sess. 12–14). Washington. June 14.

Wisotsky, S. 1983. Exposing the War on Cocaine: The Futility and Destructiveness of Prohibition. *Wisconsin Law Review* 1983:1305.

———. 1987. Crackdown: The Emerging "Drug Exception" to the Bill of Rights. *Hastings Law Journal* 38:889.

11

Linking Substance-Abuse Treatment and Primary Health Care

Thomas D'Aunno

Individuals with a history of chronic substance abuse often suffer from a variety of health problems. Indeed, the AIDS epidemic has strengthened the connection between substance abuse and the need for health care (Schlenger, Kroutil, and Roland 1992). An estimated 30,000 substance-abuse clients in treatment are HIV positive and they need health care (U.S. Department of Health and Human Services 1993). In addition to health problems stemming from AIDS, other medical complications from substance abuse (including syphillis, tuberculosis, and hepatitis) increased across the nation through the 1980s (Haverkos and Lange 1990). In many cases, early medical intervention could halt the progression of the infectious diseases that affect drug users and also prevent the transmission of such diseases (Stein, Samet, and O'Connor 1993).

Further, there is some evidence that meeting the health and social needs of substance-abuse clients can improve treatment outcomes. For example, a recent study of 649 opiate, alcohol, and cocaine patients from 22 public and private programs found that favorable social adjustment at a six-month post-discharge follow-up was associated with the number of medical, psychiatric, family, and employment services received during treatment (McLellan et al. 1994).

Given clients' need for primary health care and social services, and the benefits associated with such services, it is generally agreed that treatment programs should assess a variety of client needs and arrange to meet those needs effectively (Allison, Hubbard, and Rachal 1985; Hubbard et al. 1989; Haverkos and Lange 1990; Stein et al. 1993). Nonetheless, we know relatively little about the medical services that clients receive in substance-abuse treatment units or from other sources.

The purpose of this chapter is to examine ways to promote more effective links between substance-abuse treatment and primary health care. To meet this purpose, the chapter is organized into three sections. The first reviews what is known about links between substance-abuse treatment and primary health care. More specifically, I examine two types of approach that now exist to link substance-abuse clients with primary health care. One is to provide primary health-care services and substance-abuse treatment services at a *single site*. The second approach is to link substance-abuse clients with health services by means such as referral agreements and case management; these approaches are intended to bridge gaps between substance-abuse treatment units and primary health-care providers.

The second section of the chapter examines alternative approaches to promote effective links between substance-abuse treatment and health-care services. This section examines several mechanisms to link substance-abuse clients with health services. It also discusses the advantages and disadvantages of these approaches and factors that are likely to influence their use. Finally, the chapter concludes with a discussion of implications for policymakers and planners concerned with promoting effective links between substance-abuse treatment and health services.

Links between Substance-Abuse Treatment and Primary Health Care: A Review

Primary health-care services address the common health problems that individuals experience. In contrast, secondary and tertiary health-care services (often provided in hospitals) address problems that are less common and often more severe, such as various forms of cancer. Thus, primary health care includes care provided by practitioners in internal medicine, general and family medicine, and pediatrics.

As just noted, there are two types of approaches to link substance-abuse clients with these services. One is to provide health-care and substance-abuse services at a single site (most typically, the single site is a substance-abuse treatment unit). Federal and state planners have encouraged this approach historically simply because substance-abuse clients often have difficulty gaining access to independent health and social services. In other words, providing "one-stop shopping" for substance-abuse clients in treatment units helps them to overcome barriers to the access of health services, such as cost, transportation, and social stigma.

Nonetheless, one-stop shopping has become rarer (D'Aunno and Vaughn 1995) and, as a result, alternative approaches have been developed to link substance-abuse clients with health services. These approaches use various mechanisms intended to make it easier for substance-abuse clients to gain access to primary health-care providers. For example, case managers may be assigned to clients to help them arrange transportation to health services and find sources (such as Medicaid) to pay for such services. Below, I review what is known about both basic approaches (single-site services in substance-abuse treatment units and mechanisms to link clients to health-care providers).

Primary health services provided in substance-abuse treatment units. There are very few empirical studies that examine the kind or amount of health-care services that substance-abuse clients receive in treatment units. Of the available studies, most rely on convenience samples of relatively few treatment units. But, there are three national surveys of treatment units that do include some questions about the percentage of clients receiving medical care and related services on-site. These surveys, typically completed by unit directors, are: (1) the Drug Abuse Treatment System Survey (DATSS) conducted by the Institute for Social Research at the University of Michigan (Price and D'Aunno 1992); (2) the National Drug and Alcohol Treatment Unit Survey (NDATUS) conducted by NIDA (and now the Substance Abuse and Mental Health Services Administration); and (3) the Drug Services Research Survey (DSRS) conducted by Brandeis University (Batten et al. 1992; 1993). Unfortunately, the most recent data from two of these surveys (DATSS and DSRS) is from 1990, and DATSS includes only outpatient treatment units.

The percentage of units that report providing at least some medical care for their clients varies across the three surveys (using

1990 data for outpatient units only). Fifty-eight percent of DATSS units report providing some medical care (excluding mental health care) for clients compared with 27 percent of NDATUS units and 30 percent of DSRS units. In the DATSS units that do provide medical care, an average 25 percent of clients received some care in 1990. Data for HIV testing show that 39 percent of DATSS units conduct some testing compared with 27 percent of NDATUS units and 30 percent of DSRS units. Even using the more favorable DATSS estimates, it is clear that not many clients are receiving health-care services in substance-abuse treatment units.

Differences in the results from the three surveys should be noted. These differences could stem from the use of different sampling frames and different definitions of a "treatment unit." The DATSS survey is based on a much more comprehensive sampling frame (see Flyer 1990) than either NDATUS or DSRS (which used the same sampling frame as NDATUS) (see Schmidt and Weisner 1993, and Prottas and Elliott 1992, for a discussion of weaknesses in the NDATUS sampling frame). Further, the DATSS focused on single treatment units. In contrast, both NDATUS and DSRS collected data from treatment programs that could include multiple treatment units and, thus, aggregate data. In short, differences in sampling frames and data collection might explain why the NDATUS and DSRS results reported above are similar, while both differ from the DATSS results.

D'Aunno and Vaughn (1995) recently analyzed the DATSS data to examine changes between 1988 and 1990 in the percentage of clients receiving physical exams and medical care. The results show that the percentage of clients receiving these services decreased significantly from 1988 to 1990. Specifically, the percentage of clients receiving physical exams decreased from 39 percentage to 33 percent, and medical care decreased from 38 percent to 25 percent.

Multiple regression analyses were also conducted to identify factors related to the decrease in these services. More specifically, D'Aunno and Vaughn examined the extent to which client characteristics (age, gender, type of drug use) and organizational factors (funding, staffing patterns, ownership) are associated with changes in the percentage of clients receiving physical exams and medical care. In these analyses, the dependent variables were change scores (1988 to 1990) of the percentage of clients receiving services. The predictor variables, that is, client characteristics and organizational factors, were also change scores for 1988 to 1990 (e.g., percentage decrease in a unit's budget).

The results for physical exams indicate that units which had an increase in physician staff members also had an increase in clients who received physical exams. In contrast, units that had an increase in unemployed clients and client fees as a percentage of total funds decreased physical exams.

The results for medical care show that as client-to-FTE ratios increased, clients were less likely to receive medical care. Clients in hospital-based units were less likely to receive medical care. This result is counterintuitive; one would expect that hospital-based units would be able to provide more medical care for clients simply because they are owned by hospitals. But perhaps financial constraints that hospitals face affected their units' provision of medical care to substance-abuse clients.

Finally, contrary to the results for physical exams, units that had an increase in the percentage of their budgets that came from clients funds were likely to have more clients receive medical care. Perhaps clients only pay for health-care services that they are certain they need. That is, clients may be less likely to pay for physical exams that often yield uncertain results; when the need for medical care is clear, they may feel that they must pay for it.

Summary. The DATSS data indicate that between 1988 and 1990 substantially fewer substance-abuse clients received primary health-care services on-site in treatment units. Has this trend continued? If so, it may signal serious problems for substance-abuse clients who need primary health care. That is, these clients often have difficulties gaining access to health care when it is provided in traditional sites (hospitals, physician offices) (Umbricht-Schneiter et al. 1994). Indeed, a recent study of a county in California examined the use of substance-abuse treatment and other human services (e.g., welfare) and found that the caseloads of primary health-care clinics had the lowest percentage of individuals with drug-use problems of any type of human service agency (Weisner and Schmidt 1994a). A likely explanation is that individuals with substance-abuse problems had more difficulty gaining access to the health clinics than other service agencies (Haverkos and Lange 1990).

Further, analyses of the DATSS data suggest that decreases in primary health services were more likely to occur in substance-abuse treatment units that had decreases in resources (as measured by client-to-FTE ratio, and client unemployment and accompanying lack of funds) (D'Aunno and Vaughn 1995). Resource constraints imposed on substance-abuse treatment units, for example, by cuts in state funding may continue to erode primary health-care services on-site.

Approaches to link substance-abuse clients to health-care providers.

Recent studies have focused on two specific approaches to improve links between substance-abuse clients and health-care services: case management and referral agreements. A useful NIDA research monograph (Ashery 1992) contains several chapters that describe efforts to link drug-abuse treatment and prevention services with community-based social and medical services through the use of various case-management models. In this monograph, Ridgely and Willenbring (1992) note that definitions of case management vary widely. But it is generally agreed that, at a minimum, case management consists of efforts by a specified staff member to link clients with various services.

Many of the chapters in the monograph report work in progress but not yet completed. Further, some studies are limited by small or non-representative samples. Nonetheless, the emerging results suggest that case management is an effective tool for linking clients with services that they might otherwise have failed to obtain (Schlenger, Kroutil, and Roland 1992).

At the same time, it is important to note that case management rarely, if ever, pays for itself (Ridgely and Willenbring 1992). That is, the cost of providing case-management services often is not off-set by savings from improving (or maintaining) the health of the recipients of case management. At least two factors may account for this observation. First, hiring case managers entails personnel costs and there are often training costs as well. Second, if they are effective, case managers increase their clients' use of services. In turn, increased use of services increases costs to groups that pay for care.

On the other hand, an offset in the costs of case management may be achieved in the long run if early interventions result in savings from reducing the provision of more costly care to clients who would have become sicker if they had not been linked to services. Given these complex factors, closer analysis of the costs and benefits of case management for substance-abuse clients is clearly needed.

In contrast to the results concerning case management, a recent study of the provision of medical care to methadone clinic patients showed strong results concerning the ineffectiveness of referral agreements (Umbricht-Schneiter et al. 1994). Methadone patients were randomly assigned either to an on-site group to receive medical care or to a referral group to receive medical care at a nearby clinic. The referral group had their costs covered and arrangements were made so that staff members in the medical clinic knew in advance about the referrals. In other words, efforts were made to make the referral linkage as effective as possible. But, only 35 percent of patients in the referral group received medical treatment compared with 92 percent who received medical treatment in the on-site group.

Why are the results for case management more promising than the results from the arrangement that relied on referral agreements and covered costs? Several factors may account for the difference in results. First, case managers do more than simply make referral arrangements. For example, case managers follow-up with clients and service providers to assure that the two have connected. Further, case managers are in a strong position to take into account the practical as well as clinical needs of individual clients. For example, clients often need transportation to and from service agencies, and case managers can help them arrange for it.

Summary. There are relatively few studies that directly examine the problem of how to link substance-abuse clients with primary health-care services (Stein et al. 1993). Nonetheless, the available data raise several important concerns. First is the apparent decline in health services available to clients on-site in substance-abuse treatment units (D'Aunno and Vaughn 1995). Second, this decline is linked in part to decreases in treatment-unit resources that may well have continued since 1990. Third, recent evidence indicates that referral agreements are not effective mechanisms to link substance-abuse clients with health services (Umbricht-Schneiter et al. 1994). Fourth, though case management appears to be a useful tool for linking clients with health services (Schlenger, Kroutil, and Roland 1992), cost concerns remain a problem insofar as case management does not typically pay for itself.

In short, we need to examine alternative ways to improve links between substance-abuse clients and primary health-care services. Below, I examine a range of approaches that can be used to reach this goal. I discuss their advantages and disadvantages and, importantly, I examine factors that can influence the use of these approaches.

A Survey of Approaches to Link Substance-Abuse and Primary Health-Care Services

Figure 11.1 shows six approaches to integrate or link substance-abuse services and primary health-care services. The approaches vary in two important ways. First, they vary in how likely it is that they will effectively integrate services for substance-abuse clients.

	Ad Hoc referrals	Referral agreements	Case management	Contracts	Joint programs/Alliances/Federations	Single-site (merged) services
Definitions:	• Efforts by one agency to send clients to another agency for services	• Rues to guide referral-making	• Integration of client services by a designated coordinator	• Formal agreements to integrate service provision	• Service programs shared by two or more provider organizations	• Common ownership and single site for providing divers services
Strengths:	• Low cost	• Low cost • Reduces some barriers to access	• Focused on reducing barriers to access	• May include incentives/punishments to enforce agreements	• Cost-sharing • Commitment by member organizations • Pooled expertise	• Highest degree of service integration
Weaknesses:	• Does not typically reduce barriers to access (e.g., transportation for clients)	• No means to enforce agreements	• Relatively expensive • Does not obviate need for service availability	• Costs involved in negotiating and enforcing contracts • Cost of services remains a barrier for clients and other payers	• Same or greater transaction costs as contracts • Politics involved in managing programs	• Lack of management expertise • Resource constraints

Figure 11.1 Approaches to link substance-abuse and primary health-care services.

On the one hand, as discussed below, ad hoc referrals between substance-abuse treatment units and health-care providers typically offer the least service integration. On the other hand, single-site organizations typically provide highly integrated services for clients.

Second, the six approaches to service integration vary in the extent to which they cost the participating organizations or individuals autonomy that they value highly. That is, the integration approaches range from those that involve little interdependence between service providers (ad hoc referrals and referral agreements) to those that involve much interdependence between service providers, with a corresponding loss of autonomy (joint programs and single-site service organizations). In short, service organizations that want to integrate, link, or coordinate services for clients must often do so at the cost of their autonomy. The result for policy-makers, of course, is that the most desired level of integration is also the most difficult to achieve. I return to this key point below.

Figure 11.1 does not provide a complete list of approaches for integrating or linking services (two prominent approaches for integrating services, self-referral and managed-care programs, are discussed below). Neither does the discussion below provide a complete description of these approaches. Rather, I selected these approaches because they cover a range of options available to policy-makers, planners, and managers concerned with improving service integration. The discussion below follows the figure and focuses on the strengths and weaknesses of each approach. Factors that affect the use of the approaches are also discussed (see figure 11.2).

Ad hoc referrals. Ad hoc referrals between substance-abuse treatment units and health-care providers are probably the predominant means used to link services for substance-abuse clients. Unfortunately, as indicated above, they are probably the least effective linkage mechanism. That is, though referrals are relatively inexpensive for staff members to make, they often fail to connect clients to needed services. There are, of course, several reason why this is the case. Among the most important factors are the fact that individuals with substance-abuse problems often lack medical insurance or funds to pay for care; they are often unable to use public transportation or don't own vehicles; and they face stigma and rejection by medical care providers. As a result of these and other factors, merely referring a client to a health-care provider is simply not enough to ensure that the client will receive a needed service.

To increase the effectiveness of referral-making, the Joint Commission on the Accreditation of Health Care Organizations (JCAHO) developed a set of guidelines for referral-making. The suggested guidelines include the following: referring agencies should send a written case summary or complete chart to the agency receiving the client; in addition to, or in place of, a written case record, the referring agency should provide an oral case summary (using phones for direct conversations between clinicians); referring agencies should make a follow-up call to the receiving agency to check on the completion or progress of the referral.

In the 1990 DATSS, we asked clinical supervisors to report how often staff members used the procedures listed above when making referrals. On average, they reported using these practices "sometimes" to "often." In other words, the recommended practices are not followed consistently. Thus, a straightforward recommendation for practitioners is that they rely more consistently on the JCAHO practices for referral-making.

Referral agreements. Referral agreements are typically non-contractual oral or written guidelines that specify the conditions under which client referrals will be made between two or more service providers. Such agreements differ from ad hoc referrals in that the service providers have agreed to follow a set of rules for dealing with client exchanges. It is assumed that developing such agreements and following them will increase service integration. The study by Umbricht-Schneiter et al. (1994), reviewed above, provides a useful example of a relatively comprehensive referral agreement between a substance-abuse treatment unit and a medical clinic. In the agreement, a methadone unit arranged to pay for the costs of care for its clients at the clinic; further, staff members in the clinic were alerted that methadone clients would be coming to them for care. As noted, the results were disappointing.

Nonetheless, a strength of referral agreements is that, similar to ad hoc referrals, they are relatively inexpensive. In addition, referral agreements can reduce some barriers to service integration. For example, rules between agencies could specify how much and how clients will pay for services, and thus reduce the number of times that clients are turned away.

On the other hand, it is difficult for service organizations to enforce referral agreements. Agreements made between agency directors often are not even communicated to staff members, and, if they are, they are not emphasized as a part of standard operating procedures. In short, there are often not enough incentives to make referral agreements work.

Case management. Ridgely and Willenbring (1992) note that case management is a loosely defined service. They provide a useful discussion of the dimensions along which case-management models vary. Such dimensions include the site of service, duration and frequency of contact with clients, the content or focus of the case-management service (e.g., how broad or narrow the service is), and the training and authority held by the case managers. Though case-management approaches differ, they typically have in common the goal of attempting to integrate services for clients.

The strength of this approach clearly lies in the specialized role of the case manager. This individual or group focuses specifically on service integration and often acts as an advocate for clients, helping them to gain access to needed services. This, in turn, often entails identifying service providers, contacting them, and making arrangements to suit the particular needs of clients (e.g., identifying clients' transportation or child-care needs and resources to meet them). As noted above, the weight of the evidence presented in the NIDA research monograph on case management (127) suggests that it is an effective mechanism to integrate services for substance-abuse clients.

But, case management is not a panacea. It is clear that additional evaluations of case management are needed in the substance-abuse field. Further, case managers cannot link clients to services that do not exist; nor can they reduce the costs of services. Indeed, case management itself typically adds costs to a service system (e.g., the costs of case managers and their activities).

Contracts. Contracts between two or more organizations are yet another means to integrate or coordinate services. In this context, contracts are formal agreements that indicate what services the participating organizations will provide as well as how such services will be delivered. Further, contracts may include incentives and punishments to enforce rules. In other words, contracts are similar to referral agreements in that they identify roles for the participating organizations in service delivery, and rules to govern their working relationships. But, contracts are often taken more seriously than agreements, because of the rewards and punishments they may involve. An example of the use of contracts is when an HMO contracts with a substance-abuse treatment unit to provide services for its members who need them. The contract might specify several important aspects of the substance-abuse treatment services (e.g., duration).

An important weakness of contracts is that it is costly to develop, monitor, and enforce the agreements and rules they entail. That is, there are relatively high transaction costs (Williamson 1981) involved in such exchanges. Further, contractual agreements may not require the participating organizations to pool resources – to the extent that they do not, it is unlikely that contracts alone will reduce the costs of care. There are no efficiencies gained in merely specifying what work each agency will do and how it will be done. Finally, contracts may not take clients' needs into account very well. In other words, contracts may entail rules that make it easier for organizations to work with each other (e.g., agreement on common use of certain assessment instruments), while paying little attention to clients' needs for transportation, child care, or ways to pay for care.

Joint programs/alliances/federations. The term alliance or federation is used to refer to two or more organizations that agree to pool resources to achieve stated objectives, while maintaining their status as independent entities (D'Aunno and Zuckerman 1987a, b). Joint programs are service programs (e.g., HIV testing and counseling) developed by members of alliances or federations. Joint programs differ from contracts because, by definition, the participating organizations pool some resources. In contrast, contracts most often just clarify the roles and responsibilities that the participating organizations have with respect to each other. To be sure, such clarification can promote service integration, but not as clearly as a joint program which involves more interdependence between two organizations. Joint programs between health-care providers and substance-abuse treatment units might involve, for example, rotating or sharing personnel between two sites on a regular basis. In this way, each site (a medical clinic and a substance-abuse treatment unit) would gain access to the expertise of staff members from the two types of service providers.

A major strength of joint programs is that they share costs involved in producing a service, thus making it possible for two or more organizations to do more than one agency working alone. Similarly, pooled expertise may lead to higher quality in services. Because joint programs involve shared resources, there is often more commitment to making the jointly-provided service effective.

The transaction costs involved in developing joint programs are, however, either equal to or greater than the transaction costs involved in developing contracts. This is because the organizations involved in joint programs have a greater stake in them than in contracts. Further, there are more politics involved in joint programs than in contracts because the participants share responsibility for managing the services offered.

Single-site (merged) services. Single-site organizations are those which provide diverse health and substance-abuse treatment services under a common owner and manager at a single geographic location. Thus, single-site organizations are distinctive in that they integrate services by both location and control (i.e., common ownership and management). It is the single location and unified control that give these organizations the potential to provide high levels of service integration. As indicated above, this is the model that many policymakers have espoused in the substance-abuse treatment field.

Nonetheless, the potential for single-site organizations to integrate services for substance-abuse clients is often undercut by two important factors. One is that managers lack expertise to effectively control a wide array of services. That is, different knowledge and skills are needed to be effective in managing health-care vs. substance-abuse services. Indeed, research on health-care organizations shows that diversification is not a successful strategy (Clement, D'Aunno, and Poyser 1993). Organizations and managers do better when they focus on what they know and do best. Second, as discussed above, the costs involved in providing multiple services at a single site (especially health-care services) may be prohibitive.

Finally, two approaches not listed in the figure above merit some discussion. These are self-referral and managed-care programs. Self-referral is important to note simply because it is a major means by which clients obtain both substance-abuse treatment services and primary health care. There are many reasons to believe, however, that self-referral is an ineffective linkage mechanism (it is similar to ad hoc referral). Individuals with health problems caused by illicit drug use, for example, are reluctant to seek primary health care because they fear legal implications. Further, self-referral, by definition, means that individuals with drug-abuse problems must overcome barriers to receiving health care (e.g., lack of funds and transportation). In short, as discussed above, assisted referrals are not very effective in linking substance-abuse clients with primary health-care, and there is not a strong basis for believing that self-referrals will be more effective.

Some managed programs have control (through ownership) of multiple clinics that provide either primary health care or substance-abuse treatment. It seems that such control combined with managed-care arrangements (e.g., case managers) would promote service integration for substance-abuse clients. To date, however, no studies have examined the effects of managed-care programs on coordination of services for substance-abuse clients.

Weisner and Schmidt (1994b) argue that managed-care programs could have advantages and disadvantages for access to services. A potential advantage is that care providers have an incentive to save money by early intervention. Potential disadvantages include the incentive to save money by not providing a full range or adequate amount of services. At this point, it is not clear that there are adequate incentives for primary-care physicians working in managed-care settings to consistently screen and refer patients to substance-abuse services. Given the apparent increase in managed-care programs, this is certainly a pressing issue for research.

Factors that promote/inhibit the use of the integration approaches. We have relatively little information about the various approaches to service integration discussed above. As a result, descriptive studies are certainly needed to identify the prevalence of each approach, how it works in practice, and how organizations mix the various approaches. But we also need to move quickly from description to analysis of approaches to link substance-abuse treatment and primary health care. More specifically, we need to ask, Under what conditions do organizations rely on one or more of these approaches? That is, what can be done to promote or inhibit the use of these approaches?

This section attempts to hasten the move from description to analysis by examining factors that promote or inhibit the use of various integration approaches (see table 11.1). Oliver's (1990) excellent review of previous research on the determinants of interorganizational relations provides a starting point for this analysis (see also Hasenfeld 1992; Morrissey, Tausig, and Lindsey 1986).

Oliver's review indicates that organizations form various types of relationships with each other for five key reasons. These are to: (1) exercise power or control over other organizations (asymmetry); (2) pursue common or mutually beneficial goals or interests (reciprocity); (3) improve operating efficiency (efficiency); (4) maintain predictable flows of information and other valued resources (stability); (5) maintain or enhance their public image or acceptability (legitimacy). These factors form one axis of table 11.1, while the six approaches to service integration form the other axis.

Of course, it is rarely the case that organizations and their managers are motivated by only one of the above factors. Indeed, it is most often the case that organizations and managers have multiple, sometimes conflicting, motives and objectives in pursuing relationships with external groups. Nonetheless, it is helpful to begin by thinking about each factor independently.

As noted above, closer coordination or integration of services necessarily means that organizations must give up some autonomy. In the course of working more closely with other service providers, organizations forgo, to some extent, the option of making

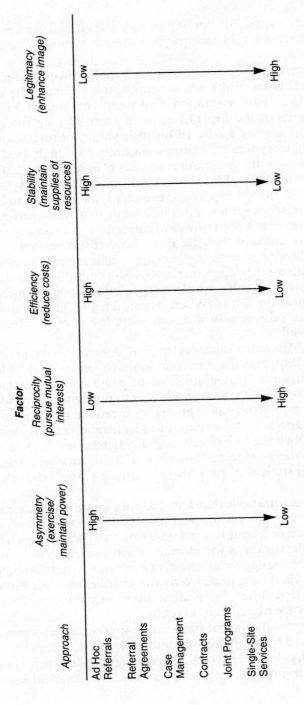

Figure 11.2 Factors that affect the use of approaches to service integration

Approach	Factor					
	Asymmetry (exercise/ maintain power)	Reciprocity (pursue mutual interests)	Efficiency (reduce costs)	Stability (maintain supplies of resources)	Legitimacy (enhance image)
Ad Hoc Referrals	High	Low	High	High	Low
Referral Agreements					
Case Management					
Contracts					
Joint Programs					
Single-Site Services	Low	High	Low	Low	High

independent choices. Further, it is widely agreed that organizations, like individuals, are reluctant to yield their autonomy (Pfeffer and Salancik 1978).

On the basis of these assumptions, I make several arguments about the conditions under which organizations will use the various approaches to service integration. The arrows in table 11.1 indicate expected effects of the five factors on the use of each integration approach. The arrows are based on high values of the factors. For example, when asymmetry among organizations is high, I expect ad hoc referrals to be the integration approach used most often (indicated by the label "high"). In contrast, when reciprocity among organizations is high, I expect the use of ad hoc referrals to be low and that more service integration will occur (e.g., joint programs).

Power asymmetries. When power asymmetries exist among service providers it is unlikely that the more powerful organizations will voluntarily develop more integrated approaches to service delivery. This is because such approaches involve yielding autonomy. Powerful organizations have little motivation to trade autonomy for service integration. Thus, when asymmetries exist or increase among service providers in a community, less service integration will be observed.

Reciprocity. The more that service providers value reciprocity in their relationships and share mutual goals, the more likely it is that high levels of service integration (joint programs and single-site agencies) will occur. One important way to promote norms of reciprocity among service organizations is to reduce overlap in their missions and goals. To the extent that organizations see themselves as symbiotically linked, they are more likely to support reciprocity. In contrast, when organizations do not share mutual goals, less service integration will be observed and ad hoc referrals will predominate.

Efficiency. Organizations that are efficiency-driven will attempt to coordinate services by means that involve fewer transaction costs (i.e., ad hoc referrals and referral agreements) (Williamson 1981). In other words, concerns for efficiency will override concerns for close service integration. In contrast, organizations that do not focus on efficiency will be less deterred by the transaction costs involved in approaches that closely integrate services; in such circumstances, joint programs are more likely to occur.

Stability. Organizations that have stable supplies of resources will not be motivated to pursue service integration approaches that cost them autonomy. In other words, if resources are secure, organizations have little need to trade their autonomy for an increase in certainty regarding the acquisition of resources (Thompson 1967). In contrast, organizations that have unstable supplies of resources will be more motivated to work closely with other organizations and, hence, more service integration will be observed (joint programs).

Legitimacy. Organizations that are secure about their legitimacy in a community will be less likely to pursue approaches to service integration that cost their autonomy. Only when legitimacy concerns are high will organizations seek to gain community acceptance by conforming to social norms about collaboration. Even so, conformity to social norms about collaboration is often only "skin deep." Organizations often attempt to give the appearance of collaborating while continuing to pursue their own interests (Scott 1990).

Summary. In sum, policymakers and planners who want to promote particular approaches to service integration can benefit by understanding the multiple, complex motives of organizations and their managers. Organizational concerns to maintain autonomy and power and to protect efficiency are likely to produce resistance to service-integration approaches that involve higher levels of interdependence. On the other hand, organizations that are concerned with legitimacy, reciprocity, and stability in resource flows will be motivated to trade autonomy for higher levels of interdependence and service integration.

Discussion

This chapter has important implications for policymakers and managers concerned with integrating substance-abuse treatment and primary health-care services. First, the DATSS data suggest that clients in substance-abuse treatment are not receiving enough health care and social services, at least relative to clients' self-reported needs. The TOPS data, for example, show that mental health problems were cited by between 33 and 50 percent of outpatient clients. D'Aunno and Vaughn (1995) report that, on average, only 25 percent of clients are receiving mental health care from their treatment units. This gap is especially significant given the results from previous studies that indicate that mental health treatment increases the effectiveness of drug-abuse treatment, particularly for methadone clients (Joe, Simpson, and Hubbard 1991; Woody 1983).

Further, TOPS data show that, though medical problems were

least frequently cited by outpatient clients, they were still cited by about one-third of clients. The DATSS data indicate that only 25 percent of outpatient clients are receiving medical care from their substance-abuse treatment units.

Perhaps more important than the level of services in 1990 is the significant decrease from 1988 to 1990 in services that clients receive in treatment units. Have decreases in services persisted? This pressing question needs to be addressed. The results from D'Aunno and Vaughn (1995) indicate that organizational resources play an important role in service levels, even after taking client characteristics into account. My interpretation of these results is relatively straightforward: clients are more likely to receive various health-care (and social) services they need when their treatment units have adequate resources.

Similarly, more research is needed that examines pathways into substance-abuse treatment and primary health-care clinics (see Weisner and Schmidt 1994a). Researchers should collect data on the paths that clients take as they find their way, either assisted or independently, through the complex maze of services in their communities. What factors or arrangements promote or hinder service integration?

Further, managers of substance-abuse treatment units may need to define their goals more broadly to include the provision of medical and social services. A broader definition of goals does not necessarily mean that units could or should provide a range of services themselves. Rather, broader treatment goals can be met first by conducting adequate assessments of a range of client needs (using, for example, the Addiction Severity Index or the Treatment Services Review, McLellan, Alterman, Cacciola, Metzger, and O'Brien 1992) and, second, by making effective connections with other service providers, using the approaches discussed here.

It also appears that primary health-care providers do not adequately link substance-abusing individuals with substance-abuse treatment (Stein et al. 1993; Haverkos and Lange 1990). Three factors contribute to this problem. First, primary health-care providers are often not trained to identify substance-abuse problems. Second, even after recognizing substance-abuse problems, primary care providers often avoid confronting their patients owing to the stigma associated with substance abuse. Third, if referrals are made to substance-abuse treatment, they often are not completed (Marwick 1992).

Case management appears to be a more promising linkage mechanism than referrals and referral agreements, but it is also more expensive. We need analytic studies of the effectiveness of various linkage mechanisms as soon as possible. At the present time, referral networks may be the best that many substance-abuse treatment units can provide for their clients given limited resources.

Federal, state, and regional planners can also support an expanded mission for substance-abuse treatment units, for example, through training. Indeed, there has been an ongoing effort by the Center for Substance Abuse Treatment (CSAT) and NIDA to strengthen the linkages between the primary health-care and alcohol, drug-abuse, and mental health treatment systems (Lehman 1990; Schlenger, Kroutil, and Roland 1992). This initiative began several years ago with the convening of primary care and substance-abuse treatment providers in regional workshops across the country to discuss barriers to the integration of services (Marwick 1992). This chapter supports the need for this initiative and provides directions for its work.

References

Allison, M., R.L. Hubbard, and J.V. Rachal. 1985. Treatment Process in Methadone, Residential, and Outpatient Drug Free Programs. *Treatment Research Monograph* (DHHS pub. no. (ADM) 85-1388). Rockville, Md.: National Institute on Drug Abuse.

Ashery, R.S. (Ed.) 1992. *Progress and Issues in Case Management* (NIDA Research Monograph No. 127). Rockville, Md.: National Institute on Drug Abuse.

Batten, H.L., C.M. Horgan, J.M. Prottas, et al. 1993. *Drug Services Research Survey, Phase I Final Report: Non-Correctional Facilities*, revised edition. Report submitted to the National Institute on Drug Abuse. Waltham, Mass.: Institute for Health Policy, Brandeis University.

Batten, H.L., J.M. Prottas, C.M. Horgan, et al. 1992. *Drug Services Research Survey, Final Report: Phase II*. Report submitted to the National Institute on Drug Abuse. Waltham, Mass.: Institute for Health Policy, Brandeis University.

Clement, J., T. D'Aunno, and B.L. Poyser. 1993. The Financial Performance of Diversified Hospital Subsidiaries. *Health Services Research* 27(6):741–64.

D'Aunno, T. and T. Vaughn. 1995. An Organizational Analysis of Service Patterns in Drug Abuse Treatment. *Journal of Substance Abuse* 7:27–42.

D'Aunno, T. and H.S. Zuckerman. 1987a. The Emergence of Hospital Federations: An Integration of Perspectives from Organizational Theory. *Medical Care Review* 44(2):323–43.

———. 1987b. A Life-Cycle Model of Organizational Federations: The Case of Hospitals. *Academy of Management Review* 25(8):781–95.

Flyer, P. 1990. *Final Weighting Documentation*. Ann Arbor, Mich.: University of Michigan, Institute for Social Research.

Ginzberg, H., M. Allison, and R.L. Hubbard. 1983. Depressive Symptoms in

Drug Abuse Treatment Clients: Correlates, Treatment and Changes. In *Problems of Drug Dependence* (Research Monograph 49. DHHS 1984 pub. no. (ADM) 84-1316) ed. L.S. Harris, 313–19. Rockville, Md.: National Institute on Drug Abuse.

Hasenfeld, Y. (Ed.) 1992. *The Organization of Human Services: Structure and Processes*. Beverly Hills: Sage.

Haverkos, H.W. and W.R. Lange. 1990. Serious Infections Other than Human Immunodeficiency Virus among Intravenous Drug Abusers. *Journal of Infectious Diseases* 161:894–902.

Hubbard, R.L., M.E. Marsden, J.V. Rachal, E.R. Cavanaugh, and H.M. Ginzburg. 1989. *Drug Abuse Treatment: A National Study of Effectiveness*. Chapel Hill, N.C.: The University of North Carolina.

Joe, G.W., D.D. Simpson, and R.L. Hubbard. 1991. Treatment Predictors of Tenure in Methadone Maintenance. *Journal of Substance Abuse* 3:73–84.

Lehman, M.K. 1990. Linking Primary Care and Substance Abuse Treatment. *ADAMHA News* 16:1.

Marwick, C. 1992. Effort under Way to Enlist More Primary Care Physicians in Treatment of Substance Abuse. *Journal of the American Medical Association* 267(14):1887–8.

McLellan, A.T., A.I. Alterman., D.S. Metzger, et al. 1994. Similarity of Outcome Predictors across Opiate, Cocaine and Alcohol Treatments: Role of Treatment Services. *Journal of Consulting and Clinical Psychology* 62(6):1141–58.

McLellan, A.T., L. Luborsky, G.E. Woody, and C.P. O'Brien. 1980. An Improved Diagnostic Evaluation Instrument for Substance Abuse Patients: The Addiction Severity Index. *Journal of Nervous and Mental Disorders* 168:26–33.

Morrissey, J.P., M. Tausig, and M.L. Lindsey. 1986. Interorganizational Networks in Mental Health Systems: Assessing Community Support Programs for the Chronically Mentally Ill. In *The Organization of Mental Health Services*, ed. W.R. Scott and B.L. Black. Beverly Hills: Sage

O'Brien, C.P., G.E. Woody, and A.T. McLellan. 1984. *Psychotherapeutic Approaches in the Treatment of Drug Abuse* (DHHS pub. no. (ADM) Research Monograph 51). Rockville, Md.: National Institute on Drug Abuse.

Oliver, C. 1990. Determinants of Interorganizational Relationships: Integration and Future Directions. *Academy of Management Review* 15:241–65.

Pfeffer, J. and G.R. Salancik. 1978. *The External Control of Organizations*. New York: Harper & Row.

Price, R.H. and T. D'Aunno. 1992. The Organization and Impact of Outpatient Drug Abuse Treatment Services. In *The Treatment of Drug and Alcohol Abuse*, ed. R.R. Watson. Alcohol and Drug Abuse Reviews, vol. III: 37-60. Clifton, N.J.: The Humana Press.

Prottas, J.M. and E.A. Elliott. 1992. The Substance Abuse Facility Identification System: Reevaluation in Two Communities. Unpublished report submitted to the National Institute on Drug Abuse by the Institute for Health Policy, Brandeis University, July 1.

Ridgely, M.S. and M.L. Willenbring. 1992. *Application of Case Management to Drug Abuse Treatment: Overview of Models and Research Issues* (DHHS pub. no. ADM 92-1946). Washington: U.S. Government Printing Office.

Schlenger, W.E., L.A. Kroutil, and E.J. Roland. 1992. Case Management as a Mechanism for Linking Drug Abuse Treatment and Primary Care: Preliminary Evidence for the ADAMHA/HRSA Linkage Demonstration. In *Progress and Issues in Case Management* (NIDA Research Monograph #127; DHHS Pub. No. (ADM) 92-1946), ed. R.S. Ashery, 316–330. Rockville, Md.: National Institute on Drug Abuse.

Schmidt, L. and C. Weisner. 1993. Developments in Alcohol Treatment. In *Recent Developments in Alcoholism, Volume II: Ten Years of Progress*, ed. M. Galanter, 369–396. New York: Plenum Press.

Scott, W.R. 1990. *Organizations: Rational, Natural, and Open Systems*, 3d ed. Englewood Cliffs, N.J.: Prentice-Hall.

Stein, M.D., J.H. Samet, and P.G. O'Connor. 1993. The Linkage of Primary Care Services with Substance Abuse Treatment: New Opportunities for Academic Generalists. *Journal of General Internal Medicine* 8 (February):106–7.

Thompson, J. 1967. *Organizations in Action*. New York: McGraw-Hill.

Umbricht-Schneiter, A., D.H. Ginn, K.M. Pabst, and G.E. Bigelow. 1994. Providing Medical Care to Methadone Clinic Patients: Referral vs On-Site Care. *American Journal of Public Health* 84:(2):207–10.

U.S. Department of Health and Human Services. 1993. *National Drug and Alcoholism Treatment Unit Survey (NDATUS): 1991 Main Findings Report*. DHHS pub. no. (SMA) 93-2007. Washington DHHS.

Weisner, C. and L. Schmidt. 1994a. Health and Social Services in the Community: Pathways into Drug Treatment. Paper presented at National Institute on Drug Abuse Technical Review Conference: Organization and Financing of Care for Drug Abuse, Bethesda, Md., June.

Weisner, C. and L. Schmidt. 1994b. A Framework for Evaluating Research on Access and Utilization of Drug Abuse Services. Alcohol Research Group, University of California, Berkeley. Paper presented at National Institute on Drug Abuse Conference on Health Services Research, Bethesda, Md., January.

Williamson, O.E. 1981. The Economics of Organization: The Transaction Cost Approach. *American Journal of Sociology* 87:233–61.

Woody, G.E. 1983. Treatment Characteristics Associated with Outcome. In *Research on the Treatment of Narcotic Addiction* (DHHS 1983 Pub No. (ADM) 83-1282), ed. J.R. Cooper, R. Altman, B.S. Brown, and D. Czechowicz (541–64). Rockville, Md.: Department of Health and Human Services.

Index